Radiation Oncology: Clinical, Translational and Laboratory Research

nova
Medicine & Health
New York

Radiation Oncology: Clinical, Translational and Laboratory Research

Stereotactic Radiosurgery (SRS): Procedure, Results and Risks (2 Volume Set)
Antonio Meola, MD, PhD (Editor), Steven D. Chang, MD (Editor)
2020. ISBN: 978-1-53617-679-7 (Hardcover)
2020. ISBN: 978-1-53617-680-3 (eBook)

More information about this series can be found at
https://novapublishers.com/product-category/series/radiation-oncology-clinical-translational-and-laboratory-research/

Sibel Karaca
Editor

Frontiers in Intensity-Modulated Radiotherapy Research

nova
Medicine & Health
New York

DOI: https://doi.org/10.52305/OQEG7796

Library of Congress Cataloging-in-Publication Data

ISBN: 979-8-88697-252-8

Published by Nova Science Publishers, Inc. † New York

Contents

Preface

Effective application of tumour treatment with high-dose radiation in radiotherapy provides an increase in the treatment rate and quality of life. Intensity-modulated radiotherapy (IMRT) can conform the radiation dose to the target while minimising the dose given to the surrounding healthy tissue. IMRT was started to be used in radiotherapy about 40 years ago and it is applied in almost all radiotherapy centers today. The IMRT technique, which has been strengthened with new software and applications (such as image-guided radiotherapy and adaptive radiotherapy) has increased the advantages of treatment.

The book consists of 18 chapters covering important topics of IMRT. Chapter 1 begins with the brief history of IMRT. Chapter 2 introduces RT devices using the modern IMRT technique. Chapter 3 focuses on the radiobiological basis and clinical implementation. Chapter 4 and Chapter 5 present the scope of imaging (CT, PET, MRI) and contouring in IMRT. Chapter 6 focuses on the algorithms used in the IMRT planning system. IMRT delivery techniques and IMRT verification and geometric uncertainties are covered in Chapters 7 and 8. Quality assurance of IMRT is in Chapter 9, and the image guide IMRT is in Chapter 10. Respiratory movement management in IMRT is described in Chapter 11. Treatment modalities and adaptive RT in IMRT are discussed in Chapters 12 and 13. Challenges in IMRT from a clinician are outlined in Chapter 14. Possible secondary cancer risk and re-irradiation after IMRT are explained in Chapters 15 and 16. Radiation protection in the IMRT approach is reported in Chapter 17. Chapter 18 describes patients' quality of life after IMRT.

Over the past four decades, thousands of patients have been treated with the IMRT technique. Hundreds of articles with dosimetric and clinical results of the IMRT technique have been published. The frontiers of IMRT research are explored in a general scope in this book. Emphasis is placed on current dosimetric and clinical articles in the book. In the conclusion of the chapters, possible future innovations for IMRT are considered. Contributions to this book are made by both medical physicists and radiation oncologists. Readers will find this book an ideal source of up-to-date information for IMRT. This book, in general terms, is a reference book for medical physicists, dosimetrists, and radiation oncologists in that it contains the basic principles of IMRT. I hope that students, teachers, clinicians, researchers, and all professionals interested in radiotherapy will benefit greatly from this book.

As a result, this book has been a valuable work in compiling comprehensive information on IMRT from the past to the present. I would like to thank the authors for their important contributions during the creation of the book. I would like to express my thanks and gratitude to the staff of Nova Science Publishers for their support.

Sibel Karaca
Assist. Prof., Dr., Akdeniz University, Turkey

Chapter 1

Historical Development of IMRT

Sibel Karaca[1,*] and Kadriye Aysenur Karacam[2]
[1]Department of Radiation Oncology, Akdeniz University Faculty of Medicine, Antalya, Turkey
[2]Department of Radiation Oncology, VM Medikal Park Hospital, Istanbul, Turkey

Abstract

In the inventions that started with the discovery of x-rays, scientists found the effect of radiation in destroying cancer cells and started to design radiation-producing devices. Radiological discoveries, imaging modalities, and advances in computer-based treatment planning systems have led to great advances in cancer treatments. For over a century radiation therapy (RT) has been an effective treatment for cancer patients. Technological advances have created a new method called intensity-modulated RT (IMRT). The IMRT method uses multiple beams of radiation of different sizes and intensities to precisely and accurately irradiate the targeted area. Since the intensity and shape of each beam used in IMRT can be controlled, the protection of healthy tissues around the target can be achieved more. It took some time for IMRT to become commercially available and widespread. RT centres around the world have adopted the IMRT method after 2002. Today, almost all RT centres are familiar with IMRT and it is used as a treatment method. The point reached in the IMRT method in the last forty years is a revolution. The purpose of this chapter is to review the development of the history of IMRT from 1895 to the present day.

---

[*]Corresponding Author's Email: sibeltuzlaci@gmail.com.

In: Frontiers in Intensity-Modulated Radiotherapy Research
Editor: Sibel Karaca
ISBN: 979-8-88697-252-8

Keywords: historical development, intensity-modulated radiation therapy, radiotherapy

1. Introduction

Before 1885, the methods of treatment used by scientists in the treatment of cancer diseases were limited. The discovery of x-rays and many subsequent discoveries have made radiotherapy (RT) an indispensable practice for cancer patients. RT had largely adopted a two-dimensional (2D) approach from the 1950s to the late 1980s. From the beginning of the 1990s, technological developments have significantly reflected on RT applications and the transition from 2D to three-dimensional (3D) approach has taken place. Compared to 2D, 3D conformal RT (3DCRT) can reduce the dose taken up by surrounding tissues and vital organs by delivering a uniform dose to the target volume. A major limitation of 3DCRT is that it cannot account for indentations in the target where critical structures enter the target volume. Intensity-modulated radiation therapy (IMRT) largely eliminates the lack of 3D-CRT with enhanced functions. Although conceptual attempts were made for IMRT in the 1960s, a new conceptual foundation was established in 1982 by Swedish medical physicist Anders Brahme. Inclusion of computed tomography (CT) images in RT planning was considered the most exciting development for radiation oncology. After the concept of IMRT was introduced, scientists investigated how to deliver the highest dose to the target with the least damage. Many optimisation algorithms available in the literature throughout history have been proposed to provide more perfect dose distribution. The improved dose distribution provides an important opportunity to reduce the overall toxicity profile associated with RT. This results in an increase in the effective success rate of RT in cancer treatment (Bentzen, 2005; Bortfeld, 2006; Brahme, 1987; Elith et al. 2011; Galvin and de Neve, 2007).

The use of IMRT has made rapid progress worldwide with the development and spread of medical technology. By the 2000s, IMRT became an indispensable part of RT. This chapter of the book will be reviewed in the history of IMRT.

2. First Discoveries (1895-1948)

The discovery of x-rays, which formed the basis of RT, was in 1895. Wilhelm Conrad Roentgen, while working as a professor at the University of Würzberg, found that a beam passing through a cardboard-lined Crookes tube glowed on barium platinocyanide paper while dealing with cathode rays from a vacuum tube. He named this unknown ray the x-ray, but after this discovery, most scientists referred to it as the Roentgen-ray. A simple x- ray tube is shown in Figure 1. The hand photographs of Wilhelm Conrad's wife Anna Bertha Roentgen were also recorded in the literature as the first image of x-rays. Wilhelm Conrad Roentgen presented this discovery on December 28, 1895, in the Physical Society. He received the Nobel Prize for Physics in 1901 for this invention that revolutionised diagnosis and treatment. Shortly after the discovery (6 months), x-rays began to be used for diagnostic purposes (Goodman, 1995; Halperin et al. 2018; Reed, 2011).

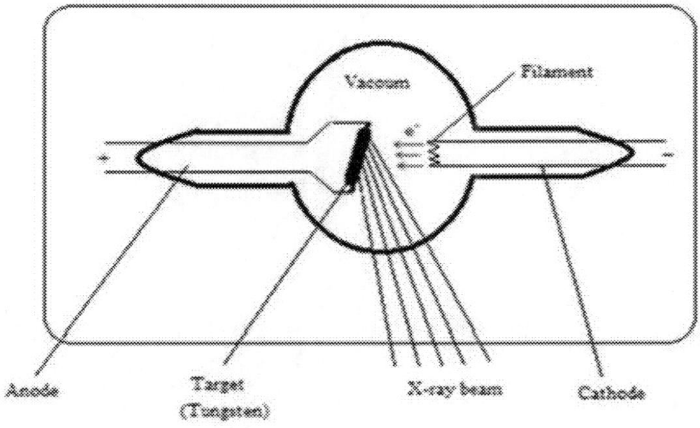

Figure 1. A simple x-ray tube.

After the discovery of x-rays, the French scientist Henri Becquerel, who worked with the photoluminescence of uranium salts, discovered radioactivity. He found that when uranium salts and mineral salts are exposed to sunlight, they emit fluorescence, which also leaves an image on photographic plates. Henri Becquerel received half the Nobel Prize for Physics in 1903, sharing it with Marie and Pierre Curie (Reed, 2011). French physicist and scientist Pierre Curie and his Polish wife Marie Curie discovered Radium and Polonium and their radioactivity after the discovery of Henri Becquerel.

The discovery of Polonium was announced in July 1898, followed by the discovery of Radium in December 1898. The rays emitted by these elements were also called Becquerel rays. Ernest Rutherford investigated the absorption of uranium radiation by increasing aluminium thickness and stated that there are at least two different types of radiation, one called γ (Gamma) radiation and the other β (Beta) radiation, which has a more penetrating character (Radvanyi and Villain, 2017). X-rays and gamma rays are short wavelength electromagnetic radiation. With a short wavelength, they have the power to penetrate matter. At the same time, electromagnetic waves can break chemical bonds in tissues with their high energies. This may cause changes in the structure or functions of cells (Reed, 2011). All these discoveries started the process of using radiation in therapy.

Shortly after these discoveries, x-rays began to be used in the treatment of benign lesions such as eczema and lupus. A medical student named Emil Grubbe started using x-rays to treat cancer in Chicago. French doctor Victor Despeignes used x-ray in the treatment of stomach cancer patients in 1986. Afterward, the use of x-rays in medicine continued to spread, including for skin cancers and sarcoma. In 1911, Claudius Regaud showed that a ram's testicles could be sterilised without causing major burns to the scrotal skin when three irradiations were made 15 days apart. As a result of this application, the basis of fractionated RT was established. The first treatment devices used in RT used low-energy x-rays obtained from x-ray tubes or radium glass tubes. These devices were mostly used in the treatment of tumours near the surface. Orthovoltage x-rays using tube voltages of 200-500 kV began to be used in the 1920s. High voltage generators were developed by Van de Graaff and Trump, and the first megavolt (MV) level x-ray was used in cancer treatment in the 1930s (Connell and Hellman, 2009). In this way, the skin dose toxicity was reduced and the treatment of deep-seated tumours was facilitated until the 1940s (Dyk et al. 2020). While all these developments were taking place, scientists gradually began to understand the nature of radiation, and the International Commission on Radiological Protection (ICRP) was established in 1928 (Gianfaldoni et al. 2017).

3. Transition to IMRT (1948- 1982)

In the historical process, RT began to spread rapidly with the discovery of x-rays and radium (Connell and Hellman, 2009). As a result of the studies, the 6-MV accelerator was developed at Stanford. Betatrons were invented by an

American, Donald Kurst, in the late 1940s. The first electron linear accelerator for RT was developed in 1948 and was installed in London. 1 to 3 Mega Electron Volt (MeV) electrons were used for RT of superficial fields. High-energy electrons produced by Betatron devices were used in the 1960s to irradiate deeply located tumours in the lungs and pelvic region (Bernier, 2004). Cobalt-60 therapy device was developed and the first cancer patient was treated in 1951. The first patient with 8 MV medical linear accelerators was treated at Hammersmith Hospital, London in 1953. The use of linacs started to become widespread throughout the world, and the number, which was 15 in 1962, reached 79 in 1968. Gamma knife device was produced using Cobalt 60 source by Swedish professors Borje Larsson of the Gustaf Werner Institute, University of Uppsala, and Lars Leksell at the Karolinska Institute in Stockholm, and stereotactic RT applications were started in 1967 (Bewley 1985; Dyk et al. 2020; Thwaites and Tuohy, 2006). The practice of RT has devolved markedly over the last 40 years. In earlier days classical 2D RT was used in the treatment of patients. 2D treatment planning consisted of simple parallel opposing or orthogonal simulation films guided by bone anatomy. Treatment areas were planned manually and a single beam of one to four beams were generated (Sanghani and Mignano, 2006). However, 2D RT plans could not adapt to the different structures of the tumour by creating rectangular areas. New approaches targeting the whole tumour were needed. The first clinical application of computer tomography (CT), developed by Godfrey Newbold Hounsfield, was used in brain imaging in 1971 at Atkinson Morley Hospital. The use of CT in imaging has been highly successful in the diagnostic process. CT was quickly used in RT planning in the following process (Bhattacharyya, 2016; Sittig et al. 2006). The revolution in RT has been accelerated by advances in imaging technology.

Research has increased to reduce the large volume irradiated with the 2D method during RT. In order to solve this problem, the 3DCRT was developed by combining computer-controlled multileaf collimators (MLCs) and computer-controlled medical systems, where high-dose radiation with equal intensity is properly delivered to the target (Rehman et al. 2018). Studies on the 3DCRT application were made in 1948 by Takahaski et al. In addition, studies have been initiated by different scientists such as the Monitoring Cobalt Project in England to put RT on an automatic basis. Over time, linear accelerators were designed on a computer-based basis (Fraass et al. 1995). 3D dose calculation and isodose distribution with a computer-based 3D planning programme were developed by Sterling and Weinkam in 1972. Although treatment plans with the 3DCRT method provided a more accurate irradiation area compared to 2D RT, there were still some limitations (Goitein and Abrams, 1983).

Emerging as the advanced form of 3DCRT, IMRT is a specific technique with superior radiation distribution. 2D RT, 3D-CRT and IMRT treatment plan scheme is shown in Figure 2. IMRT is a method that allows modulation of the intensity or flux of the radiation beam. In this way, each field can have one or more high-intensity radiation fields and any number of low-intensity areas within the same field. With IMRT, the radiation beam can be divided into many "beamlets" and the intensity of each beam can be adjusted individually. By modulating the intensity of radiation in each area and the number of areas, there are many possibilities to shape the radiation dose (Intensity Modulated Radiation Therapy Collaborative Working Group, 2001).

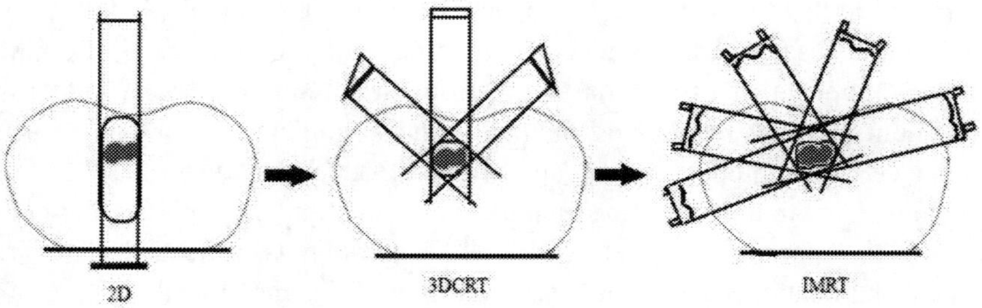

Figure 2. Schematic representation of 2D RT, 3DCRT and IMRT.

The concept of IMRT first appeared in the 1960s. Proimos created a gravity-focused therapy device that allows for dynamic preservation of critical structures as the beam rotates around the patient (Proimos, 1960). Takahashi developed a model in Japan that allowed MLC-based dual-density modulation (on-off) similar to this approach. However, this model failed to provide the complex density modulation needed (Takahashi, 1965). In these years, IMRT studies slowed a down due to technology inadequacies and cost problems. The formation and development of the methods we use in modern times took place in the 1980s and 1990s, that is, in a period of about 10 years (Bortfeld, 2006). With the spread of CT imaging in the early 1970s and magnetic resonance imaging (MRI) in the late 1970s, imaging of cancer tissue became easier. The IMRT method was used to obtain better dose distribution by taking the innovations in imaging and by increasing the number of treatment beams. In the early 1980s, IMRT was developed by several laboratories, enabling radiation oncologists to deliver treatment tailored to the contours of the tumour. MLC systems that can act independently to allow modulation of radiation field intensity began to be developed in the 1980s. The leaves of the MLC could also be precisely controlled with the developing computer technology. In this way, it would be possible to irradiate the target tissue more homogeneously and protect the normal tissues.

The 3DCRT method and computer-controlled RT systems, which developed after the 1980s, could be insufficient in dose wrapping and organ protection in concave-shaped treatment targets. Wedges and compensating filters were used to provide beam fluency. All these systems pioneered the development of IMRT (Intensity Modulated Radiation Therapy Collaborative Working Group, 2001).

4. Beginning of Modern IMRT (1982-1992)

Before modern IMRT came to the stage of implementation, Shinji Takahashi's primitive creation of beam shaped by MLC in the 1950s and the use of jaws for shaping fields in a linac made a significant contribution (Webb, 2003). Although attempts were made in the 1960s to create conceptual innovations in IMRT, a more advanced conceptual basis was developed in 1982 by Anders Brahme et al. In their study, they showed that the circular dose distribution to be blocked centrally can be transmitted by a rotating beam with an irregular fluidity profile. After that, inverse planning was put into practice (Bentzen, 2005). Brahme further contributed to the development of inverse planning by developing his thesis published in 1982 with his new study in 1988 (Brahme, 1987; Webb, 2003). In this method, the desired dose distribution can be obtained by converting the dose desired to be delivered to the target into point dose nuclei, and the backward projection of the density of these point dose nuclei can provide the necessary flux for each beam (Brahme, 1987). Thus, inverse planning, which started with Brahme in 1982 and was well-formed, was further shaped by 1989 Steve Webb and other scientists' work on inverse planning optimisation. Bortfeld et al.'s work on the algorithm of the inverse planning system in 1990 was notable (Bortfeld, 2006). Numerical IMRT optimisation algorithms were further developed in the early 1990s. These analytical approaches have had a significant impact on the emergence of the idea of IMRT rotation (Wang et al. 1995). In this period, many optimisation algorithms that can be found in the literature have been proposed to enable the desired dose distribution in RT. In their independent work, Brahme and

Cormack presented many of the basic concepts of using non-uniform density distributions to generate a series of advanced dose distributions. Scientists have produced reports discussing both planning/optimisation issues and treatment delivery issues (Brahme, 1987; Cormack, 1987). Most of the IMRT studies that followed focused on plan optimisation. By the mid-1990s (and before there was much discussion in the literature about IMRT delivery methods), other delivery techniques related to modern IMRT had developed (Bortfeld et al. 1990). The basic algorithm types developed in the 1990s are still used in reverse treatment planning practice.

Modern IMRT applications are based on plans created with MLCs and linear accelerators. Modern IMRT required both computer-controlled field shaping and precision spaced fit. Unfortunately, the metal compensators that were produced could not provide this precision. The first commercial MLC was developed and produced by Brahme in 1984. The discovery of MLCs made of tungsten has been the most suitable tool for field shaping in IMRT. This produced MLC is in binary MLC form and was used in the first tomotherapy. In addition, the basis of the first IMRT clinical application and the use of the first MLC was with tomotherapy (Anders et al. 2006; Cho, 2018).

5. Developments in the Transition to Modern IMRT (1992-2002)

Although the IMRT concept and early planning algorithm was developed in Sweden in 1982, they could be applied clinically after 1993 with the invention of the IMRT planning and management system called NOMOS Peacock (Carol et al. 1996). The Peacock system required the use of a beam modulating device known as a dynamic multi-vane intensity-modulating collimator (MIMiC). The NOMOS MIMiC system was first introduced in 1992. It was first used in 1994 and IMRT applications using the developed techniques took about three years (Huh and Kim, 2020). Convery and Rosenbloom found that varying dose intensity can be adjusted by sliding MLC, which is the basis of IMRT administration in 1992. They designed to adjust the dose intensity with the leaf sweeping action. Solutions for optimisation problems were developed in 1994 by 3 groups working in different parts of the world. These groups were the Memorial Sloan Kettering Cancer Centre (MSKCC) group in New York (Spirou and Chui, 1998), the Deutsches Krebsforschungszentrum (DKFZ) group in Heidelberg (Stein et al. 1994), and the Karolinska group in Stockholm (Svensson et al. 1994). The first patient considered to be treated with this system had brain metastases and three tumours were to be treated simultaneously in 1993 using IMRT. Quality Assurance (QA) testing performed before the day of treatment revealed an error in the MIMiC collimator. Therefore, the planned treatment was cancelled. Later the first patient was then able to be treated with the Peacock system in 1994, after replacing the sensors for the MIMiC's moving wings and correcting the malfunction. The introduction of the NOMOS Peacock IMRT system took place in the summer of 1995. After IMRT was implemented by various institutions such as Tufts-New England Medical Centre, University of Connecticut and Washington University, many treatment centres became a method used to treat patients (Mills and Woo, 2015).

Step-and-shoot is a multi-static field technique in which several treatment fields are used to deliver RT to the target, with each treatment field divided into sub-fields. These subdomains are transmitted in a specific sequence and in separate steps, only one at a time. The beam is delayed as the MLC takes the next position. Boyer et al. (1991) used a small number of monitor units (MUs) to implement the IMRT method, in each segment for the step-and-shoot technique. The MLC sequencing algorithm was developed in 1993 for step-and-shoot IMRT to obtain a minimum amount of MU and thus reduce stray radiation (Bortfeld et al. 1994).

After 1995, fixed-field IMRT techniques were developed that produced high RT dose distributions using several fixed-angle radiation fields produced by linacs. These techniques quickly became the most common form of IMRT, and the traditional linacplus multi-leaf combination can therefore be considered the standard IMRT delivery system. Using techniques developed at the Memorial Sloan Kettering Cancer Institute, IMRT applications took about three years (1994-1997). Although there are studies for the development of MLC, clinical IMRT applications from step-and-shoot mode or dynamic mode could not be performed before 1997 (Huh and Kim, 2020).

Stereotactic radiosurgery (SRS) is the use of single high-dose radiation directed stereotactically to a relevant intracranial site. The SRS was developed by a team of doctors, physicists, and engineers at Stanford University, and the first patient was treated in 1994. This system consists of a small, lightweight linac with six degrees of freedom supported by a robotic arm. Thanks to the camera system used, it can monitor any change in patient setup and target movement during treatment, and then notify the robot to transmit radiation accordingly. Since the cyberknife is not a fixed concentric, radiation can be transmitted gradually in any direction in a step-shoot manner (Rehman et al. 2018).

A form of arc therapy, called intensity-modulated arc therapy (IMAT), was first introduced by Yu in 1995 (Yu et al. 2002). IMAT uses dynamically moving MLCs of the linac to shape the overlapping rotating cone beams to generate the intensity modulation. However, due to its inadequacy in some subjects (reverse planning, distribution techniques, etc.), IMAT did not gain much fame on a commercial basis, although it treated about 50 patients in 2000 (Rehman et al. 2018).

Axial or serial tomotherapy was started to be applied clinically as early as 1994 (Fenwick et al. 2006). First helical tomotherapy was recommended by Mackie et al. (Mackie et al. 1993). Both axial and helical forms of tomotherapy emit radiation using a rotating intensity-modulated fan beam; the modulation changes according to the portal angle. This approach, called helical tomotherapy, required a newly designed device as many major system components had to be placed in a ring cradle combined with the remaining non-rotating components by slip ring technology to achieve continuous beam return. TomoTherapy Hi-Art devices were developed, manufactured, and commercialised in 2002 by Tomotherapy Inc (Madison, WI) at the University of Wisconsin (Fenwick et al. 2006).

Researchers at Memorial Sloan Kettering Cancer Institute began treating prostate cancer with IMRT in 1995 using dynamic MLC. Until 1997, the number of patients treated with the IMRT technique increased some centres in the United States and Europe have begun investigating the clinical use of IMRT. Initial reports from studies of clinical outcomes of IMRT provided tentative evidence of reduced toxicity with IMRT (Mills and Woo, 2015). Actual IMRT was applied clinically in 2000 (Huh and Kim, 2020).

6. Innovations of IMRT from 2002 to Present

Arc therapy developed more rapidly in the 2000s and took its place among the modern IMRT applied. Today, arc therapy is classified into two types.

The first of modern arc therapy is called Tomotherapy is an RT device that combines dynamic IMRT and an embedded imaging system (Mackie, 2006). TomoHelical (Hi-Art), an original system from TomoTherapy, provides rotational transmission of a fan beam similar to CT. TomoDirect is also a type of TomoTherapy IMRT system and uses a fixed portal angle instead of rotating-beam distribution (Franco et al. 2011). In the tomotherapy system called TomoHDA, both helical (H) and static portal direct (D) treatments have increased as well as advanced dynamic jaw planning capabilities. As of 2013, Tomotherapy HDA units started to replace Tomotherapy Hi-Arts. The system, called Radixact, is the newest of the Tomotherapy delivery systems and was created as a result of the redesign of both the gantry and the treatment planning system, and the Radixact research unit was established in 2015. The dosimetric change added to Radixact is its ability to treat at a higher dose rate than that of TomoHDA units (Smilowitz et al. 2017).

The second novel form of arc therapy is called volumetric modulated arc therapy (VMAT) was introduced in 2007. In the VMAT, the slide is rotated when the beam is on, and three parameters can be changed while the beam is rotated: dose rate, beam shape, and speed of rotation (Otto, 2008). VMAT differs in that it can treat the entire tumour volume at once rather than in slices and can be delivered using a standard linear accelerator. There are several variations on VMAT with names such as RapidArc (Varian), SmartArc (Phillips) and Elekta VMAT (Elekta) (Fenwick et al. 2006; Teoh et al. 2011).

The MR-Linac is a hybrid RT device that combines an MRI scanner and a linear accelerator. The first technical prototype MR-Linac was developed and installed in Utrecht, the Netherlands. It has been used to develop, evaluate and validate clinical procedures in collaboration with Elekta and Philips since 2008 (Kerkmeijer et al. 2016). This technology of MR-Linac provides continuous monitoring of patients with high soft-tissue contrast, allowing tumour monitoring during treatment (Corradini et al. 2019).

Hall, introduced refinements in the design of the multi-leaf collimator for IMRT after raising the possibility of an increase in second malignancy (especially in children) with the high-monitor unit used in IMRT, in 2006. Varian introduced the straightening, filter less RT device with a significantly higher monitor unit output per minute in 2010 (Mills and Woo, 2015). Following this, Electa unveiled the new Versa HD™ linear accelerator in March 2013. Later, Varian introduced the Hycon Linac, which IMRT developed further in almost every aspect, to the market in 2017. Halcyon Linacs are designed with a closed, ring-mounted gantry with a straightening flattening filter-free (FFF) beam and a dose rate of 800 MU/min (Li et al. 2019). A brief history of IMRT is shown in Table 1.

Table 1. A brief history of the IMRT

Year	Name	Developments
1895	Wilhelm Conrad Roentgen	Discovered the X-rays
1930	Robert J. Van de Graaff and John George Trump	Developed the high voltage generators
1960	Basil Proimos	Created the devices to modulate the intensity of beams during rotational therapy
1965	Shinji Takahashi et al.	Developed a model MLC based dual-density modulation
1971	Godfrey Newbold Hounsfield	Developed the CT
1972	James J. Weinkam and Theodor D. Sterling	Developed the 3D dose calculation and isodose distribution with a computer-based 3D planning programme
1982	Andres Brahme et al.	Introduced the IMRT
1983	Michael Goitein et al.	Described a Beam Eye View
1984	Andres Brahme	Patented the first commercial MLC
1988	Andres Brahme	Presented a theory for modulating the flow of beam radiation by the inverse planning
1989	Steve Webb	Described the optimisation problem for IMRT planning by simulated annealing
1990	Thomas Bortfeld et al.	Developed the optimisation for IMRT planning
1991	Art Boyer et al.	Reconfigured the multiple segmented field IMRT
1992	David J. Convery and M. E. Rosenbloom	Founded the varying dose intensity with sliding MLC movement
1993	Thomas Mackie et al.	Designed the Helical Tomotherapy
1994	Thomas Bortfeld et al.	Practiced an initially multiple static fields IMRT
1994	Mark Carol et al.	Performed a primary IMRT treatment with serial tomotherapy
1995	Cedric X. Yu et al.	Developed the IMAT
2007	Karl Otto et al.	Developed the VMAT

Conclusion

After the discovery of the lethal effect of radiation on cancer cells, RT applications began in the treatment of cancer. New RT methods have been developed in the last century's adventure and IMRT has managed to stand out among these methods. IMRT has made incredible progress from its initial conception in the early 1980s to the present day. Although its development seems to be slow in the initial stages, it has been a method that started to rise rapidly between 1990 and 2000 and increased in prevalence after the 2000s. Today, almost all RT centres have included the IMRT method in their clinical routines. It is envisaged that the IMRT method will continue to make progress in the future and develop beyond what has been achieved so far.

References

Anders, A., Hårdemark, B., Isacsson, U., and Montelius, A. (2006). The IMRT Information Process - Mastering the Degrees of Freedom in External Beam Therapy. *Physics in Medicine and Biolology*, 51: 381-402.

Bentzen, S. M. (2005). Radiation Therapy: Intensity Modulated, Image Guided, Biologically Optimized and Evidence Based. *Radiotherapy and Oncology,* 77(3): 227-230.

Bernier, J., Hall, E. J., Giaccia, A. (2004). Radiation oncology: a century of achievements. *Nature Reviews Cancer,* 4: 737-747.

Bewley, D. K. (1985). The 8 MeV Linear Accelerator at the MRC Cyclotron Unit Hammersmith Hospital, London. *The British Journal of Radiology*, 58(687): 213-217.

Bhattacharyya, K. (2016). Godfrey Newbold Hounsfield (1919-2004): The Man Who Revolutionized Neuroimaging. *Annals of Indian Academy of Neurology*, 19(4): 448-450.

Bortfeld, T., Bürkelbach, J., Boesecke, R., and Schlegel, W. (1990). Methods of Image Reconstruction from Projections Applied to Conformation Radiotherapy. *Physics in Medicine and Biology,* 35: 1423-1434.

Bortfeld, T. R., Kahler, D. L., Waldron, T. J. and Boyer, A. L. (1994). X-Ray Field Compensation with Multileaf Collimators. *International Journal of Radiation Oncology Biology Physics*, 28: 723-730.

Bortfeld, T. (2006). IMRT: A Review and Preview. *Physics in Medicine and Biology*, 51: 363-379.

Boyer, A. L., Desobry, G. E. and Wells, N. H. (1991). Potential and limitations of invariant kernel conformal therapy. *Medical Physics,* 18: 703-712.

Brahme, A. (1987). Design Principles and Clinical Possibilities with a New Generation of Radiation Therapy Equipment: A Review. *Acta Oncologica*, 26(6): 403-412.

Carol, M., Grant, W. H., Bleier, A. R., Kania, A. A., Targovnik, H. S., Butler, E. B. and Woo, S. W. (1996). The Field-Matching Problem as It Applies to The Peacock Three-Dimensional Conformal System for Intensity Modulation. *International Journal of Radiation Oncology Biology Physics*, 34: 183-187.

Cho, B. (2018). Intensity-Modulated Radiation Therapy: A Review with a Physics Perspective. *Radiation Oncology Journal,* 36(1): 1-10.

Connell, P. P. and Hellman, S. (2009). Advances in Radiotherapy and Implications for the next Century: A Historical Perspective. *Cancer Resarch*, 69(2): 383-392.

Convery, D. J. and Rosenbloom, M. E. (1992). The generation of intensity- modulated fields for conformal radiotherapy by dynamic collimation. *Physics in Medicine and Biology*, 37: 1359-1374.

Cormack, A. M., and Cormack, R. A. (1987). A Problem In Rotation Therapy With X-Rays: Dose Distributions With An Axis Of Symmetry. *International Journal Of Radiation Oncology Biology Physics*, 13(12): 1921-1925.

Corradini, S., Alongi, F., Andratschke, N., Belka, C., Boldrini, L., Cellini, F., Debus, J., Guckenberger, M., Hörner-Rieber, J., Lagerwaard, F. J., Mazzola, R., Palacios, M. A., Philippens, M. E. P., Raaijmakers, C. P. J., Terhaard, C. H. J., Valentini, V. and Niyazi, M. (2019). MR-Guidance in Clinical Reality: Current Treatment Challenges and Future Perspectives. *Radiotherapy and Oncology*, 14.

Dyk, J. V., Battista, J. J. and Almond, P. R. (2020). A Retrospective of Cobalt-60 Radiation Therapy: "The Atom Bomb That Saves Lives. *Medical physics international Journal, Special Issue, History of Medical Physics,* 4: 327-350.

Elith, C., Dempsey, S. E., Findlay, N., and Warren-Forward, H. M. (2011). An Introduction to the Intensity-Modulated Radiation Therapy (IMRT) Techniques, Tomotherapy, and VMAT. *Journal of Medical Imaging and Radiation Sciences*, 42(1): 37–43.

Fenwick, J. D., Tomé, W. A., Soisson, E. T., Mehta, M. P., and Mackie. T. R. (2006). Tomotherapy and Other Innovative IMRT Delivery Systems. *Seminars in Radiation Oncology*, 16 (4): 199–208.

Fraass, B. A., Mcshan, D. L., Kessler, M. L., Matrone G. M., Lewis, J. D. and Weaver, T. A. (1995). A Computer-Controlled Conformal Radiotherapy System I: Overview. *International Journal of Radiation Oncology Biology Physics*, 33.

Franco, P., Catuzzo P., Cante D., La Porta, M. R., Sciacero, P., Girelli, G., Borca, V. P., Pasquino, M., Numico, G., Tofani, S., Meloni, T., Ricardi, U. and Ozzello, F. (2011). TomoDirect: An Efficient Means to Deliver Radiation at Static Angles with Tomotherapy. *Tumori Journal,* 97(4): 498-502.

Galvin, J. M., and Wilfried, N. (2007). Intensity Modulating and Other Radiation Therapy Devices for Dose Painting. *Journal of Clinical Oncology*, 25(8): 924-930.

Gianfaldoni, S., Gianfaldoni, R., Wollina, U., Lotti, J., Tchernev, G. and Lotti, T. (2017). An Overview on Radiotherapy: From Its History to Its Current Applications in Dermatology. *Open Access Macedonian Journal of Medicine Sciences*, 5(4): 521–525.

Goitein, M., and Abrams, M. (1983). Multi-Dimensional Treatment Planning: I. Delineation of Anatomy." *International Journal of Radiation Oncology Biology Physics*, 9(6): 777-787.

Goodman, P. C. (1995). The New Light: Discovery and Introduction of the X-Ray. *American Journal of Roentgenology*, 165(5): 1041-1050.

Halperin, E. C., Perez, C. A., & Brady, L. W. 2018. The Discipline of Radiation Oncology. In *Principles and Practice of Radiation Oncology*, 64-254. Philedelphia: Wolters Kluwer.

Huh, H. and Kim S. (2020). History of Radiation Therapy Technology. *Progress in Medical* Physic*s*, 31(3): 124–34.

Intensity Modulated Radiation Therapy Collaborative Working Group. (2001). Intensity-modulated radiotherapy: current status and issues of interest. *International Journal of Radiation Oncology Biology Physics*, 51(4), 880–914.

Kerkmeijer, L. G. W., Clifton, D. F., Verkooijen. H. M., Verheij, M., Choudhury, A., Harrington, K. J., Schultz, C., Sahgal, A., Frank, S. J., Goldwein, J., Brown, K. J., Minsky, B. D. and Vulpen, Marco van, On Behalf of the MR-Linac Consortium Clinical Steering Committee. (2016). The MRI-Linear Accelerator Consortium: Evidence-Based Clinical Introduction of an Innovation in Radiation Oncology Connecting Researchers, Methodology, Data Collection, Quality Assurance, and Technical Development. *Frontiers Oncology*, 6: 215.

Li, C., Chen J., Zhu, J., Gong, G., Tao, C., Li, Z., Lu, J. and Yin, Y. (2019). Plan Quality Comparison for Cervical Carcinoma Treated with Halcyon and Trilogy Intensity-Modulated Radiotherapy. *Journal of Cancer*, 10(24): 6135-6141.

Mackie, R. T, Holmes, T., Swerdloff, S., Reckwerdt, P., Deasy, J. O., Yang, J., Paliwal, B. and Kinsella, T. (1993). Tomotherapy: A New Concept for the Delivery of Dynamic Conformal Radiotherapy. *Medical Physics*, 20(6): 1709–1719.

Mackie, R. T. (2006). History of Tomotherapy. *Physics in Medicine and Biology*, 51(13).

Mills, M. D., Woo, S. Y. (2015). History of IMRT. In *Intensity-Modulated Radiation Therapy*, edited by Komaki R, Nishimura Y, 3–14. okyo: Springer.

Nutting, C. (2003). Intensity-Modulated Radiotherapy (IMRT): The Most Important Advance in Radiotherapy since the Linear Accelerator? *British Journal of Radiology*, 76(910): 673.

Otto, K. (2008). Volumetric Modulated Arc Therapy: IMRT in a Single Gantry Arc. *Medical Physics*, 35(1): 310–317.

Proimos, B. S. (1960). Synchronous Protection and Field Shaping in Cyclotherapy. *Radiology*, 77(4).

Radvanyi, P., and Villain, J. (2017). The Discovery of Radioactivity. *Comptes Rendus Physique*, 18: 544-550.

Reed, A. B. (2011). The History of Radiation Use in Medicine. *Journal of Vascular Surgery*, 53(1): 3S-5S.

Rehman, J., Zahra, N. A., Khalid, M., Asghar, H. M., Gilani, Z. A., Ullah, I., Nsar, G., Akhtar, M. M. and Usmani, M. N. (2018). Intensity Modulated Radiation Therapy: A Review of Current Practice and Future Outlooks. *Journal of Radiation Research and Applied Sciences,* 11(4): 361–367.

Sanghani, M., and Mignano, J. (2006). Intensity Modulated Radiation Therapy: A Review of Current Practice and Future Directions. *Technology in Cancer Resarch and Treatment*, 5 (5): 447–50.

Sittig, D. F., Joan, S. A., and Ledley, R. S. (2006). The Story Behind the Development of the First Whole-Body Computerized Tomography Scanner as Told by Robert S. Ledley. *Journal of the American Medical Informatics Association*, 13(5): 465–469.

Smilowitz, J. B., Dunkerley, D., Hill, P. M., Poonam, Y., and Mark, W. G. (2017). Long-Term Dosimetric Stability of Multiple TomoTherapy Delivery Systems. *Journal of Applied Clinical Medical Physics*, 18(3): 137–143.

Spirou, S. V. and Chui, C. S. (1998). A Gradient Inverse Planning Algorithm with Dose-Volume Constraints. *Medical Physics*, 25(3): 321-333.

Stein, J., Bortfeld, T., Dörschel, B. and Schlegel, W. (1994). Dynamic X-Ray Compensation for Conformal Radiotherapy by Means of Multi-Leaf Collimation. *Radiotherapy and Oncology*, 32(2): 163-173.

Svensson, R., Killman, P. and Brahme, A. (1994). An Analytical Solution for the Dynamic Control of Multileaf Collimators. *Physics in Medicine and Biology*, 39(1).

Takahashi, S. (1965). Conformation Radiotherapy Rotation Techniques as Applied to Radiography and Radiotheraphy of Cancer. *Acta Radiologica: Diagnosis* (Stockh), 242.

Teoh, M., Clark, C. H., Wood, K., Whitaker, S. and Nisbet, A. (2011). Volumetric Modulated Arc Therapy: A Review of Current Literature and Clinical Use in Practice. *British Journal of Radiology*, 84.

Thwaites, D. I. and Tuohy, J. B. (2006). Back to the Future: The History and Development of the Clinical Linear Accelerator. *Physics in Medicine and Biology*, 51(13): 343-362.

Wang, X. H., Mohan, R., Jackson, A., Leibel, S., Fuks, Z. and Ling, C. C. (1995). Optimization of Intensity-Modulated 3D Conformal Treatment Plans Based on Biological Indices. *Radiotherapy and Oncology*, 37(2): 140-152.

Webb, S. (2003). The Physical Basis of IMRT and Inverse Planning. *British Journal of Radiology.*

Yu, C. X. (1995). Intensity-modulated arc therapy with dynamic multileaf collimation: an alternative to tomotherapy. *Physics in Medicine and Biology*, 40: 1435-49.

Yu, C. X., Li, X. A., Ma, L., Chen, D., Naqvi, S., Shepard, D., Sarfaraz, M., Holmes, T. W., Suntharalingam, M., & Mansfield, C. M. (2002). Clinical implementation of intensity-modulated arc therapy. *International Journal of Radiation Oncology Biology Physics*, 53(2): 453-463.

Chapter 2

Treatment Devices for IMRT

Ercan Balci*
Depatment of Radiation Oncology, Ataturk University, Erzurum,Turkey

Abstract

In the second half of the twentieth century, in parallel with the technological developments, significant developments were also made in radiotherapy (RT). As a result of the application of developments in technology, RT devices that can best protect normal tissues and deliver high doses to tumour tissues have been developed. Thanks to the Intensity Modulated Radiotherapy (IMRT) method, which started to be used in the 1990s, more advanced treatment planning has begun. The Image-Guided Radiotherapy (IGRT) technique became widespread in the 2000s, so the fourth dimension was added to the treatment by considering the movements of the tumour in the treatment volume and the moving organs. These developments have led to the development of new generation devices by adapting them to RT devices. In this chapter, new generation RT devices with IMRT ability (Linear accelerator, Tomotherapy, MR-Linac and CyberKnife) and their features will be explained.

Keywords: cyberknife, IMRT, linear accelerator, MR-Linac, radiotherapy, tomotherapy

*Corresponding Author's Email: ercanbalci08@hotmail.com.

In: Frontiers in Intensity-Modulated Radiotherapy Research
Editor: Sibel Karaca
ISBN: 979-8-88697-252-8

1. Introduction

In recent years, significant developments have been achieved in radiotherapy (RT) with the production of modern RT devices (Linear accelerator, MR-Linac, Tomotherapy and CyberKnife) and the use of these devices in patient treatment. The medical linear accelerator (Linac) is the primary workforce for radiation oncology. With these devices, there has been a transition from traditional RT using simple rectangular treatment areas to modern RT methods such as three-dimensional conformal radiotherapy (3D-CRT), intensity modulated radiotherapy (IMRT), and image-guided radiotherapy (IGRT). These changes in RT practice increase the dose given to tumour tissues, increase the therapeutic rate of RT, and provide better protection by lowering the dose of organs at risk (OAR). Reducing the dose to the OAR using techniques such as IMRT, along with reducing the size of the planning target volume (PTV) using image-guided radiotherapy (IGRT), allows increasing the radiation dose to improve treatment outcomes.

IMRT is a more advanced approach compared to 3D-CRT and two-dimensional (2D) RT. It optimises delivery of irradiation to irregularly shaped volumes and has the ability to form concaves in radiation therapy volumes. IMRT can be performed using linear accelerators with static multi-leaf collimators (MLC, step and shoot IMRT) or dynamic leaf MLC, tomotherapy machines or volumetric arc modulated therapy (VMAT). Simultaneous boost IMRT allows the delivery of varying doses to various target volumes in a single-phase and minimises dosimetric uncertainties by eliminating the need for field mapping and electron utilisation.

2. Linear Accelerator (Linac)

Linear accelerators (linacs) are devices that can provide kinetic energy from 4 to 25 MeV to charged particles such as electrons by using high-frequency electromagnetic waves (Figure 1). Linacs have two different designs, standing wave and moving wave accelerators. In traveling wave accelerators, a finisher is needed at the end of the tube to absorb the increased power. Thus, the back reflection of the wave is prevented. In standing wave accelerators, on the other hand, at the end of the tube, the advancing and reflected wave overlaps to form the standing wave, which will ensure the maximum reflection of the wave. Standing wave accelerators, although more effective than moving wave accelerators, are more expensive than the other and require the use of a circulator or isolator.

The structure of the linear accelerator consists of basic and auxiliary components as shown in Figure 2.

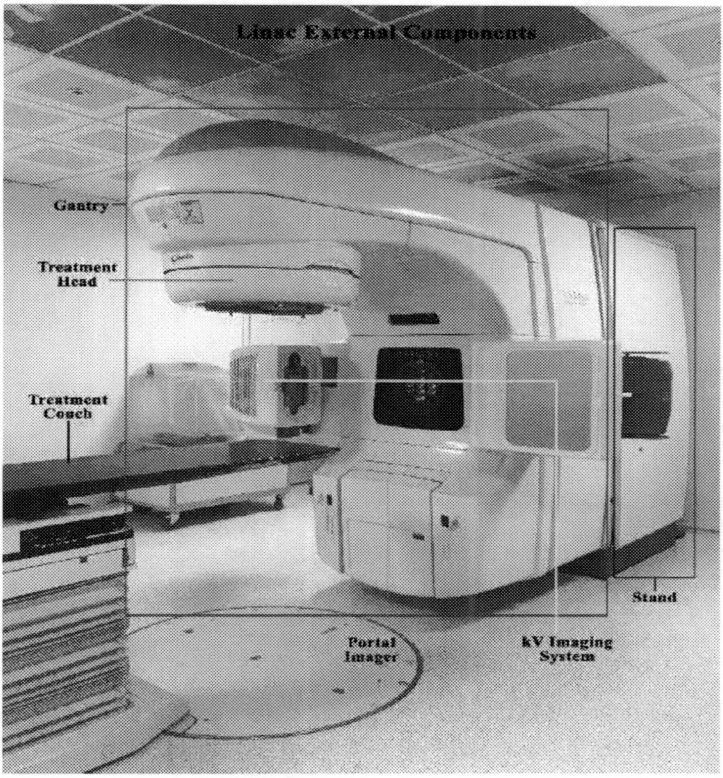

Figure 1. Linear accelerator main components.

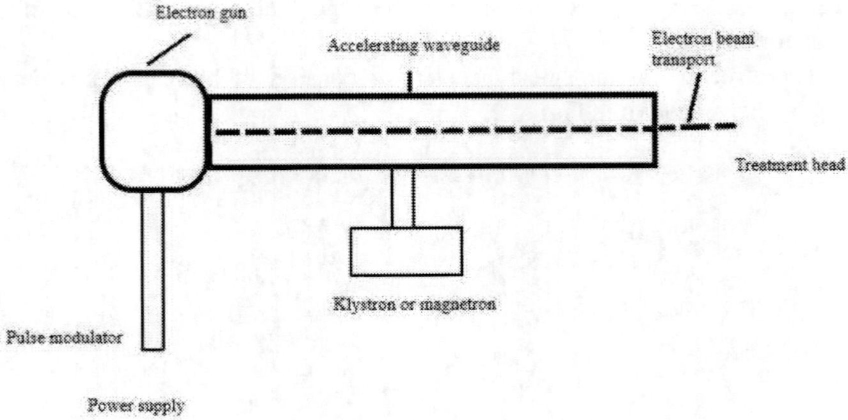

Figure 2. Linear accelerator block diagram.

2.1. Power Supply

In the power supply, the cathode in the centre gives direct current (DC) to the modulator, which includes a mesh network that creates a cylindrical pulse (pulse) with the anode around it, and hydrogen thyratron lamps.

2.2. Modulator

The high-voltage DC electrical current supplied to the device is stored in the modulator. A control system periodically vibrates with this current (microwave). High voltage pulses from the modulator are transmitted to the magnetron or klystron tubes and also to the electron gun.

2.3. Electron Gun

The electron gun is the electron source for the accelerator, which is obtained from a heated cathode by thermionic emission of electrons at high temperature. It is an electron source for the waveguide. Generally, the cathode consists of a spiral-shaped tungsten filament. The electron beam obtained with the electron gun is injected into the accelerator tube with an energy of about 50 kV. Electrons detached from the streamer are accelerated from the cathode to the anode by applying a potential difference and move towards the accelerator. Electrons are injected into the accelerator guide simultaneously with high-power microwaves. The electron gun is controlled by a gun driver subsystem. Functions of this system; to provide power to heat the gun streamer, to provide high voltage for the gun cathode, to provide a pulse programme and waveform in the correct phase (Khan, 2003; Podgorsak, 2005).

2.4. Magnetron/Klystron

2.4.1. Magnetron

A magnetron is a device that generates electromagnetic microwaves. It functions as a high-power oscillator that produces microwave pulses at microsecond intervals with a repetition rate of several hundred pulses per second. The frequency of the microwaves in each pulse is about 3,000 MHz. The magnetron has a cylindrical structure with a central cathode and an outer anode with resonant cavities machined from a solid piece of copper (Figure 3). The space between the cathode and the anode is vacuumed. The cathode is heated by an inner filament and electrons are generated by thermionic emission. A static magnetic field is applied perpendicular to the cross-sectional plane of the cavities, and a pulsed DC electric field is applied between the cathode and the anode. Electrons emitted from the cathode are accelerated towards the anode under the influence of the pulsed DC electric field. Under the simultaneous action of the magnetic field, the electrons move in complex spirals towards the resonant cavities and radiate energy in the form of microwaves. The generated microwave pulses are directed to the accelerator structure through the waveguide. Typically, magnetrons operate at a peak power output of 2 megawatt (MW) to power low-energy linacs (6 MV or less). Although most high-energy linacs use klystrons, energy accelerators as high as 15 MeV are designed to use magnetrons of about 5 MW (Podgorsak, 2005).

2.4.2. Klystron

Klystron is actually a microwave amplifier, not a microwave generator. Klystrons require a low power microwave unit. Klystron consists of two electron cavities and a beam collector, separated from each other by a drag tube. Electrons produced by the cathode are energised by low-power microwaves and accelerated by a negative voltage pulse into the primary cavity, called the beaming cavity. Microwaves create an electric field between spaces. The speed of electrons is related to the effect of this electric field. Some electrons accelerate, while others slow down, while others do not. The accelerating electrons catch up with the slowing electrons. In this case, bundles of decelerated electrons passing through the drag tube are formed. Klystron is used to obtain electrons with energies greater than 15 MeV (Figure 4) (Khan, 2003; Podgorsak, 2005).

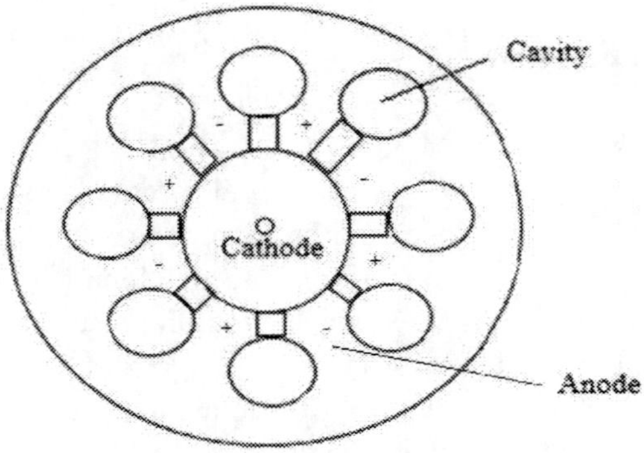

Figure 3. Cross sectional diagram showing principle of magnetron operation.

2.5. Accelerator Waveguide

The main component of linear accelerators is the waveguide. Waveguides generally consist of a series of cylindrical copper tubes with a diameter of about 10 cm and a metallic disk or diagram at ¼ wavelength intervals, which have high electrical conductivity at microwave frequencies to prevent energy loss. The internal structure of this copper guide is horizontally divided into discs (cavities). Powerful microwaves create electric and magnetic fields in each cavity of the accelerator. The first few cavities are more widely spaced and the next cavities are evenly spaced to allow the microwaves to keep up with the phase velocities of the electrons transmitted to the guide. Microwave pulses are transmitted to the waveguide by means of an electron gun. Electrons are accelerated by two-fifths the speed of light. To prevent electron loss, the guide is kept under a high vacuum, and a focusing solenoid coil is placed around the guide to prevent the electrons from focusing, losing their orientation and position in the guide. Thus, very little power loss occurs when microwaves are reflected off the cavity walls. There are two types of guides, traveling wave and stationary wave (Kutsaev et al., 2011). In the traveling waveguide, the microwave is given from the end of the electron gun and absorbed at the end of the tube. The electrons injected into the grid are captured by the traveling moving microwaves and begin to move in phase. On the other hand, in standing waveguides, unlike traveling ones, microwave power is not absorbed at the end of the guide, on the contrary, standing waves are created by superimposing the incident and reflected waves with maximum reflection.

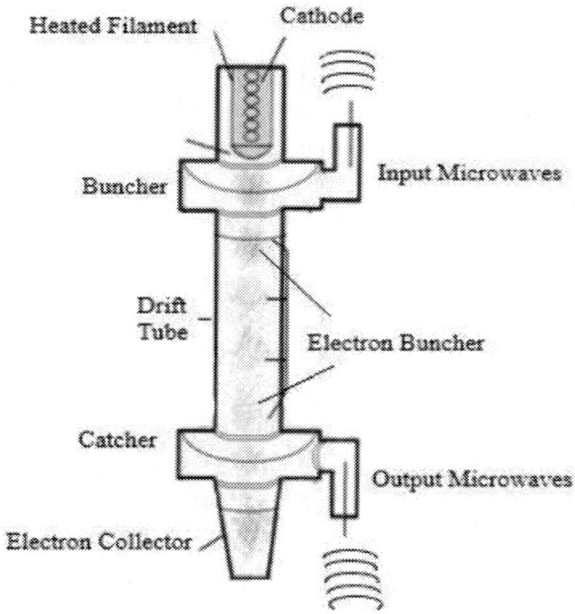

Figure 4. Cross- sectional drawing of a two -cavity klystron.

Microwaves with a frequency of about 3000 MHz coming out of the magnetron or klystron come to the accelerator tube with the waveguide system. Meanwhile, the electrons obtained by heating the tungsten filament in the electron gun are energised under the potential difference and sent into the accelerator tube. When the electrons enter the accelerator tube, their initial energies are around 50 keV. Electrons interacting with the electromagnetic field of microwaves in the tube gain energy in a sinusoidal electric field like a surfer on a wave. Thus, electrons are superimposed on the top of the electromagnetic wave and are delivered to high speeds (Khan, 2003; Cakır, 2012).

2.6. Electron and X-Ray Beam of Linear Accelerator

While electron beams are used in the treatment of superficial and medium depth tumours according to their energies, X-ray beams are used in the treatment of deeply located tumours. The focal point of the rays emanating from linear accelerators is very small (2-3 mm). Therefore, the boundaries of the radiation beam are sharp. Before the rays are sent from the linear accelerator to the patient, the x-rays formed pass through the flattening filter, and the electrons pass through the scattening foil (Mikhailichenko, 1995). A vacuum pump is used to ensure that all the vibrations transmitted to the linear acceleration foci are at the same frequency, to keep the ions that may occur in the frequency regulator and the linear accelerator tube and to provide the vacuum created before. Magnetic focusers are used to collect the electrons in a bundle and send them to the target in this state. High-energy electrons gain their highest energy from the exit window of the accelerator and exit as a pencil beam with a diameter of 3 mm. Their energies are about 5 MV/meter. In order to obtain higher energy beams, they are deflected by the bending magnet (90° bending magnet, 270° bending magnet and slalom system bending magnet) between the tube and the target and directed to the head part of the electron beam, where the electron beam will emerge (Figure 5). From here, the target is hit or the electron beam is sent out of the structure.

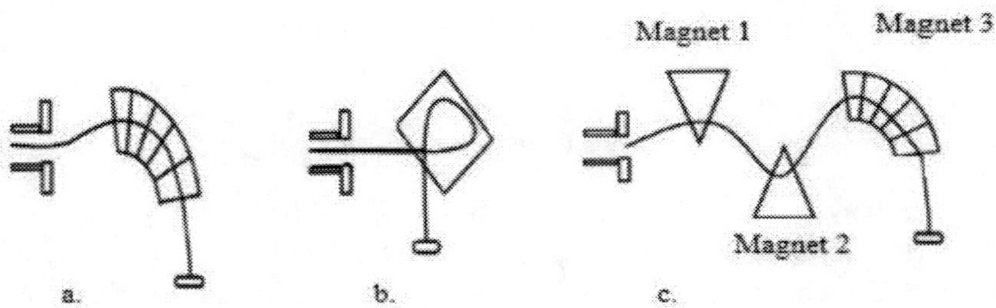

Figure 5. a. 90 bending magnet b. 270 bending magnet c. Slalom system bending magnet.

Megavoltage x-rays are obtained from bremsstrahlung rays, which are formed by striking high-energy electrons on a metal target with a high atomic number of tungsten or a copper-tungsten alloy. The target must be thick enough for the incoming electron to be absorbed. X-ray beams in linear accelerators have heterogeneous distribution. However, as the energy increases, the bremsstrahlung emission increases forward, so the target acts as a transmission target at megavoltage energies (Mayles, 2007).

2.7. Treatment Head of Linear Accelerator

The Gantry is formed from high-density shielding materials, either lead or tungsten alloy, against radiation leaks. It acts as a sufficient shield against radiation leakage. Gantry tungsten target (for x-ray formation), scattering foil, flattening filter, ion chambers, fixed and mobile collimator and light localised systems. Straightening filters are composed of uranium, tungsten, steel, aluminium, lead or an alloy of these metals. In order to homogenise the x-ray beam, a cone-shaped filter called "equalizer" is used (Figure 6).

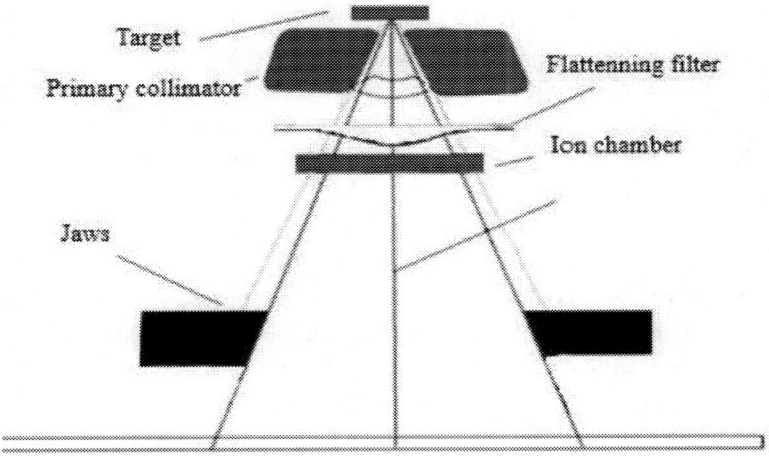

Figure 6. Components of treatment head (x ray therapy mode).

The beam, which becomes homogeneous with the straightening filter, passes through two multi-channel parallel ion chambers. By measuring the delivered dose in two separate ion chambers, the physical parameters of the beam such as dose, dose rate, smoothness and symmetry are measured. Ion chambers are usually made of Kapton. Mica was used before, and in recent years, Kapton has been widely used. There is also less bremsstrahlung x-ray contamination from Kapton ion chambers in electron mode. The two ions are closed to external influences in order to avoid the necessary corrections for gas density changes in the ion chamber due to pressure and temperature fluctuations in the environment (Khan, 2010). Linacs are designed in such a way that the radiation source can be rotated on the horizontal axis. The gantry rotates about a horizontal axis while it rotates about the vertical axis passing through the collimator field. The point where the axis of rotation of the gantry and the axis of rotation of the collimator intersect is called the isocentre. The focus-skin (SSD) distance is usually 100 cm. Modern linacs rotate 360 degrees in the gantry axis and are made in accordance with the isocentric rotation irradiation technique (Flinton, 2019).

2.7.1. Collimator Systems

Collimator systems takes place in three different forms as primary fixed collimator, secondary collimator and multi-leaf collimator.

2.7.1.1. Primary Fixed Collimator

Primary fixed collimators are mounted above flattening filters and are usually made of tungsten. This apparatus, which is open at both ends, cone-shaped and has a low slope, only allows forward scattering electrons to exit the linear accelerator. The beam is formed by the first collimator. The dimensions of the primary collimators are usually placed around 50 cm in diameter on a 100 cm source skin distance (SSD) (Madcalse, 2002).

2.7.1.2. Secondary Collimator

Secondary collimator systems consist of two opposite pairs of blocks, approximately 8 cm, made of a mixture of lead or tungsten. Treatment areas are also created with the movable X and Y jaws in the second collimator. Figure 2.6 General collimator structure (Madcalse, 2002).

2.7.1.3. Multileaf Collimator

Only rectangular or square areas can be created with conventional collimators. A multi-leaf collimator (MLC) has been developed to irradiate areas with different geometric shapes. MLCs allow the beam field to be shaped quickly and easily in accordance with the shapes of tumours and risky organs that need protection. They are composed of 80 or more tungsten leaflets instead of a single block and can move independently. Tungsten; It is used as MLC material because it is a material with high density, easy to process, very hard, and low stretching coefficient (Greer, 2000; Madcalse, 2002).

MLCs consist of many individual fibers that can move perpendicular to the radiation beam and are designed to match the fiber edges. This design of MLCs is known as the "tongue and groove" and is a design developed to reduce leakage radiation between adjacent fibers. Although it varies according to MLC designs, the width of the fibers is 0.5-1 cm at the isocentre (Podgorsak, 2005).

2.8. Patient Couch

In linacs, there is a treatment table that can make horizontal, vertical and rotational movements to ensure the correct positioning of the patient during the treatment. The treatment table is usually made of carbon fiber to reduce scattered radiation and minimise photon beam attenuation (Cakır, 2012).

3. Tomotherapy

Tomotherapy device is one of the most advanced RT devices performing IMRT today (Figure 7). Tomotherapy literally means "slice therapy" and provides continuous transmission of radiation beams. New generation tomotherapy devices can perform 360-degree helical section RT in an integrated and compact manner. Tomotherapy system was created by combining three different functions in a single device. Inspired by computed tomography (CT), instead of tomography tube, a continuously rotating linear accelerator with 6 MV energy is placed on the slide. This device also has the ability to take CT images of the patient in the treatment position. It uses MV energy to display. While performing IGRT, the treatment beam is used and the energy of the treatment beam, which is 6 MV, automatically decreases to 3 MV. For this reason, the images taken on the device are called MVCT (Yartsev et al., 2007).

Tomotherapy is divided into two groups as serial tomotherapy and helical tomotherapy (Van Dyk et al., 2002).

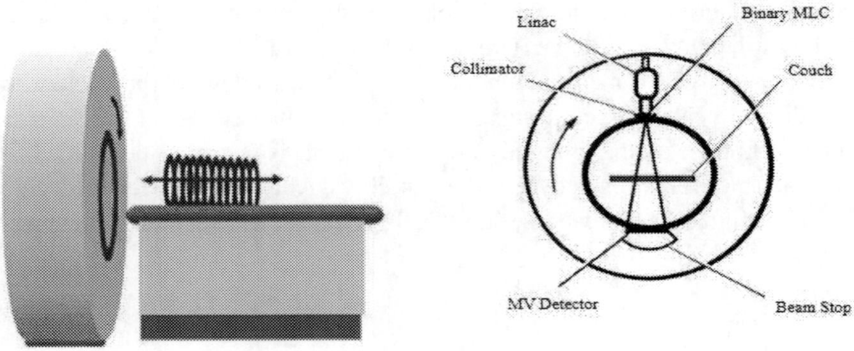

Figure 7. A schematic overview of the tomotherapy device.

3.1. Serial Tomotherapy

Serial tomotherapy is based on the technique of simultaneous irradiation of two sections using a narrow radiation beam modulated by two sets of binary collimators. With the 360-degree rotation of the gantry once, two sections are irradiated without the table moving. This system was named "Peacock" and binary collimator "MIMiC" (Mackie, 2006; Yang, 2006).

3.2. Helical Tomotherapy

Helical tomotherapy uses the IMRT method to deliver high-dose therapeutic doses. Gantry, couch movement and working style is similar to CT (Mackie, 2006). Helical tomotherapy has dynamic fast-moving multi-leaf collimators that can move with the gantry rotation together with the couch movement (Murthy et al., 2010). Helical tomotherapy combines the accuracy of CT scanning technology with the advanced, IMRT form in a single machine. Before each treatment, it takes a three-dimensional (3D) image of the treatment forehead. During the treatment, it adjusts the intensity and direction of the radiation beams in real time and performs irradiation according to the size, shape and location of the tumour area with the 3D image of the target volume. With this method, less radiation reaches the healthy tissues and organs around the tumour. Accordingly, side effects related to RT are minimised (Van Dyk et al. 2002). The comparison of the conventional linear accelerator and helical tomotherapy device is shown in Table 1.

Table 1. Distinguishing features of the Helical Tomotherapy device from the conventional linear accelerator

Conventional Linear Accelerator	Helical Tomotherapy
Source-to-skin distance (SSD) is 100cm	Source-to-skin distance (SSD) is 85 cm
Different photon beams (ranged 4 MV to 18 MV)	Only one photon beam option (6 MV)
There are electron beams (4 to 25 MeV)	None
Wedge filter, comparator and block options	None
None	The treatment couch moves
Have an area light	None
2D RT, 3D RT and IMRT treatment	Only IMRT
Port films, electronic portal imaging, KV or MV cone beam CT	MVCT
Different MLC	Binary MLC
Several angles	360 degrees rotate
Non-coplanar	Strictly coplanar

3.2.1. Specific Parameters of Tomotherapy Device

3.2.1.1. Treatment Slice Thickness (Jaw Width)

Jaw width is the width of the treatment area in the Y axis. Tomotherapy device has three different thicknesses (1.0, 2.5 and 5.0 cm) chin width.

3.2.1.2. Pitch Factor (PF)

The ratio of table movement per gantry rotation for treatment area width. Pitch factors used in treatment vary between 0.10 and 0.50.

3.2.1.3. Modulation Factor (MF)

The ratio of the maximum fiber opening time to the average fiber opening time. It describes the speed of movement and dose distributions of binary MLC. It is a factor that adjusts the opening and closing speed of MLC. The larger the MF, the higher its intensity and the slower the gantry rotation. With the slowing of the gantry rotation, the dose volume histogram (DVH) improves in planning, but the treatment period is prolonged (Langen, 2010; Mackie, 2006).

4. MR-Linac

RT is the discipline most affected by the positive effects of technological developments. Technological advances have led to innovations in RT. Today, RT focuses on increasing the effectiveness of the treatment as well as providing patient comfort and shortening the treatment period. The soft tissue contrast obtained by magnetic resonance imaging (MRI) facilitated the identification of organ at risk (OARs) and tumours compared to CT. Due to the invasive nature of X-rays, continuous monitoring of tumour movement during treatment was not possible. The idea for the MR-Linac device came from the idea of integrating MRI into a linear accelerator, which is non-invasive and gives excellent tissue contrast (Kerkmeijer et al., 2016).

The MR-Linac device is the latest technological device used in RT today. MR-Linac is an MRI guided RT device that can both take images and perform treatment during treatment. The first version of the device, which was used for the first time in the world in 2015, was created by integrating the MRI system into the cobalt 60 teletherapy device (Pollard et al., 2017). Later, the MRI (magnetic resonance imaging) system was integrated into linear accelerators and the MR-Linac device was created (Figure 8). MRI is based on sending electromagnetic waves to the body in a magnetic field and converting the received signals into images. The excitation and the collection of information are obtained from the spin movements of the protons in the cell atoms. Giant magnets located outside the device create a constant magnetic field. Superconducting materials are used to prevent high heat to occur. However, liquid helium and nitrogen called cryogen are used to provide the necessary cooling. The homogeneity of the magnetic field is ensured by the shim windings inside the main magnet. Radiofrequency (RF) coils, which act as both a signal generator and collector, surround the body and form the image (Slotman and Gani, 2019).

MR images with superior soft tissue contrast have been used in RT planning for many years. To facilitate online adaptive MR-guided RT, the MR-Linac device was created by combining a linac and MRI in a single device. With the MRI device, high quality images are obtained in the abdomen, brain, prostate and breast. Changes may occur in the patient's weight, tumour volume, and visceral movements during treatment sessions. Considering these changes, the treatment plan can be adapted according to the current situation. Imaging, marking and plan preparation processes are done again for each session. With the new plan, safe RT is applied to the patient with image (Corradini et al., 2019).

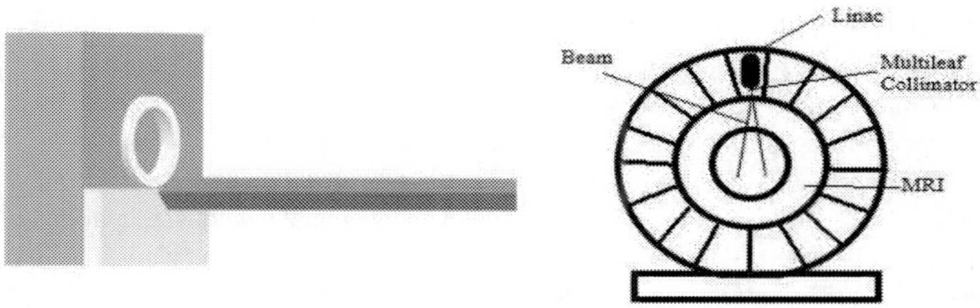

Figure 8. A schematic overview of the MR-Linac device.

The MR-Linac therapy device can take fast and clear images and can detect organ movement and perform online adaptive RT. With the online adaptive RT feature of MR-Linac, if there is a difference from the original plan after the IGRT of the session, the necessary planning is done again while the patient is waiting on the table, and the treatment is completed in accordance with the criteria initially accepted (Thorwarth, and Low, 2021). With high-dose radiation to the tumours with high-quality MR images taken during and after the treatment, the tumour can be destroyed and the surrounding healthy tissues can be protected in the best way (Frantzen, 2019; Slotman and Gani, 2019).

There are two different MR-Linac produced by two different companies in the market. One was created by integrating a 0.35 Tesla MRI system into a 6 MV linear accelerator. The other is created by integrating a 1.5 Tesla MRI system into a 7 MV linear accelerator. (Slotman and Gani, 2019).

5. CyberKnife

The CyberKnife system can perform stereotactic radiosurgery (SRS) and stereotactic body radiation therapy (SBRT) treatments without the need for a mechanical fixation frame. CyberKnife system consists of 6 MV mobile linear accelerator, robotic arm, 2 diagonal X-ray imaging systems, image detectors and treatment bed (Gibbs, 2006). CyberKnife is mounted on a 6-joint robotic arm that produces 6MV energy X-rays and consists of a mobile and 140 kilograms linear accelerator (Figure 9). It is smaller and lighter than the linac used in conventional RT. It has a computer-controlled, 1 mm precision robotic arm with six degrees of freedom of movement. The purpose of the robotic arm in the device is to irradiate the target with 1200 different angles. The robotic arm can repeat the movement between 0° and 45° with an accuracy of about 0.2 mm with 6 axes. The robotic arm moves in a specific and limited coordinate space. The movements of the robotic arm are constrained by a spherical frame in 3D spatial coordinates. The robotic arm's workspace is a configuration array of points where the treatment robot can be positioned without entering a prohibited area. The forbidden zone is an obstacle and any defined coordinate plane around the obstacle. Obstacles defined in the treatment area include patient, bed, cameras, floor and ceiling coordinates (Ding, 2018; Langen, 2010; Mackie, 2006; Pollomet al., 2019).

X-ray sources are placed in the ceiling of the room at concentric angles of 45° on both sides of the treatment bed and there is an aluminium filter with a thickness equivalent to 2.5 mm. The power of X-ray generators is 37.5 kW, energy is between 40 and 125 kV, current intensity is between 25 and 300 mA, and X-ray is produced in a time between 1 and 500 ms (Kilby, 2020).

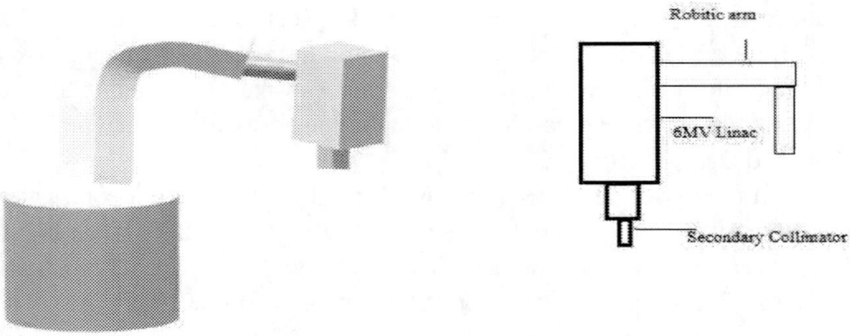

Figure 9. A schematic overview of the CyberKnife device.

5.1. CyberKnife Collimator Systems

5.1.1. Fixed Collimator

Source Axis Distance (SAD) are secondary collimators with 12 fixed circular area sizes ranging from 5 mm to 60 mm in diameter at a distance of 80 cm. These have diameters of 5 to 60 mm, and the treatment plan is made by choosing the appropriate collimator for the tumour size (Echner et al., 2009).

5.1.2. Iris Collimator

The iris collimator is the secondary collimator providing the same 12 apertures as the fixed collimator. Alternatively, a computer-controlled iris variable diaphragm collimator can be used. It allows twelve field sizes in the same set to be achieved with a single variable aperture and therefore provides the flexibility to apply any field size in any beam position without the need to swap collimators during treatment. It consists of two fans, consisting of 6 tungsten segments with a hexagonal opening (Echner, 2009)

5.1.3. Multileaf Collimator (MLC)

MLC is the secondary collimator that creates a radiation field for the treatment of larger non-uniformly shaped tumours. In MLC, independently movable leaves are used to shape the radiation field and optimisation is provided by treatment planning. In the latest devices, MLC system can also be found in order to ensure that the device is used for different purposes. Features of MLC; Non-coplanar beam targeting, maximum geometric field size is 115x100 mm. In its structure; It consists of 41 pairs of tungsten MLCs with a slope of 0.5°, 2.5 mm wide, and normalised for 3.85 mm leaf spacing at 800 mm SAD (Pollomet al., 2019).

5.2. CyberKnife Tracking Systems

Depending on the location of the tumour, different tracking systems are used in the cyberknife device. These tracking systems are:

5.2.1. D Skull Tracking System

It is a follow-up system used in head and neck treatment up to the intracranial and C3 vertebra level. The CyberKnife system determines the bone structure of the patient's skull, and the location of the reference tumour. A thermoplastic head and neck mask are applied to the patient in order to restrict patient movements and reduce the margin of error in the treatment. The device periodically takes digitally reconstructed radiograph (DRR) and matches these images with the images from the Treatment Planning System (TPS). When a difference is detected between the images, the table moves automatically, the images overlap, and the treatment continues. During the treatment, irradiation is continued by tracking the target in this way. Thus, the errors that may occur during the treatment are minimised (Kilby et al.,2010).

5.2.2. X-Sight Lung Tracking System

This system is the follow-up system used in the treatment of lung tumours larger than 2 cm. It detects the image of tumours by making use of the contrast difference. During the treatment, care should be taken not to overshadow the tumour images taken at 45° angles by bone structures. In order for the treatment to be performed, it is essential to see the tumour in the images taken during the treatment (Jordan et al.,2010).

5.2.3. Fiducial Follow-up System

This monitoring system is used when treating soft tissue (such as prostate, pancreas, liver) tumours. Gold markers pre-inserted into the tissue are used as a reference. At least 3 references are needed to calculate the axes of rotation (X, Y, Z) and rotations. For this, at least 3 to 5 gold markers are placed. During planning, the markers are localised in the CT image, and the DRRs are recorded at the corresponding locations in the snapshots, and the tracking algorithm is created. A correlation is established by comparing x-ray images and DRR images. The patient is treated by considering the displacements in the positions of the fiducial markers in the DRR images and correcting the position (Kilby et al.,2010).

5.2.4. X-Sight Vertebra Tracking System

This system is used in the treatment of tumours adjacent to or near the vertebra. While preparing the plan, the vertebra closest to the tumour is taken as reference. This system calculates how much the position of the patient's skeletal system has changed during the treatment. The x-sight spine tracking system was integrated with the CyberKnife unit to provide radio-surgical treatments for spine tumours without reference placement. However, the tracking system can also be used in the treatment of abdominal tumours located at a certain distance from the spine (Eken et al., 2019).

Conclusion

RT is a form of treatment that has proven its efficacy and adequacy in cancer treatment. Since the early 1900s, scientists have made many attempts to improve RT. In this direction developed new techniques and devices. The IMRT method has been developed since 1990. After 2000, IGRT was developed and put into practice. Along with these, with the widespread use of robotic arm devices, high-tech linac-based RT devices (such as Modern Linac, Tomotherapy, MR-Linac and CyberKnife) have been developed. Technology is rapidly changing and developing day by day. The develop-ment of the devices used was directly reflected in the treatment techniques and planning systems. Thanks to these developments, superior treatments can be made that ensure that the tumour tissues receive the maximum dose by preserving the normal tissues, which is the basic principle of RT. It is thought that this rapid change in technology will bring RT devices closer to perfection in the future.

References

Cakır, A., and Bilge, H. (2012). Çok yapraklı lineer hızlandırıcılarda kolimatör tasarımlarının klinik önemi. *Türk Onkoloji Dergisi*, *27*(1), 46-54.

Corradini, S., Alongi, F., Andratschke, N., Belka, C., Boldrini, L., Cellini, F., Debus, J., Guckenberger, M., Hörner-Rieber, J., Lagerwaard, F. J., Mazzola, R., Palacios, M. A., Philippens, M., Raaijmakers, C., Terhaard, C., Valentini, V., & Niyazi, M. (2019). MR-guidance in clinical reality: current treatment challenges and future perspectives. *Radiation oncology* (London, England), 14(1), 92.

Ding, C. S. (2018). Cyberknife Stereotactic Radiosurgery and Radiation Therapy Treatment Planning System. *Medical Dosimetry*, 43(2), 129–140.

Echner, G. G., Kilby, W., Lee, M., Earnst, E., Sayeh, S., Schlaefer, A., ... & Schlegel, W. (2009). The design, physical properties and clinical utility of an iris collimator for robotic radiosurgery. *Physics in Medicine & Biology*, 54(18), 5359.

Eken, S., Zorlu, F., Yeginer, M., and Ozyigit, G. (2019). Performance evaluation of the X-sight spine tracking system for abdominal tumors distal to spine: A 2D dosimetric analysis. *Medical Dosimetry*, 44(4), 370-374.

Flinton, D. (2019). Radiotherapy Beam Production. *Practical Radiotherapy: Physics and Equipment*, 145.

Frantzen-Steneker, M., Astreinidou, E., & Nowee, M. E. (2019). MRI basics for radiation oncologists. *Clinical and translational radiation oncology*, 18, 74-79.

Gibbs, I. C. (2006). Frameless image-guided intracranial and extracranial radiosurgery using the Cyberknife™ robotic system. *Cancer/Radiotherapie*, 10(5), 283-287.

Greer, P. (2000). *A dual Assembly multileaf collimator for radiathearpy, Thesis (PhD), Adelaide University.*

Jordan, P., West, J., Sharda, A., & Maurer, C. (2010). SU-GG-J-24: Retrospective Clinical Data Analysis of Fiducial-Free Lung Tracking. *Medical Physics*, *37*(6Part9), 3150-3150.

Kerkmeijer, L. G., Fuller, C. D., Verkooijen, H. M., Verheij, M., Choudhury, A., Harrington, K. J., Schultz, C., Sahgal, A., Frank, S. J., Goldwein, J., Brown, K. J., Minsky, B. D., van Vulpen, M., & MR-Linac Consortium Clinical Steering Committee. (2016). The MRI-Linear Accelerator Consortium: Evidence-Based Clinical Introduction of an Innovation in Radiation Oncology Connecting Researchers, Methodology, Data Collection, Quality Assurance, and Technical Development. *Frontiers in oncology*, 6, 215.

Khan F. M. (2003). Linear Accelerator. *The Physics of Radiation therapy.* 3rd Edition. Philadelphia, USA: Lippincott Willams & Willkins, pp.42-47

Khan F. M. (2010). *The Physics of Radiation Theraphy. Forth Edition,* USA: Lippincott Wilkins, USA, pp 560.

Kilby, W., Dooley, J. R., Kuduvalli, G., Sayeh, S., & Maurer Jr, C. R. (2010). The CyberKnife® robotic radiosurgery system in 2010. *Technology in cancer research & treatment*, 9(5), 433-452.

Kilby, W., Naylor, M., Dooley, J. R., Maurer Jr, C. R., & Sayeh, S. (2020). A technical overview of the CyberKnife system. *Handbook of robotic and image-guided surgery*, 15-38.

Kutsaev, S. V., Sobenin, N. P., Smirnov, A. Y., Kamenschikov, D. S., Gusarova, M. A., Nikolskiy, K. I., ... & Lalayan, M. V. (2011). Design of hybrid electron linac with standing wave buncher and traveling wave structure. *Nuclear Instruments and Methods in Physics Research Section A: Accelerators, Spectrometers, Detectors and Associated Equipment*, *636*(1), 13-30.

Langen, K. M. (2010). QA for Helical Tomotherapy: Report of the AAPM Task Group 148. *Medical Physics 37 (9)*, 4817–53.

Mackie, T. (2006). History of Tomotherapy. *Phys. Med. Biol. 51*, 427- 453.

Madcalse, P. K. (2002). The Physics of Radiotherapy X-Ray From Linear Accelerators. *Medical Physics*, 493.

Mayles, P. N. (2007). *Handbook of Radiotherapy Physics, Theory and Practice*, 1st ed. London, UK: Taylor & Francis Group.

Mayles, P. R. (2010). *Handbook of Radiotherapy Physics.* New York: Taylor&Francis.

Mikhailichenko, A. A. (1995, May). A beam focusing system for a linac driven by a traveling laser focus. In *Proceedings Particle Accelerator Conference* (Vol. 2, pp. 784-786). IEEE.

Murthy, V., Master, Z, Gupta, T, Ghosh Laskar, S. (2010). Helical tomotherapy for head and neck squamous cell carcinoma: dosimetric comparison with linear accelerator-based step-and-shoot IMRT. *J Cancer Res Ther*, 6, 194-8.

Podgorsak, E. (2005). *Treatment Machines for External Beam Radiotherapy Chapter 5.* Department of Medical Physics, Vienna: IAEA, pp.136-151

Pollard, J. M., Wen, Z., Sadagopan, R., Wang, J., & Ibbott, G. S. (2017). The future of image-guided radiotherapy will be MR guided. *The British journal of radiology*, *90*(1073), 20160667.

Pollom, E., Wang, L., Gibbs, I. C., & Soltys, S. G. (2019). CyberKnife Robotic Stereotactic Radiosurgery. In *Stereotactic Radiosurgery and Stereotactic Body Radiation Therapy* (pp. 67-76). Springer, Cham.

Slotman, B., & Gani, C. (2019). Online MR-guided radiotherapy - A new era in radiotherapy. *Clinical and translational radiation oncology*, 18, 102–103. https://doi.org/10.1016/j.ctro.2019.04.011

Thorwarth, D., & Low, D. A. (2021). Technical challenges of real-time adaptive MR-guided radiotherapy. *Frontiers in Oncology*, 11, 332.

Van Dyk, J., Kron, T., Bauman, G., & Battista, J. J. (2002). Tomotherapy: a 'revolution' in radiation therapy. *Physics in Canada*, 58(2), 79-86.

Yang, J. (2006). *Arc binary intensity modulated radiation therapy (AB IMRT).* University of Miami.

Yartsev, S., Kron, T., & Van Dyk, J. (2007). Tomotherapy as a tool in image-guided radiation therapy (IGRT): theoretical and technological aspects. *Biomedical imaging and intervention journal*, *3*(1), e16.

Chapter 3

The Radiobiological Basis of Intensity Modulated Radiation Therapy and Clinical Implementations

Meltem Kirli Bolukbas*
Department of Radiation Oncology, Health Sciences University Bakirkoy Dr. Sadi Konuk Training and Research Hospital, Istanbul, Turkey

Abstract

Radiation therapy has a vital role in almost every stage of different cancer types. Tolerance of organs at risk (OAR) limits the dose of radiation; tumour unresponsiveness shows that the given dose is insufficient, and a higher dose should be given. With more sophisticated radiotherapy (RT) techniques, it is possible to give a higher dose to the tumour while protecting the normal tissue. Over the past decades, there has been a transition from two-dimensional (2D) treatments for tumours, first to three-dimensional (3D) conformal treatments and then to intensity-modulated RT (IMRT). With IMRT, the transition to the 'inverse' RT planning technique has been made. The common goal of all volumetric arc therapy (VMAT) and stereotactic radiosurgery (SRS) or stereotactic RT (SRT) derived from IMRT is to increase the target dose while reducing toxicity in normal tissues. In addition to the benefit obtained with the technique, more effective treatments can be given using radiobiology information. This chapter will give information about how radiobiological principles affect IMRT planning and how they are used.

*Corresponding Author's Email: meltemkrl@gmail.com.

In: Frontiers in Intensity-Modulated Radiotherapy Research
Editor: Sibel Karaca
ISBN: 979-8-88697-252-8

Keywords: hypoxia, intensity-modulated radiation therapy, redistribution, radiobiology, radiotherapy, reoxygenation, repair, repopulation, secondary cancer

1. Introduction

Radiotherapy (RT) aims to damage the cell's genetic material by applying high-energy radiation and killing cancer cells by preventing the cells from dividing (Jackson and Bartek, 2009). RT is a technology-dependent treatment modality, and there have been significant developments in this field in the last few decades. A transition was made from 2D conventional treatments to 3D conformal treatments and then to IMRT. With IMRT, the 'inverse' RT planning technique has entered our lives. Contrary to the 'forward' treatment planning in 2D and 3D conformal RT, programmes with complex computer algorithms are used in IMRT to provide target dose distribution and coverage while preserving normal tissues. In the conformal RT planning, the dose distribution can be changed by modifying the weight of the fields, the ganry angle and the table angle by the physicist. Whereas in the IMRT, the treatment planning systems (TPS) find the best dose distribution according to the dose-volume constraints. This type of backward planning is called 'inverse planning.' In IMRT, the desired dose is achieved by dividing the radiation beams into smaller divisions called beamlets and arranging each beamlet independently with up and down-regulation. The development of IMRT techniques has made it possible to apply the treatment with a continuous rotating gantry instead of plans containing multiple static fields (Jin et al., 2011; Otto, 2008).

The common goal of all IMRT, VMAT, SRS, and SRT techniques is to increase the target dose while reducing toxicity in normal tissues. By virtue of these techniques, RT is administered with shorter-lasting schemes, and larger doses per fraction are given more safely. Alternatively, it may be possible to increase to higher treatment doses with the same fraction dose which may lead to improved treatment results and reduced toxicity (Kachnic et al., 2012; Klopp et al., 2018; Nutting et al., 2011).

The RT planning success depends on the dose given, the duration of treatment, and the characteristics of the irradiated organs (radiosensitivity, parallel or serial organ status, total irradiated volume). While high doses of radiation kill the cancerous cell, it can also kill the normal cell in its immediate vicinity. While highly proliferating tissues such as the intestine and bone marrow are at risk of early side effects, normal tissues with slow repopulation are at risk of late side effects. The sharp dose distribution obtained with IMRT plans may increase the dose in the tumour while allowing more protection of normal tissue. This may reduce the early side effects that result in the prolongation of the treatment by causing treatment breaks (Bockbrader and Kim, 2009).

In all RT techniques with increased conformality, there is a risk of geographical missing the dose due to the organ movement and set-up errors. Because of the sharp dose distribution obtained with IMRT and increased inhomogeneity compared to 3D dimensional plans, complications might occur if the hot spots on the plane coincide with the normal tissue and if the cold spots coincide with the tumour, resulting in treatment unresponsiveness. In addition, IMRT plans typically have a longer execution time than 3D conformal plans. With the prolonged fraction time, the movement of the tumour and normal tissue comes to the fore. This may negatively affect local tumour control and survival. Finally, in IMRT plans, the dose distribution is created with small areas from multiple angles, which means that more tissues in the body are exposed to low-dose radiation. This low-dose region, which is well below the limits for acute or chronic side effects, may increase the risk of secondary cancer in long-term survivors (Welsh et al., 2005).

In fractionated RT, OAR toxicity decreases as the therapeutic effect increases. This situation occurs with the sum of the positive and negative effects of radiobiological events during the treatment. These radiobiological events can be counted as repair, reoxygenation, redistribution, and repopulation (Egeland et al., 2006; Trott, 1982). This chapter will discuss the advantages and disadvantages of IMRT from a radiobiological point of view and how the radiobiological events change the clinical practice.

2. Repair

Elkind et al., reported surviving fraction of the mammalian cells after RT. They showed an increased survival between fractions. The increase in surviving cells has been shown to reach the coat 2 hours after the RT dose (Elkind et al., 1965; Elkind and Sutton 1959). This situation is called sublethal damage.

Ionising radiation causes two types of damage to deoxyribonucleic acid (DNA). One of these is double chain breaks, which mainly result in cell death, and the other is single chain breaks. Single chain breaks cause sublethal damage. Sublethal damage can often be repaired during treatment. However, as their number increases, they may be lethal to the cell. It is known that tumour cells also repair sublethal damage between treatments (Dale, 1985).

The cell surviving fraction is 0.09 after 4 Gray (Gy) radiation dose. However, if this dose is divided in 2 Gy and sufficient time is given for repair between fractions, it is seen that the surviving fraction increases to 0.02. Subletal damage repair is greatest immediately after the application of radiation. A characteristic shouldering is seen in the cell survival curves due to repair (Niemierko, 2006).

As we progress from the conventional techniques to the conformal techniques, the treatment fraction times get longer. In IMRT with static fields, the total treatment time to deliver 2 Gy can be 30 min (or more), while it takes only 6 minutes with conventional RT. Because accurate patient positioning is required in IMRT, a longer time is required for RT fractions (Niemierko, 2006; Shibamoto et al., 2004). It should be kept in mind that current treatment results come from conventional techniques. It should not be forgotten that if we adapt these results to IMRT techniques, the same dose will be administered for a longer time, and this may cause worse clinical results with the sublethal repair of damage (Niemierko, 2006).

Although there are not many studies on the clinical reflection of prolonged treatment periods, this issue has been investigated in the literature with cell, animal, brachytherapy, and modelling studies (Fowler and Van Limbergen, 1997; Mu et al., 2003; Shibamoto et al., 2004; Steinberger et al., 2015; Wang et al., 2003)

In the study of Mu et al., on Chinese hamster fibroblasts (V79-379-A), the effect of changing the delivery time for each fraction was studied. In this study, each fraction was divided into different subfractions, simulating the delivery of a complicated treatment. This study showed that prolonging the fraction time was underestimated in treatments given as 2Gy/fraction (Mu et al., 2003).

In the study of Shibamoto et al., with EMT6 and SCCVII cell lines, it was determined that the biological effect decreases by 9-14% due to sublethal damage repair in total RT periods lasting 20-30 minutes, and the dose should be increased by 8-16% in order to achieve the same biological effect in the given radiotherapy (Shibamoto et al., 2004).

The study of Benedict et al., compared gamma-ray SRS and multiple arch SRS techniques. The intermittent radiation is delivered with the SRS arc by dividing the total dose (6, 9, 12, and 18 Gy) into equal fractions (1.5, 2.0, 3.0, and 6 Gy). It was shown that the cell survival rate increased as the irradiation time increased (Benedict et al., 1997).

Wang et al., investigated the effect of total treatment duration on cell death in prostate cancer. It has been shown that cell death is significantly reduced at treatment times ranging from 15 minutes to 45 minutes. The equivalent dose of an IMRT dose of 81 Gy administered in 30 minutes decreases to 69 Gy. Their study showed that the total delivery time for a single fraction might significantly impact IMRT treatment outcomes (Wang et al., 2003).

Especially when respiratory control is used in the treatment of lung and liver patients when there is a linac breakdown, and it is desired to continue the treatment on another device, the treatment is applied intermittently (Hoogeman et al., 2008; Linthout et al., 2009). Interruptions in the treatment and the prolongation of the duration of treatment were investigated by Kawahara et al., using a microdosimetric kinetic model. Their study showed that the biological dose difference with and without interruption was over 3% at the interruption (>3 minutes) (Kawahara et al., 2020).

Paganetti studied the effects of single-fraction and fractionated irradiation for different dose rates in 9 cell lines (8 human tumour xenografts and a C3H10T1/2 cell line). When the application of 2 Gy over 30 minutes per fraction and the application of 2 Gy over 1 minute per fraction were compared, it was determined that the equivalent dose decreased by 1.3-12%. Even more significant differences are detected when the dose rate is lower than 0.1 Gy/min (Paganetti, 2005).

According to studies, if the duration of treatment is close to 20 minutes and a loss of more than 10% of the biologically effective dose is predicted, adjustments in effective dose by increasing the fracton dose may be necessary for IMRT (Kawahara et al., 2020; Paganetti, 2005). Therefore, some models, such as the microdosimetric kinetic model, should be used.

3. Reoxygenation and Hypoxia

Tumour hypoxia is a well-known biological event that is commonly seen in solid tumours (Walsh et al., 2014). Thomlinson and Gray showed that hypoxic and well-oxygenated cells coexist in the tumour (Thomlinson and Gray, 1955). Tumour hypoxia causes changes in DNA repair mechanisms and cell death/survival signal pathways in the cell, resulting in increased radioresistance and treatment failure. Besides, hypoxia may trigger angiogenesis and cause metastatic spread (Bindra et al., 2007). The hypoxia-inducible factor 1 (HIF-1) has a very important role in hypoxia-induced tumour radioresistance (Harada, 2016; Walsh et al., 2014).

A wide variety of treatment strategies have been tried over the years to address hypoxia. Strategies used to combat tumour hypoxia are divided into two categories: overcoming hypoxia by increasing reoxygenation and sensitising hypoxic areas to RT by applying an additional dose of RT to hypoxic areas.

One of the underlying goals of fractionation in RT is to reduce tumour hypoxia. With the death of well-oxygenated cells after RT fractions, cells that were previously hypoxic in the tumour begin to become well-oxygenated (Okamoto et al., 2016; Trott, 1982).

Another strategy that has been used in the last decade to prevent hypoxia is the simultaneous integrated boost (SIB) technique, which allows simultaneously administering different doses to different parts of the tumour in IMRT and IMAT techniques (Mohan et al., 2000). Today, as an alternative to conventional fractionated RT, dose-escalation methods with SIB are tested in many cancer types: breast (Hamilton et al., 2016; Nitsche et al., 2015), head and neck (Franceschini et al., 2013; Orlandi et al., 2010), prostate (Fonteyne et al., 2008; Timon et al., 2016).

To create a non-homogeneous dose distribution in the tumour in IMRT, the areas where additional doses will be applied must be well defined and contoured. This has led to advances in radiology and nuclear medicine imaging techniques. We are currently assisting with the multiparametric magnetic resonance imaging (mpMRI) and positron emission tomography (PET) with hypoxia-specific radioisotopes such as CuATSM, 18F-FRP170, and 18F-MISO to identify radioresistant regions within the tumour and to identify subregions to be increased to higher doses (Gaertner et al., 2012). Contouring and targeting of radioresistant regions detected by imaging methods are also possible thanks to fusion and registration algorithms developed in treatment planning systems (Brock et al., 2017). Thus, radiation oncologists determine the areas where they want to increase the dose or where they want to do SIB. Through IMRT's inverse treatment planning algorithms, higher doses are given to these areas by considering the balance of the Probability of Normal-Tissue Complications (NTCP) and Tumour Control Probability (TCP) (Nahum and Uzan, 2012).

In the study of Chao et al., with 165 Head and neck (HNC) patients, it was determined that only 28% of the relapses occurred outside the area, most of the remaining relapses were within the area (53%), and some of them were marginal misses (12%) at the edge of the area (Chao et al., 2003). Similar locoregional recurrence rates (56% to 82%) were found in other series in the literature at high dose sites (Chen et al., 2009; Santa Cruz et al., 2018;

Silvoniemi et al., 2018). The predominance of intra-area recurrences indicates the presence of radioresistant subvolumes (such as hypoxic regions) for the tumour.

PET has been studied with different radioisotopes to show hypoxic areas, especially in HNC cancers where hypoxia is very important (Silvoniemi et al., 2018). FMISO (fluoromisonidazole) is a 2-nitroimidazole that can be labelled with the positron emitter 18F for PET imaging. It is the most extensively studied radioisotope for hypoxia imaging in vitro and preclinical models and has also been used in many patient studies (Gaertner et al., 2012). In vitro studies have shown the accumulation of FMISO in hypoxic cells. Rasey et al.,'s study of Chinese hamster lung cells showed that FMISO marked hypoxic cells, but it was found that normoxic or necrotic cells accumulation was not observed (Rasey et al., 1985). A study conducted in rat myocytes showed that FMISO accumulated 26 times more than normal in anoxic cells and 15 times more than normal in hypoxic cells (Martin et al., 1990). While increased FMISO accumulation was correlated with lower pO2 levels in some human studies, some studies also found low FMISO accumulation in regions with low pO2 levels. These lesions are generally necrotic lymph nodes (Bentzen et al., 2003). Other hypoxia-specific radioisotopes used in PET include [18F] fluoroazomycin- arabinofuranoside ([18F] FAZA), etanidazole pentafluoride (EF5), 18F-FPR170, and Cu (II)-diacetyl-bis(N4-methylthiosemicarbazone) (Cu-ATSM) (Gaertner et al., 2012). These isotopes can give us metabolic information about the tumour, helping us to decide on the radioresistant regions (Lopes et al., 2021).

Chao et al., studied the feasibility of Cu-ATSM-guided IMRT application in HNC. An ATSM-avid or hypoxic tumour subvolume was determined using Cu-ATSM, and this sub-volume was planned with 80 Gy/35 fractions and 70 Gy/35 fractions SIB for normal gross tumour volume (Chao et al., 2001). In a study with FAZA-PET in HNCs, hypoxia was detected in 63% of the patients. Moreover, it was determined that this hypoxia continued during RT in some patients (Mortensen et al., 2012). Since hypoxia has been determined to be a dynamic process, it is recommended to use FAZA-PET taken in the second week of the treatment instead of baseline FAZA-PET for dose escalation (Bollineni et al., 2014). Lee et al., studied IMRT planning with 18F-FMISO-PET imaging in HNC patients. The hypoxic regions detected by FMISO-PET received a 20% dose increase (84 Gy), while OAR doses were kept below tolerance doses (Lee et al., 2008). A meta-analysis comparing SIB-IMRT with sequential IMRT to increase radiobiological efficiency showed that the treatment results and effect profile are comparable (Jiang et al., 2019).

In lung cancer, hypoxia-specific radioisotopes can be used to overcome the effect of hypoxia. FMISO PET/CT-guided hypoxic tumour volume was determined in 5 non-small cell lung cancers, and SIB of 72 Gy, 78, and 84 Gy doses were defined in 30 fractions to this volume. Normal tissue dose tolerances met the tolerance criteria without compromising the original target volume dose distribution (Li et al., 2018).

In patients with single brain metastases, the tumour was determined by the fusion of contrast-enhanced CT and T1W images, and the tumour was divided into high- and low-perfusion areas according to the difference in cerebral blood flow. In this study, in which hypoxic volume was detected in half of the patients, 60 Gy RT was planned for normoxic GTVs, while 72 Gy RT could be planned for hypoxic metastases without compromising normal tissue doses (Hou et al., 2020).

Hypoxia is also an important issue in breast cancer (Lundgren et al., 2007). Hypoxic areas are present in 25–40% of patients (Vaupel et al., 2004). Therefore, boosting with SIB and hypofractionated treatments in breast cancer are being investigated (Hamilton et al., 2016; Nitsche et al., 2015).

MpMRI can help to define the hypoxic area distribution in prostate cancer (Her et al., 2021). One of the major causes of prostate cancer resistance is intratumoral hypoxia. Currently, dose-escalation studies are carried out with SIB to the prostate. In the Hypo-FLAME study, intermediate or high-risk prostate cancer patients were treated with extreme hypofractionated schedules doses of 35 Gy in 5 weekly fractions to the whole prostate gland with a SIB up to 50 Gy to the mpMRI-defined tumours. Ninety days after the initiation of treatment, the acute grade 2 GU and GI toxicity rates were found at 34.0% and 5.0%, respectively (Draulans et al., 2020). In the FLAME study, 571 prostate cancer patients with intermediate- and high-risk diseases were included. Patients in the standard arm received 77 Gy (fractions of 2.2 Gy) to the entire prostate. The focal boost arm received an additional SIB boost up to 95 Gy (fractions up to 2.7 Gy) to the intraprostatic lesion visible on MpMRI. In this study, no difference was found between the standard and study arms in terms of toxicity and quality of life (Kerkmeijer et al., 2021). Hypo-FLAME and FLAME studies showed that SIB to the primary tumour (s) while respecting OAR dose constraints is effective and safe. Currently, there are ongoing clinical studies on dose escalation and IMRT in the case of tumour hypoxia.

4. Redistribution

Redistribution during the cell cycle has a critical role in radiotherapy, given that cells present various radiosensitivities along with the four phases of the cell cycle (G1, S, G2, M). The cells in the synthesis (S) phase are three times more radioresistant than the cells in the mitosis (M) phase. Since the S phase constitutes one-third of the cell cycle, many tumour cells manage to escape death in a single radiotherapy fraction. One of the underlying factors of fractional radiotherapy is to ensure the redistribution of cells towards more sensitive phases by progressing in the mitotic cell cycle between fractions (Marcu et al., 2015). A phase-specific radiosensitivity occurs between the RT fractions as the cells progress through the mitotic cycle (Withers, 1975).

Zhao et al., examined the DNA repair and cell apoptosis mechanisms after irradiation at different doses of X-ray irradiation (0, 2, 4, 6, 8, 10, 12.5, 15, and 20 Gy) in cervical cancer cell line HeLa. While there was a significant decrease in cells in the S phase within 24 hours after RT, a significant increase was detected after 30 hours. Moreover, this situation was similar for all fraction doses (Stark and Taylor, 2006; Yan et al., 2007). An increased dose of irradiation resulted in a greater G2/M delay. Also, it was shown in this study that the cells returned to their normal cycles later with increasing doses. While the return to normal cycle pattern at <10 Gy doses occurs in 48 hours, when the RT dose exceeds 10 Gy, it has been shown that the return to normal cycle pattern is prolonged because the DNA repair capacity of the cell is exceeded (Zhao et al., 2019).

The cell cycle changes after RT actually occur through the changes in the levels of some proteins and enzymes. A decrease in CDK1 protein expression and an increase in the expression of CHK1 and g-H2AX were detected in HeLa cells due to irradiation at different doses (Zhao et al., 2019).

It has been tried most in HNCs in fractionation studies. Different advantages are obtained with different fractionation schemes. In hyper fractionated regimens, radiotherapy is administered in two or more fractions per day. The time given between RT fractions allows cells to progress towards radiosensitive phases by redistribution. While this allows the tumour to be given RT more than once a day, it provides a protective effect on non-proliferating normal tissues as the fraction doses decrease (Withers, 1975). The MARCH meta-analysis compared the hyper fractionated, accelerated, and accelerated with total dose reduction regimens in HNCs. However, overall survival contribution was achieved in all alternating fractionation schemes compared to conventional fractions; it was shown that the greatest contribution was made with hyper fractionated regimens (Bourhis et al., 2006).

In hypofractionated regimens that aim to give a higher dose in one fraction, the tumouricidal effect increases due to an increase in DNA double-strand breaks, increase in reactive oxygen products, prolongation of G2/M arrest in the cell cycle, and induction of apoptosis. In cell studies, this biological effect has been shown to occur at doses greater than 4 Gy (Zhao et al., 2019).

5. Repopulation

Repair and redistribution occur in a short time throughout the cell cycle. Since these factors are completed until the end of the daily fractions, they are important in hyperfractionated treatments where more than one fraction per day is applied. On the other hand, there are reoxygenation and repopulation factors that play a role for a longer time. For these factors, the term 'time' comes to the fore (Gasinska et al., 2004).

Repopulation is a factor that directly affects treatment response because any cell increase that may occur during treatment reduces the effectiveness of radiotherapy (Marcu et al., 2015).

Conventional RT is delivered in 1.8-2.0 Gy doses in five fractions per day/a week. This type of fractionation allows the repair of sublethal damage at OAR (Kim and Tannock, 2005). In many studies, it has been shown that in some cancer types, for example, HNC cancer, cervical cancer, bladder cancer, the tumour control rate decreased when overall treatment time was prolonged (Maciejewski and Majewski, 1991; Petereit et al., 1995; Withers et al., 1995). Withers et al., found that there is a non-linear, two-component relationship between the tumour control dose of 50% (TCD50) and overall treatment time, there being no consistent change in TCD50 between overall times of about 11 to 30 days but a steep rate of increase thereafter. In order to avoid the negative effects of repopulation, it is necessary to give an additional dose of 0.6 Gy for each day of prolonged treatment five weeks after the start of RT (Withers et al., 1988).

Besides historical results, human breast and rectal cancer revealed similar results with some labelling indices. In Ki 67, S phase fraction (SPF) and bromodeoxyuridine (BrdUrd) stainings showed repopulation, a decrease was observed at the beginning of RT, and an increase was observed later on

(Gasinska et al., 2011; Kovarík et al., 1996; Ramsay et al., 1988; Thames et al., 1996).

The cell cycle is fast in the HNCs. Repopulation affects the success of treatment in HNCs. Altered fractionation schemes such as hypofractionated or hyperfractionated schemes have been studied in the literature and demonstrated a statistically significant benefit of 2% on survival at five years (Bourhis et al., 2006; Overgaard et al., 2003).

Ferraira et al., compared four RT techniques by calculating the tumour response according to the Poisson Linear-Quadratic-Time model (Fowler, 1989). In this study, forward planning RT and two IMRT techniques (conventional and SIB) were used for comparison with the conventional RT technique. Compared to the conventional technique, a 42% increase in TCP was obtained in forward planning RT. On top of this benefit, an additional 5% benefit was obtained with IMRTcon and an additional 9% benefit with IMRTsib. In the IMRTsib technique, the NTCP rates of the ipsilateral parotid, contralateral parotid, the oral cavity, and the mandible decreased to 20%, 9%, 4%, and 3%, respectively (Costa Ferreira et al., 2010). Today inverse IMRT planning is standard in HNCs.

For patients with HNC undergoing definitive RT, a significant increase in delivered dose was obtained with the clinical implementation of SIB-IMRT. Costa Ferreira et al., examined 181 HNC patients treated with radical RT (68.0-70.6 Gy, 1.8-2.15 Gy fraction dose). The doses received by the groups were converted from 2 Gy to an equivalent dose and divided into two as <70 and ≥ 70 Gy. The mean overall treatment time (OTT) was shorter in the ≥ 70 Gy group, and the main reasons for the prolongation of OTT were RT toxicity and recurrence of the disease (26.6% and 21.9%, respectively). In the ≥ 70 Gy with SIB group, primary tumour doses were significantly higher, while parotid doses were significantly lower. This biological dose escalation resulted in an acceptable treatment outcome with similar rates of survival and late toxicity (Costa Ferreira et al., 2017).

Radioisotope imaging may also be useful to demonstrate tumour repopulation. 3′-deoxy-3′-18F-fluorothymidine (18F-FLT), which detects repopulation by showing thymidine kinase activity in cells, is one of the imaging methods used for this purpose (Idema et al., 2012; Herrmann et al., 2011). For example, in the study of Yue et al., two patients out of 21 had unplanned interruptions during RT and then underwent 18F FLT PET/CT scans, which had a corresponding increase in 18F FLT uptake, indicating tumour repopulation (Yue et al., 2010).

6. Radiosensitivity and Linear-Quadratic Model

Radiosensitivity is the tumour feature that aims to account for the fact that tumours respond differently to radiation therapy in a manner correlated with the intrinsic and individual radiosensitivity (Marcu et al., 2015). The linear-quadratic model represents the basis for predicting the clinical effects of alternative fractionation schemes in RT. In this model, the tissue response to altered fractionation (i.e., different from the standard 2 Gy/fraction) is determined by the tissue α/β ratio. In clinical practice, most tumours have a high α/β ratio (about 10 Gy); therefore, these tumours are treated with the standard fractionation of 2 Gy/fraction or with a hyper fractionated regimen (dose/fraction <2 Gy, two times a day).

In recent years, hypofractionation has been increasingly tried and studied in tumours with low α/β (Brenner and Hall, 1999; Miralbell et al., 2012). Prostate cancer is one of the cancers with a low α/β ratio (1.5) (Tree et al., 2014). The hypofractionated regimens have not been shown to be superior to conventional regimens in randomised studies in prostate cancer today, and it has been proven to be non-inferior (Incrocci et al., 2016; Henderson et al., 2015). In the CHHiP trial, instead of conventional fractionation (74 Gy/37 fractions), hypofractionated RT (60 Gy/20 fractions) is recommended (Dearnaley et al., 2016). Since it is possible to apply regimens at these doses with a sharp accuracy only with RT techniques such as IMRT and SBRT, IMRT and SBRT are increasingly being applied to patients with prostate cancer today.

Dose reduction is not always necessary to reduce NTCP. Bansal et al., compared 3D-CRT followed by an IMRT boost with a SIB-IMRT. Compared to sequential-IMRT, SIB-IMRT reduced the mean doses to both bladder and rectum by 13% and 17%, respectively, for all 30 patients (Bansal et al., 2012). In a similar study by Landry et al., with IMRT plans, a 25% reduction in intestinal doses and a 3-fold reduction in NTCP were achieved (Landry et al., 2002).

An estimate of 4 Gy for α/β value has already been reported for the fractionation sensitivity of breast cancer (Kurtz, 2005). This situation indicates that there will be benefits from hypofractionation in breast cancer. Today, hypofractionation has become standard in breast cancer (Bentzen et al., 2008; Trialists' Group, (2008)). IMRT may be considered in this treatment to increase the dose in the tumour bed with SIB. Guerrero et al., have shown that the conventional treatment of 45 Gy (1.8 Gy * 25) to the whole breast and then a boost of 20 Gy (2 Gy *10) is biologically equivalent to the 1.8 Gy * 25 to the whole breast with a 2.4 Gy * 25 SIB to the tumour bed RT (Guerrero et al., 2004). In fact, much more ambitious hypofractionated regimens are being tried for breast cancer today. Brunt et al., studied irradiation of breast cancer with different schedules of either 40 Gy/15 fractions/3-week or 27 Gy/5 fractions/1-week, or 26 Gy/5 fractions/1-week. When the repopulation-corrected BED values were calculated, it was shown that 26 Gy/5 fractions/1-week was the most balanced dose for primary tumour dose and erythema and late fibrosis side effects among hypofractionated regimens. This is consistent with the fact that the researchers saw mild side effects in patients. This study showed that the conventional scheme had the highest effective dose for erythema and fibrosis (Brunt et al., 2016).

Dose escalation can also be done by radiobiological evaluation in IMRT planning. Huang et al., showed that increasing the dose in the primary tumour by 14.8 Gy with IMRT in upper thoracic oesophagal cancers can be done without increasing radiation pneumonia and spinal cord damage. In this study, the tumour control was predicted to increase by 31.8%, 39.1%, and 40.9% for three independent TCP models. The predicted incidence of radiation pneumonitis was similar (3.9% versus 3.6%), and the estimated spinal cord injury risk was deficient (0.13%) in both groups (Huang et al., 2017).

Jones et al., found that >70 Gy doses are effective to improve RT response in high-grade glioma patients (Jones and Sanghera, 2007). Herman et al., compared 59.6 Gy in 3D-CRT with 90 Gy IMRT technique in terms of TCP and NTCP. In this study, which included ten patients with high-grade glioma, a 20% increase was obtained in TCP relative to 59.4Gy. NTCP for normal brain were negligible, 0.13% and 0.03%, whereas, at 90 Gy, the NTCP were 10.8% and 3.8% for 3DCRT and IMRT, respectively (De La Fuente Herman et al., 2010).

7. Secondary Cancer Risk with IMRT

It is possible to give different doses to the tumour and lymphatic area at the same time with IMRT. And it is possible to increase the dose to the tumour without increasing OAR toxicity, to complete the treatments in a shorter time, and to bring the NTCP and TCP balance to a more advantageous position. In the IMRT, a larger low dose region is formed due to a large number of fields compared to other RT techniques. Moreover, the low radiation dose has a potential risk of increased second malignancies (Hall and Wuu, 2003).

There are studies comparing IMRT techniques in terms of radiobiology among themselves. Tang et al., compared five techniques in Tomotherapy and IMRT for the postmastectomy radiotherapy with SIB. TomoDirect plans and hybrid -IMRT plans had better dose sparing for the lungs and heart. The fixed-field-IMRT plans had relatively higher NTCP and the second cancer complication probability for the lungs. The unblocked-helical TomoTherapy plans have the highest OAR mean dose, highest NTCP for the lungs and heart, and highest secondary cancer risk for the lungs and contralateral breast, among all techniques. Therefore, the unblocked-helical TomoTherapy should not be preferred (Tang et al., 2020). Similarly, in another breast cancer study in which RT techniques were compared, a field-in-field technique was found that the field-in-field technique had the lowest risk of secondary cancer among IMRT and VMAT techniques (Haciislamoglu et al., 2019).

Haciislamoglu et al., compared the secondary cancer risk between the sequential boost and SIB in IMRT/VMAT in nasopharyngeal cancer patients. In this study, the SIB IMRT/VMAT was found to be associated with the lowest organ equivalent doses for the oral cavity, pharynx, parotids, and submandibular glands, resulting in a secondary cancer risk reduction. It has been determined that the organ with the highest decrease in secondary cancer risk among these organs is the parotids (Haciislamoglu et al., 2020).

Jahreiß et al., compared secondary cancer risk in prostate survivors by IMRT and 3DCRT techniques. Extrapelvic secondary cancer was detected in 159 of 11,664 cases with an 8-year follow-up. When subgroup analysis was performed, the patients at risk for secondary cancer were generally found to be young patients (50-69 years) (Jahreiß et al., 2020).

Conclusion

Technological developments show progress on eliminating the deficiencies of current treatments and devices. What we need in cancer treatment is hidden in tumour biology. In the past decades, knowledge of tumour biology and radiobiology has gradually increased and deepened. When we start to use this information by reflecting it in clinical practice, the doors of personalised RT will be opened.

References

Bansal, A., Kapoor, R., Singh, S. K., Kumar, N., Oinam, A. S., & Sharma, S. C. (2012). Dosimetric comparison of standard three-dimensional conformal radiotherapy followed by intensity-modulated radiotherapy boost schedule (sequential IMRT plan) with simultaneous integrated boost–IMRT (SIB IMRT) treatment plan in patients with localized carcinoma prostate. *Indian Journal of Urology: IJU: Journal of the Urological Society of India*, 28(3), 300.

Benedict, S. H., Lin, P. S., Zwicker, R. D., Huang, D. T., & Schmidt-Ullrich, R. K. (1997). The biological effectiveness of intermittent irradiation as a function of overall treatment time: development of correction factors for linac-based stereotactic radiotherapy. *International journal of radiation oncology, biology, physics*, 37(4), 765-769.

Bentzen, L., Keiding, S., Nordsmark, M., Falborg, L., Hansen, S. B., Keller, J., ... & Overgaard, J. (2003). Tumour oxygenation assessed by 18F-fluoromisonidazole PET and polarographic needle electrodes in human soft tissue tumours. *Radiotherapy and Oncology*, 67(3), 339-344.

Bentzen, S. M., Agrawal, R. K., Aird, E. G., Barrett, J. M., Barrett-Lee, P. J., Bliss, J. M., ... & Yarnold, J. R. (2008). The UK Standardisation of Breast Radiotherapy (START) Trial A of radiotherapy hypofractionation for treatment of early breast cancer: a randomised trial. *The Lancet. Oncology*, 9(4), 331-341.

Bindra, R. S., Crosby, M. E., & Glazer, P. M. (2007). Regulation of DNA repair in hypoxic cancer cells. *Cancer and Metastasis Reviews*, 26(2), 249-260.

Bockbrader, M. and Edward K. (2009). Role of Intensity-Modulated Radiation Therapy in Gastrointestinal Cancer. *Expert Review of Anticancer Therapy* 9 (5): 637–47.

Bollineni, V. R., Koole, M. J. B., Pruim, J., Brouwer, C. L., Wiegman, E. M., Groen, H. J. M., Vlasman, R., Halmos, G. B., Oosting, S. F., Langendijk, J. A., Widder, J., & Steenbakkers, R. J. H. M. 2014. "Dynamics of Tumor Hypoxia Assessed by 18F-FAZA PET/CT in Head and Neck and Lung Cancer Patients during Chemoradiation: Possible Implications for Radiotherapy Treatment Planning Strategies." *Radiotherapy and Oncology: Journal of the European Society for Therapeutic Radiology and Oncology* 113 (2): 198–203.

Bourhis, J., Overgaard, J., Audry, H., Ang, K. K., Saunders, M., Bernier, J., Horiot, J.-C., Le Maître, A., Pajak, T. F., Poulsen, M. G., O'Sullivan, B., Dobrowsky, W., Hliniak, A., Skladowski, K., Hay, J. H., Pinto, L. H., Fallai, C., Fu, K. K., Sylvester, R., & Pignon, J. P. 2006. "Hyperfractionated or Accelerated Radiotherapy in Head and Neck Cancer: A Meta-Analysis." *The Lancet* 368 (9538): 843–54.

Brenner, D. J., & Hall, E. J. (1999). Fractionation and protraction for radiotherapy of prostate carcinoma. *International Journal of Radiation Oncology* Biology* Physics*, *43*(5), 1095-1101.

Brock, K. K., Mutic, S., McNutt, T. R., Li, H., & Kessler, M. L. (2017). Use of image registration and fusion algorithms and techniques in radiotherapy: Report of the AAPM Radiation Therapy Committee Task Group No. 132. *Medical physics*, *44*(7), e43-e76.

Brunt, A. M., Wheatley, D., Yarnold, J., Somaiah, N., Kelly, S., Harnett, A., ... & Bliss, J. M. (2016). Acute skin toxicity associated with a 1-week schedule of whole breast radiotherapy compared with a standard 3-week regimen delivered in the UK FAST-Forward Trial. *Radiotherapy and Oncology*, *120*(1), 114-118.

C Gaertner, F., Souvatzoglou, M., Brix, G., & J Beer, A. (2012). Imaging of hypoxia using PET and MRI. *Current pharmaceutical biotechnology*, *13*(4), 552-570.

Carlos-Reyes, A., Muñiz-Lino, M. A., Romero-Garcia, S., López-Camarillo, C., & Hernández-de la Cruz, O. N. (2021). Biological Adaptations of Tumor Cells to Radiation Therapy. *Frontiers in Oncology*, *11*.

Chao, K. C., Bosch, W. R., Mutic, S., Lewis, J. S., Dehdashti, F., Mintun, M. A., ... & Welch, M. J. (2001). A novel approach to overcome hypoxic tumor resistance: Cu-ATSM-guided intensity-modulated radiation therapy. *International Journal of Radiation Oncology* Biology* Physics*, *49*(4), 1171-1182.

Chao, K. C., Ozyigit, G., Tran, B. N., Cengiz, M., Dempsey, J. F., & Low, D. A. (2003). Patterns of failure in patients receiving definitive and postoperative IMRT for head-and-neck cancer. *International Journal of Radiation Oncology* Biology* Physics*, *55*(2), 312-321.

Chen, A. M., Jennelle, R. L., Sreeraman, R., Yang, C. C., Liu, T., Vijayakumar, S., & Purdy, J. A. (2009). Initial clinical experience with helical tomotherapy for head and neck cancer. *Head & Neck: Journal for the Sciences and Specialties of the Head and Neck*, *31*(12), 1571-1578.

Costa Ferreira, B., Sá-Couto, P., Khouri, L., & Lopes, M. D. C. (2017). Biological dose-escalated definitive radiation therapy in head and neck cancer. *The British Journal of Radiology*, *90*(1072), 20160477.

Dale, R. G. (1985). The application of the linear-quadratic dose-effect equation to fractionated and protracted radiotherapy. *The British journal of radiology*, *58*(690), 515-528.

Dale, R. G. (2018). Radiation repair models for clinical application. *The British Journal of Radiology*, *92*(1093), 20180070.

De La Fuente Herman, T., Ahmad, S., & Vlachaki, M. T. (2010). Intensity modulated radiation therapy versus three dimensional conformal radiation therapy for treatment of high grade glioma: A radiobiological modeling study. *Journal of X-Ray Science and Technology*, *18*(4), 393-402.

Dearnaley, D., Syndikus, I., Mossop, H., Khoo, V., Birtle, A., Bloomfield, D., ... & CHHiP Investigators. (2016). Conventional versus hypofractionated high-dose intensity-modulated radiotherapy for prostate cancer: 5-year outcomes of the randomised, non-inferiority, phase 3 CHHiP trial. *The Lancet Oncology*, *17*(8), 1047-1060.

Draulans, C., van der Heide, U. A., Haustermans, K., Pos, F. J., van der Voort van Zyp, J., De Boer, H., Groen, V. H., Monninkhof, E. M., Smeenk, R. J., Kunze-Busch, M., De Roover, R., Depuydt, T., Isebaert, S., & Kerkmeijer, L. G. W. 2020. "Primary Endpoint Analysis of the Multicentre Phase II Hypo-FLAME Trial for Intermediate and High Risk Prostate Cancer." *Radiotherapy and Oncology: Journal of the European Society for Therapeutic Radiology and Oncology* 147 (June): 92–98.

Egeland, T. A., Gaustad, J. V., Vestvik, I. K., Benjaminsen, I. C., Mathiesen, B., & Rofstad, E. K. (2006). Assessment of fraction of radiobiologically hypoxic cells in human melanoma xenografts by dynamic contrast-enhanced MRI. *Magnetic Resonance in Medicine: An Official Journal of the International Society for Magnetic Resonance in Medicine*, *55*(4), 874-882.

Elkind, M. M., and Harriet Sutton. 1959. "X-Ray Damage and Recovery in Mammalian Cells in Culture." *Nature* 184 (4695): 1293–95.

Elkind, M. M., Sutton-Gilbert, H., Moses, W. B., Alescio, T., & Swain, R. (1965). Radiation response of mammalian cells grown in culture: V. Temperature dependence of the repair of x-ray damage in surviving cells (aerobic and hypoxic). *Radiation research*, *25*(2), 359-376.

Ferreira, B. C., do Carmo Lopes, M., Mateus, J., Capela, M., & Mavroidis, P. (2010). Radiobiological evaluation of forward and inverse IMRT using different fractionations for head and neck tumours. *Radiation Oncology*, *5*(1), 1-13.

Fonteyne, V., Villeirs, G., Speleers, B., De Neve, W., De Wagter, C., Lumen, N., & De Meerleer, G. (2008). Intensity-modulated radiotherapy as primary therapy for prostate cancer: report on acute toxicity after dose escalation with simultaneous integrated boost to intraprostatic lesion. *International Journal of Radiation Oncology* Biology* Physics*, *72*(3), 799-807.

Fowler, J. F. (1989). The linear-quadratic formula and progress in fractionated radiotherapy. *The British journal of radiology*, *62*(740), 679-694.

Fowler, J. F., & Van Limbergen, E. F. (1997). Biological effect of pulsed dose rate brachytherapy with stepping sources if short half-times of repair are present in tissues. *International journal of radiation oncology, biology, physics*, *37*(4), 877-883.

Franceschini, D., Paiar, F., Meattini, I., Agresti, B., Pasquetti, E. M., Greto, D., ... & Biti, G. (2013). Simultaneous integrated boost–intensity-modulated radiotherapy in head and neck cancer. *The Laryngoscope*, *123*(12), E97-E103.

Gasinska, A., Fowler, J. F., Lind, B. K., & Urbanski, K. (2004). Influence of overall treatment time and radiobiological parameters on biologically effective doses in cervical cancer patients treated with radiation therapy alone. *Acta oncologica*, *43*(7), 657-666.

Gasinska, A., Richter, P., Darasz, Z., Niemiec, J., Bucki, K., Malecki, K., & Sokolowski, A. (2011). Gender-related differences in repopulation and early tumor response to preoperative radiotherapy in rectal cancer patients. *Journal of Gastrointestinal Surgery*, *15*(9), 1568-1576.

Guerrero, M., Li, X. A., Earl, M. A., Sarfaraz, M., & Kiggundu, E. (2004). Simultaneous integrated boost for breast cancer using IMRT: a radiobiological and treatment planning study. *International Journal of Radiation Oncology* Biology* Physics*, *59*(5), 1513-1522.

Haciislamoglu, E., Cinar, Y., Eren, M., Canyilmaz, E., Gurcan, F., Serdar, L., & Yoney, A. (2020). Comparison of radiation-induced secondary malignancy risk between sequential and simultaneous integrated boost for the treatment of nasopharyngeal carcinoma: intensity-modulated radiotherapy versus volumetric-modulated arc therapy. *Cancer Management and Research*, *12*, 2513.

Haciislamoglu, E., Cinar, Y., Gurcan, F., Canyilmaz, E., Gungor, G., & Yoney, A. (2019). Secondary cancer risk after whole-breast radiation therapy: field-in-field versus intensity modulated radiation therapy versus volumetric modulated arc therapy. *The British Journal of Radiology*, *92*(1102), 20190317.

Hall, E. J., & Wuu, C. S. (2003). Radiation-induced second cancers: the impact of 3D-CRT and IMRT. *International Journal of Radiation Oncology* Biology* Physics*, *56*(1), 83-88.

Hamilton, D. G., Bale, R., Jones, C., Fitzgerald, E., Khor, R., Knight, K., & Wasiak, J. (2016). Impact of tumour bed boost integration on acute and late toxicity in patients with breast cancer: A systematic review. *The Breast*, *27*, 126-135.

Harada, H. (2016). Hypoxia-inducible factor 1–mediated characteristic features of cancer cells for tumor radioresistance. *Journal of radiation research*, *57*(S1), i99-i105.

Henderson, D. R., Tree, A. C., & Van As, N. J. (2015). Stereotactic body radiotherapy for prostate cancer. *Clinical oncology*, *27*(5), 270-279.

Her, E. J., Haworth, A., Sun, Y., Williams, S., Reynolds, H. M., Kennedy, A., & Ebert, M. A. (2021). Biologically Targeted Radiation Therapy: Incorporating Patient-Specific Hypoxia Data Derived from Quantitative Magnetic Resonance Imaging. *Cancers*, *13*(19), 4897.

Herrmann, K., Buck, A. K., Schuster, T., Rudelius, M., Wester, H. J., Graf, N., ... & Keller, U. (2011). A pilot study to evaluate 3′-deoxy-3′-18F-fluorothymidine pet for initial and early response imaging in mantle cell lymphoma. *Journal of Nuclear Medicine*, *52*(12), 1898-1902.

Hoogeman, M. S., Nuyttens, J. J., Levendag, P. C., & Heijmen, B. J. (2008). Time dependence of intrafraction patient motion assessed by repeat stereoscopic imaging. *International Journal of Radiation Oncology* Biology* Physics*, *70*(2), 609-618.

Hou, C., Gong, G., Wang, L., Su, Y., Lu, J., & Yin, Y. (2022). The Study of Cerebral Blood Flow Variations during Brain Metastases Radiotherapy. *Oncology Research and Treatment*, *45*(3), 130-137.

Huang, B. T., Wu, L. L., Guo, L. J., Xu, L. Y., Huang, R. H., Lin, P. X., ... & Chen, C. Z. (2017). Radiobiological evaluation of simultaneously dose-escalated versus non-escalated intensity-modulated radiation therapy for patients with upper thoracic esophageal cancer. *OncoTargets and therapy*, *10*, 2209.

Idema, A. J., Hoffmann, A. L., Boogaarts, H. D., Troost, E. G., Wesseling, P., Heerschap, A., ... & Oyen, W. J. (2012). 3′-Deoxy-3′-18F-Fluorothymidine PET–Derived proliferative volume predicts overall survival in high-grade glioma patients. *Journal of Nuclear Medicine*, *53*(12), 1904-1910.

Incrocci, L., Wortel, R. C., Alemayehu, W. G., Aluwini, S., Schimmel, E., Krol, S., ... & Pos, F. (2016). Hypofractionated versus conventionally fractionated radiotherapy for patients with localised prostate cancer (HYPRO): final efficacy results from a randomised, multicentre, open-label, phase 3 trial. *The Lancet Oncology*, *17*(8), 1061-1069.

Jackson, S. P., & Bartek, J. (2009). The DNA-damage response in human biology and disease. *Nature*, *461*(7267), 1071-1078.

Jahreiß, M. C., Aben, K. K., Hoogeman, M. S., Dirkx, M. L., de Vries, K. C., Incrocci, L., & Heemsbergen, W. D. (2020). The risk of second primary cancers in prostate cancer survivors treated in the modern radiotherapy era. *Frontiers in oncology, 10,* 2519.

Jiang, L., Zhang, Y., Yang, Z., Liang, F., Wu, J., & Wang, R. (2019). A comparison of clinical outcomes between simultaneous integrated boost (SIB) versus sequential boost (SEQ) intensity modulated radiation therapy (IMRT) for head and neck cancer: a meta-analysis. *Medicine, 98*(34).

Jin, J. Y., Wen, N., Ren, L., Glide-Hurst, C., & Chetty, I. J. (2011). Advances in treatment techniques: arc-based and other intensity modulated therapies. *The Cancer Journal, 17*(3), 166-176.

Jones, B., & Sanghera, P. (2007). Estimation of radiobiologic parameters and equivalent radiation dose of cytotoxic chemotherapy in malignant glioma. *International Journal of Radiation Oncology* Biology* Physics, 68*(2), 441-448.

Kachnic, L. A., Tsai, H. K., Coen, J. J., Blaszkowsky, L. S., Hartshorn, K., Kwak, E. L., ... & Hong, T. S. (2012). Dose-painted intensity-modulated radiation therapy for anal cancer: a multi-institutional report of acute toxicity and response to therapy. *International Journal of Radiation Oncology* Biology* Physics, 82*(1), 153-158.

Kawahara, D., Nakano, H., Saito, A., Ozawa, S., & Nagata, Y. (2020). Dose compensation based on biological effectiveness due to interruption time for photon radiation therapy. *The British Journal of Radiology, 93*(1111), 20200125.

Kerkmeijer, L. G., Groen, V. H., Pos, F. J., Haustermans, K., Monninkhof, E. M., Smeenk, R. J., ... & van der Heide, U. A. (2021). *Focal boost to the intraprostatic tumor in external beam radiotherapy for patients with localized prostate cancer: results from the FLAME randomized phase III trial.*

Kim, J. J., & Tannock, I. F. (2005). Repopulation of cancer cells during therapy: an important cause of treatment failure. *Nature Reviews Cancer, 5*(7), 516-525.

Klopp, A. H., Yeung, A. R., Deshmukh, S., Gil, K. M., Wenzel, L., Westin, S. N., ... & Bruner, D. W. (2018). Patient-reported toxicity during pelvic intensity-modulated radiation therapy: NRG Oncology–RTOG 1203. *Journal of clinical oncology, 36*(24), 2538.

Kovarík, J., Skry, G. D., Mikel, J., & Svoboda, V. H. (1996). Changes of Ki67 index of various tumors during radiation therapy. *Neoplasma, 43*(2), 89-92.

Kurtz, J. M. (2005). The clinical radiobiology of breast cancer radiotherapy. *Radiotherapy and Oncology, 75*(1), 6-8.

Landry, J. C., Yang, G. Y., Ting, J. Y., Staley, C. A., Torres, W., Esiashvili, N., & Davis, L. W. (2002). Treatment of pancreatic cancer tumors with intensity-modulated radiation therapy (IMRT) using the volume at risk approach (VARA): employing dose-volume histogram (DVH) and normal tissue complication probability (NTCP) to evaluate small bowel toxicity. *Medical Dosimetry, 27*(2), 121-129.

Lee, N. Y., Mechalakos, J. G., Nehmeh, S., Lin, Z., Squire, O. D., Cai, S., ... & Schöder, H. (2008). Fluorine-18-labeled fluoromisonidazole positron emission and computed tomography-guided intensity-modulated radiotherapy for head and neck cancer: a feasibility study. *International Journal of Radiation Oncology* Biology* Physics, 70*(1), 2-13.

Li, H., Xu, D., Han, X., Ruan, Q., Zhang, X., Mi, Y., ... & Li, G. (2018). Dosimetry study of 18F-FMISO+ PET/CT hypoxia imaging guidance on intensity-modulated radiation therapy for non-small cell lung cancer. *Clinical and Translational Oncology*, *20*(10), 1329-1336.

Linthout, N., Bral, S., Van de Vondel, I., Verellen, D., Tournel, K., Gevaert, T., ... & Storme, G. (2009). Treatment delivery time optimization of respiratory gated radiation therapy by application of audio-visual feedback. *Radiotherapy and Oncology*, *91*(3), 330-335.

Lopes, S., Ferreira, S., & Caetano, M. (2021). PET/CT in the evaluation of hypoxia for radiotherapy planning in head and neck tumors: Systematic literature review. *Journal of Nuclear Medicine Technology*, *49*(2), 107-113.

Lundgren, K., Holm, C., & Landberg, G. (2007). Hypoxia and breast cancer: prognostic and therapeutic implications. *Cell Mol Life Sci*, *64*(24), 3233-3247.

Maciejewski, B., & Majewski, S. (1991). Dose fractionation and tumour repopulation in radiotherapy for bladder cancer. *Radiotherapy and Oncology*, *21*(3), 163-170.

Marcu, L. G., Dasu, I. T., & Dasu, A. (2015). The six Rs of head and neck cancer radiotherapy. *Contemporary Issues in Head and Neck Cancer Management*, 35-58.

Martin, G. V., Cerqueira, M. D., Caldwell, J. H., Rasey, J. S., Embree, L., & Krohn, K. A. (1990). Fluoromisonidazole. A metabolic marker of myocyte hypoxia. *Circulation research*, *67*(1), 240-244.

Miralbell, R., Roberts, S. A., Zubizarreta, E., & Hendry, J. H. (2012). Dose-fractionation sensitivity of prostate cancer deduced from radiotherapy outcomes of 5,969 patients in seven international institutional datasets: α/β = 1.4 (0.9–2.2) Gy. *International Journal of Radiation Oncology* Biology* Physics*, *82*(1), e17-e24.

Mohan, R., Wu, Q., Manning, M., & Schmidt-Ullrich, R. (2000). Radiobiological considerations in the design of fractionation strategies for intensity-modulated radiation therapy of head and neck cancers. *International Journal of Radiation Oncology* Biology* Physics*, *46*(3), 619-630.

Mortensen, L. S., Johansen, J., Kallehauge, J., Primdahl, H., Busk, M., Lassen, P., ... & Overgaard, J. (2012). FAZA PET/CT hypoxia imaging in patients with squamous cell carcinoma of the head and neck treated with radiotherapy: results from the DAHANCA 24 trial. *Radiotherapy and oncology*, *105*(1), 14-20.

Mu, X., Löfroth, P. O., Karlsson, M., & Zackrisson, B. (2003). The effect of fraction time in intensity modulated radiotherapy: theoretical and experimental evaluation of an optimisation problem. *Radiotherapy and oncology*, *68*(2), 181-187.

Nahum, A. E., & Uzan, J. (2012). (Radio) biological optimization of external-beam radiotherapy. *Computational and mathematical methods in medicine*, *2012*.

Niemierko, A. (2006). Biological Aspects of IMRT Planning and Delivery. In *Image-Guided IMRT* (pp. 91-96). Springer, Berlin, Heidelberg.

Nitsche, M., Dunst, J., Carl, U. M., & Hermann, R. M. (2015). Emerging role of hypofractionated radiotherapy with simultaneous integrated boost in modern radiotherapy of breast cancer. *Breast Care*, *10*(5), 320-324.

Nutting, C. M., Morden, J. P., Harrington, K. J., Urbano, T. G., Bhide, S. A., Clark, C., ... & PARSPORT Trial Management Group. (2011). Parotid-sparing intensity modulated versus conventional radiotherapy in head and neck cancer (PARSPORT): a phase 3 multicentre randomised controlled trial. *The lancet oncology*, *12*(2), 127-136.

Okamoto, S., Shiga, T., Yasuda, K., Watanabe, S., Hirata, K., Nishijima, K. I., ... & Tamaki, N. (2016). The reoxygenation of hypoxia and the reduction of glucose metabolism in head and neck cancer by fractionated radiotherapy with intensity-modulated radiation therapy. *European journal of nuclear medicine and molecular imaging*, *43*(12), 2147-2154.

Orlandi, E., Palazzi, M., Pignoli, E., Fallai, C., Giostra, A., & Olmi, P. (2010). Radiobiological basis and clinical results of the simultaneous integrated boost (SIB) in intensity modulated radiotherapy (IMRT) for head and neck cancer: a review. *Critical reviews in oncology/hematology*, *73*(2), 111-125.

Otto, K. (2008). Volumetric modulated arc therapy: IMRT in a single gantry arc. *Medical physics*, *35*(1), 310-317.

Overgaard, J., Hansen, H. S., Specht, L., Overgaard, M., Grau, C., Andersen, E., ... & Evensen, J. F. (2003). Five compared with six fractions per week of conventional radiotherapy of squamous-cell carcinoma of head and neck: DAHANCA 6&7 randomised controlled trial. *The Lancet*, *362*(9388), 933-940.

Paganetti, H. (2005). Changes in tumor cell response due to prolonged dose delivery times in fractionated radiation therapy. *International Journal of Radiation Oncology* Biology* Physics*, *63*(3), 892-900.

Petereit, D. G., Sarkaria, J. N., Chappell, R., Fowler, J. F., Hartmann, T. J., Kinsella, T. J., ... & Buchler, D. A. (1995). The adverse effect of treatment prolongation in cervical carcinoma. *International Journal of Radiation Oncology* Biology* Physics*, *32*(5), 1301-1307.

Ramsay, J., Suit, H. D., Preffer, F. I., & Sedlacek, R. (1988). Changes in bromodeoxyuridine labeling index during radiation treatment of an experimental tumor. *Radiation research*, *116*(3), 453-461.

Rasey, J. S., Grunbaum, Z., Krohn, K., Nelson, N., & Chin, L. (1985). Comparison of Binding of and in Multicell Spheroids. *Radiation research*, *101*(3), 473-479.

Santa Cruz, O., Tsoutsou, P., Castella, C., Khanfir, K., Anchisi, S., Bouayed, S., ... & Ozsahin, M. (2018). Locoregional control and toxicity in head and neck carcinoma patients following helical Tomotherapy-delivered intensity-modulated radiation therapy compared with 3D-CRT data. *Oncology*, *95*, 61-68.

Shibamoto, Y., Ito, M., Sugie, C., Ogino, H., & Hara, M. (2004). Recovery from sublethal damage during intermittent exposures in cultured tumor cells: implications for dose modification in radiosurgery and IMRT. *International Journal of Radiation Oncology* Biology* Physics*, *59*(5), 1484-1490.

Silvoniemi, A., Suilamo, S., Laitinen, T., Forsback, S., Löyttyniemi, E., Vaittinen, S., ... & Minn, H. (2018). Repeatability of tumour hypoxia imaging using [18F] EF5 PET/CT in head and neck cancer. *European Journal of Nuclear Medicine and Molecular Imaging*, *45*(2), 161-169.

Stark, G. R., & Taylor, W. R. (2006). Control of the G2/M transition. *Molecular biotechnology*, *32*(3), 227-248.

Steinberger, E., Kollmeier, M., McBride, S., Novak, C., Pei, X., & Zelefsky, M. J. (2015). Cigarette smoking during external beam radiation therapy for prostate cancer is associated with an increased risk of prostate cancer-specific mortality and treatment-related toxicity. *BJU international*, *116*(4), 596-603.

Tang, D., Liang, Z., Guan, F., & Yang, Z. (2020). Dosimetric and Radiobiological Comparison of Five Techniques for Postmastectomy Radiotherapy with Simultaneous Integrated Boost. *BioMed research international*, *2020*.

Thames, H. D., Ruifrok, A. C., Milas, L., Hunter, N., Mason, K. A., Terry, N. H., & White, R. A. (1996). Accelerated repopulation during fractionated irradiation of a murine ovarian carcinoma: downregulation of apoptosis as a possible mechanism. *International Journal of Radiation Oncology* Biology* Physics*, *35*(5), 951-962.

Thomlinson, R. H., & Gray, L. H. (1955). The histological structure of some human lung cancers and the possible implications for radiotherapy. *British journal of cancer*, *9*(4), 539.

Timon, G., Ciardo, D., Bazani, A., Garioni, M., Maestri, D., De Lorenzo, D., ... & Jereczek-Fossa, B. A. (2016). Rationale and protocol of AIRC IG-13218, short-term radiotherapy for early prostate cancer with concomitant boost to the dominant lesion. *Tumori Journal*, *102*(5), 536-540.

Tree, A. C., Khoo, V. S., Van As, N. J., & Partridge, M. (2014). Is biochemical relapse-free survival after profoundly hypofractionated radiotherapy consistent with current radiobiological models? *Clinical Oncology*, *26*(4), 216-229.

Trialists' Group, T. S. (2008). The UK Standardisation of Breast Radiotherapy (START) Trial B of radiotherapy hypofractionation for treatment of early breast cancer: a randomised trial. *The Lancet*, 371(9618), 1098-1107.

Trott, K. R. (1982). Experimental results and clinical implications of the four R's in fractionated radiotherapy. *Radiation and Environmental biophysics*, *20*(3), 159-170.

Vaupel, P., Mayer, A., & Höckel, M. (2004). Tumor hypoxia and malignant progression. In *Methods in enzymology* (Vol. 381, pp. 335-354). Academic Press.

Walsh Joseph, C., & KolbHartmuth, C. (2014). The clinical importance of assessing tumor hypoxia: relationship of tumor hypoxia to prognosis and therapeutic opportunities. *Antioxidants & redox signaling*.

Wang, J. Z., Li, X. A., D D'Souza, W., & Stewart, R. D. (2003). Impact of prolonged fraction delivery times on tumor control: a note of caution for intensity-modulated radiation therapy (IMRT). *International Journal of Radiation Oncology* Biology* Physics*, *57*(2), 543-552.

Welsh, J. S., Limmer, J. P., Howard, S. P., Diamond, D., Harari, P. M., & Tomé, W. (2005). Precautions in the use of intensity-modulated radiation therapy. *Technology in Cancer Research & Treatment*, *4*(2), 203-210.

Withers, H. R. (1975). Cell cycle redistribution as a factor in multifraction irradiation. *Radiology*, *114*(1), 199-202.

Withers, H. R., Peters, L. J., Taylor, J. M., Owen, J. B., Morrison, W. H., Schultheiss, T. E., ... & Hanks, G. E. (1995). Local control of carcinoma of the tonsil by radiation therapy: an analysis of patterns of fractionation in nine institutions. *International Journal of Radiation Oncology* Biology* Physics*, *33*(3), 549-562.

Withers, H. R., Taylor, J. M. G., & Maciejewski, B. (1988). The hazard of accelerated tumor clonogen repopulation during radiotherapy. *Acta oncologica*, *27*(2), 131-146.

Yan, Y., Black, C. P., & Cowan, K. H. (2007). Irradiation-induced G2/M checkpoint response requires ERK1/2 activation. *Oncogene*, *26*(32), 4689-4698.

Yue, J., Chen, L., Cabrera, A. R., Sun, X., Zhao, S., Zheng, F., ... & Li, Y. (2010). Measuring tumor cell proliferation with 18F-FLT PET during radiotherapy of esophageal squamous cell carcinoma: a pilot clinical study. *Journal of Nuclear Medicine*, *51*(4), 528-534.

Zhao, H., Zhuang, Y., Li, R., Liu, Y., Mei, Z., He, Z., ... & Zhou, Y. (2019). Effects of different doses of X-ray irradiation on cell apoptosis, cell cycle, DNA damage repair and glycolysis in HeLa cells. *Oncology letters*, *17*(1), 42-54.

Chapter 4

Imaging in Radiotherapy

Taylan Tuğrul*
Department of Radiation Oncology, Van Yüzüncü Yıl University, Van, Turkey

Abstract

The contribution of imaging systems in radiation therapy is not only to treat tumour volume but also to treat areas that may show microscopic spread.

Imaging methods are of great importance for the extent of the disease, the staging of the tumour and its localization to the adjacent tissues. To accurately calculate the absorbed radiation dose, the mass attenuation factor and heterogeneity of the tissue type must be accurately defined. This is only possible with the use of Computed Tomography (CT) in the planning of radiation treatments. Today, radiotherapy planning is done on CT images. The most important reason for this is that it is possible to determine the properties of the mass attenuation coefficient for high-energy radiations in CT images. The use of imaging tools such as Magnetic Resonance (MR) imaging and positron emission tomography (PET) helped to deliver the dose to the tumour with a more precise limits in radiation therapy. MR images provide better soft tissue discrimination than CT images, which allows for more accurate selection of the distinction between the area to be treated and healthy tissue. PET images are also effective in identifying regions where tumour activity is intense and low.

The aim of this chapter is to give general information about image methods used in radiotherapy treatments.

*Corresponding Author's Email: taylantugrul@gmail.com.

In: Frontiers in Intensity-Modulated Radiotherapy Research
Editor: Sibel Karaca
ISBN: 979-8-88697-252-8

Keywords: computed tomography, emission tomography, imaging, magnetic resonance, positron, radiotherapy

1. Introduction

It was soon realized that x-rays, which are frequently used in imaging methods today, have a biological effect on tissue with the discovery of their imaging properties. The discovery of the damage it caused to the tumour at the beginning of the 20th century led to the formation of the radiotherapy method (Van den Berge et al., 2000). In particular, the discovery of x-rays (1845-1923), radioactivity (1852-1908), and radium (1867-1934) led to the emergence of radiation therapy (Pereira et al., 2014). Radiotherapy is part of the treatment of the majority of cancer patients today. The contribution of imaging systems to radiation therapy is not only to treat tumour volume, but also to treat areas that may show microscopic spread. Imaging methods are of great importance for the extent of the disease, the staging of the tumour and its localisation to the adjacent tissues. The ability to obtain 3 dimensional (3D) images has greatly contributed to the dosimetry process in radiotherapy. Features such as the relationship between electron densities and 3D anatomical configuration have significantly increased the accuracy of dosimetry in radiotherapy (Van den Berge et al., 2000). In addition, the use of imaging tools such as Magnetic Resonance (MR) imaging and Positron Emission Tomography (PET) helped to deliver the dose to the tumour with more precise limits in radiation therapy (Mak et al., 2011; Schlegel, 2010). MR images provide better soft tissue discrimination than Computed Tomography (CT) images, which allows for more accurate selection of the distinction between the area to be treated and healthy tissue. PET images are also effective in identifying regions where tumour activity is intense and low (Grosu et al., 2005; Hunter and Eisbruch, 2011). Today, radiotherapy planning is done on CT images. The most important reason for this is that it is possible to determine the properties of the mass attenuation coefficient for high-energy radiations in CT images. This provides a more precise dose calculation, which leads to more accurate treatment. Another reason is that the acquisition time of CT images is much shorter than MR and PET images (Pereira et al., 2014). Important events in the interaction of radiation with tissue (Photoelectric effect, Compton effect, double formation/annihilation) depend on the atomic number, electron density of the tissue and the energy of the radiation. To accurately calculate the absorbed radiation dose, the mass attenuation factor and heterogeneity of the tissue type must be accurately defined. This is only possible with the use of CT in the planning of radiation treatments. The most important disadvantage of using CT images is the possibility of different tumour identification for each physician due to the low tissue contrast of the images. To prevent this, it is recommended to select the target region after the fusion of images such as MR and PET with CT images. The sample picture is shown in Figure 1.

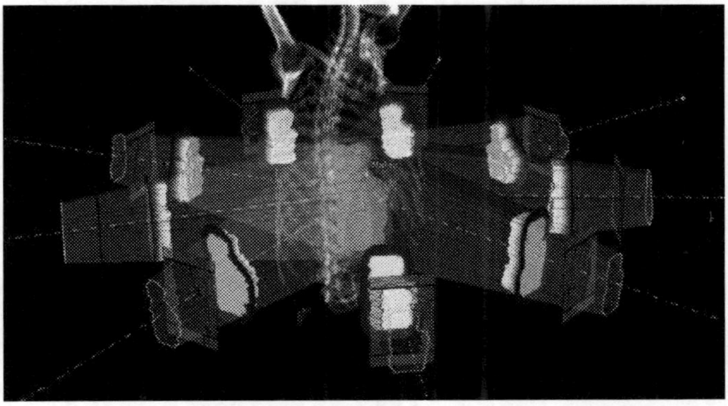

Figure 1. A sample radiotherapy plan image obtained from the treatment planning system.

2. Computed Tomography (CT)

In a modern multislice CT device used today, an image is obtained as a result of a component consisting of an X-ray generating source and detector array rotating around the patient at one to three revolutions per second (Lu and Brady, 2008). Figure 2 shows an example CT device and its components.

The voltage values in the X-ray tube vary between 80-140 kilovoltage (kV). In addition, the current of the X-ray tube, which controls the radiation exposure rate and the signal-to-noise ratio, can be between 10 Milliampere-500 Milliampere. However, in some systems, the current of the X-ray tube may be automatically limited to a maximum value for certain parameters. Scan exposure time and value of tube current are the main parameters used to determine the dose achieved. McCollough et al. showed that these dose values can be between 1-15 mSv (Mccollough et al., 2008).

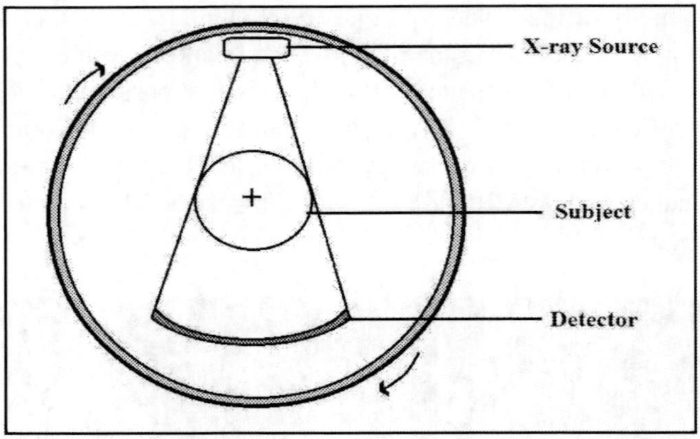

Figure 2. An example CT device and its components.

CT images are and will continue to be, one of the main equipment for radiotherapy today (Jaffray et al., 2007). CT images are used in almost all radiation treatments for pre-treatment imaging, treatment planning and treatment accuracy. Today, the number of centres that perform 2D radiation therapy is very low. In radiotherapy (RT), CT images are used to define gross tumour volume (GTV), clinic tumour volume (CTV), planning tumour volume (PTV), and normal tissues. In addition to identifying the target volume to be irradiated and healthy tissues, it is the primary method for calculating the dose of radiation and treatment simulation (Jaffray et al., 2007).

A CT simulator used in radiotherapy centres is a CT imaging system with some hardware and software for simulating and planning the radiation therapy to be applied to the patient. The CT simulator should have a flat table top for the location of the radiation therapy. The hole size of the CT device should be larger than 80 cm. In devices with smaller CT holes, it is difficult for the apparatus used in the treatment of some regions to enter the device. (For example, in breast patients). Expanded field of view reconstruction (FOV) is required in these systems, especially for large shooting fields, in order to fully capture the patient's anatomy and draw the skin contours correctly (Jaffray et al., 2007).

Moving laser systems, which radiotherapy technicians use to facilitate patient setup and immobilisation, are one of the most important equipment of CT simulators. It should have a large detector array to allow a large scanning area at high resolution. This can also be useful for breath-hold imaging and 4D imaging. Using an extended Hounsfield Unit (HU) scale is useful for imaging patients with high-density implants. In order to calculate all the values that can be obtained from the absorbed dose correctly in CT scans, the scanning region of the patient's anatomy should be selected appropriately. The main method of CT simulation; Before scanning, the isocentre of the patient is marked with a radiopaque material with the help of lasers, CT images are taken and then these images are transferred to the treatment planning system (TPS), as a result of the identification of these markers by the TPS, the system gives the differences to the centre of the radiation beam in x, y and z directions and it is based on the use of these values by the radiotherapist in the patient setup. Digitally reconstructed radiographs (DRR) images sent by the TPS are used for patient setup. As a result, the CT images taken are used in all stages of radiotherapy treatment. Guidelines for a CT simulation are given in American Association of Physicists in Medicine (AAPM) Task Group 66 (Mutic et al., 2003).

3. Four-Dimensional Computed Tomography (4DCT)

Imaging systems that allow respiratory-related patient scans are called four-dimensional computed tomography (4DCT). For treatment plans where the intensity modulated radiotherapy (IMRT) technique is used for radiotherapy treatment, it plays an important role in terms of the accuracy of the treatment. It is a method used to measure respiratory and organ movements. It is used to prevent the determination of wrong tumour location and size, which may be caused by organ movements. Such imaging systems enable the capture of various stages of the respiratory cycle and the planning of radiotherapy treatment according to these images. This, in turn, will ensure that the target area, which moves with the effect of respiration, receives a more accurate radiation dose and will cause the healthy tissues to receive less dose. 4DCT technique; it helps to reduce image artifacts that may be associated with respiration and to design a more appropriate method during radiotherapy (Van den Berge et al., 2000).

With this method, target volume limits specific to each patient can be determined. The 4DCT method can be applied by a system that monitors chest enlargement or by monitoring a reflector placed on the abdomen with a camera. An exemplary 4DCT acquisition is shown in Figure 3.

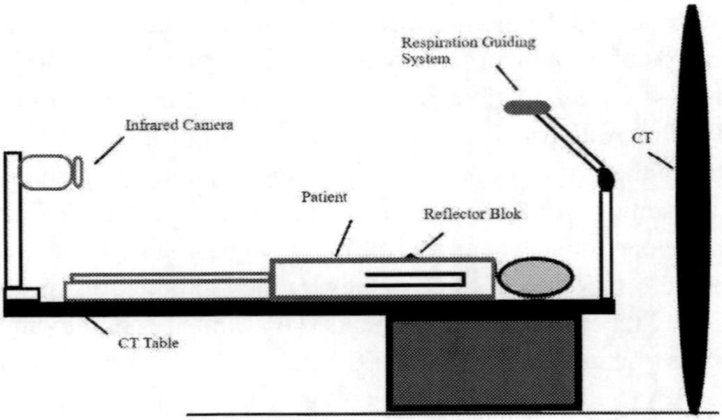

Figure 3. Image of a sample 4DCT scan including camera systems.

4DCT scan can take several times longer than a 3DCT scan, as several respiratory point data are received for different positions. After certain percentage values are assigned to the inspiration and expiratory peaks, a linear position is determined by the interpolation method. Thus, different CT data defined according to respiratory status are obtained. This forms the basis of 4D treatment planning. In the 4DCT method, the doses reaching the patient are 5-10 times higher than the standard CT shots (Li et al., 2005).

4. Cone-Beam Computed Tomography (CBCT)

The Cone-beam Computed Tomography (CBCT) method is an imaging method that uses flat panel detector technology to acquire a 3D dataset consisting of a wide-area X-ray source and detectors (Xing et al., 2006). Images are obtained as a result of the X-ray source rotating 180-360 degrees around the patient (Atalar and Özyar, 2010). Although CBCT is similar to CT, the image quality obtained from CBCT is lower than the image obtained from CT due to the detector structure and X-ray collimation that CBCT has. Compared to CT images, CBCT images may have reduced image quality at the field edges (Atalar and Özyar, 2010). The CBCT plays an important role in the accuracy of the treatment in the the IMRT technique. A kV CBCT integrated into a linear accelerator (LINAC) device consists of a source that generates an X-ray at the kV level and a flat panel detector placed opposite the source. In a LINAC device integrated with the MV CBCT, the MV therapy beam is used. In MV energies, differences in image quality occur depending on the interaction of radiation with matter (Jaffray and Siewerdsen, 2000; Pouliot et al., 2005).

The images obtained in the CBCT imaging method are used to confirm the patient setup online, correct it and decide whether a new treatment plannin is needed depending on the changes in the target organ. The resulting images are manually or automatically compared with the initial CT images. Through the software of the system, the differences in x, y and z directions (rotation movements can be included in some systems) are calculated and necessary corrections are made if necessary (Gayou and Miften, 2007; Letourneau et al., 2005; Moseley et al., 2007; Xing et al., 2006; White et al., 2007). CBCT imaging, which is frequently used in the IGRT method, provides the appropriate radiotherapy treatment as a result of comparing the imaging performed before the treatment with the images obtained in the treatment room. With the CBCT method, changes in tumour size are also examined, allowing the right decision to be made for the preparation of new treatment planning when necessary. Although the radiation dose received by the patient during CBCT increased, studies have shown that this dose is not very high (Atalar and Özyar, 2010). The guidelines and quality assurance that should be used for the CBCT method are explained in detail in the studies (Letourneau et al., 2007; Mao et al., 2008; Yoo et al., 2006).

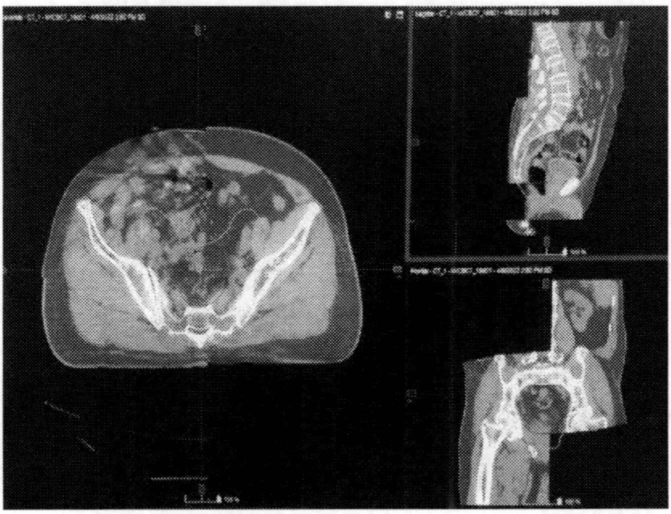

Figure 4. Comparison of the image obtained after CBCT with the planning image.

5. Positron Emission Tomography (PET)

The use of nuclear devices in imaging methods provides important information for the detection of the disease process and spread. This type of imaging uses two methods: PET and single photon emission computed tomography (SPECT). Due to the insufficient spatial resolution of SPECT images, their use in radiation therapy is very limited (Jaffray et al., 2007). PET/CT, on the other hand, has played an important role in radiation treatments since its emergence. A radioactive isotope is biologically bound to some molecules and decays through positron emission. In the meantime, the emitted positron takes some distance depending on its energy before disappearing. During extinction, it produces two photons with an energy of 511 keV in opposite directions. These photons are stopped by scintillation detectors (Jaffray et al., 2007; Van den Berge et al., 2000). The sample picture is shown in Table 1.

Table 1. Some radioisotopes used in PET imaging

Radio-Isotopes	Half life	Decay mode abundance (%)	Maximum β + energy (keV)	Mean β + energy (keV)
^{18}F	1.83	B + (96.7%)	633.5	249.8
^{11}C	0.34	B + (99.8%)	960.2	385.6
^{13}N	0.17	B + (99.8%)	1198.4	491.8
^{15}O	0.03	B + (99.9%)	1731.9	735.3

The PET/CT system is an imaging method that integrates a CT scanner and a PET scanner. PET/CT scanning accurately identifies the anatomical region where the tumour is located, allowing the physician to make more accurate diagnosis and treatment decisions. It is a more appropriate approach for the patient and the physician to examine only PET/CT images instead of performing separate PET and CT examinations. [^{18}F] 2-fluoro-2-deoxy-D glucose (FDG) is the most common molecule used for the detection, staging, diagnosis and monitoring of the treatment applied. Compared to normal tissues, there is more FDG accumulation in tumour cells (Warburg, 1956). An average of 5MBq FDG activity per kilogram of the patient is applied. Because of the use of FDG in PET scans, radiation oncologists are also focusing more on FDG.

We can list the use of PET/CT applications in RT under 3 main headings. First, by staging the cancer disease, to select patients who will receive radiotherapy more accurately and to provide a more accurate determination of the target area to be irradiated. Second, to detect environmental features related to the radiobiology and aggressiveness of the tumour. Third, it is used for evaluation of tumour response after radiation therapy. PET/CT scans repeated at regular intervals after treatment can be used to measure tumour response. The way in which radiation oncology physicians define target volumes in PET/CT images may differ. To avoid this problem, it is recommended to use algorithms that define tumour boundaries (Black et al., 2004; Erdi et al., 1997; Van Baardwijk et al., 2006). However, many studies are still needed to determine the borders of a standard tumour by algorithms. In conclusion, the use of PET/CT scan in radiation oncology: to prepare an appropriate radiotherapy plan before treatment, to determine target volumes during treatment, and to evaluate tumour response after treatment. The 4DPET imaging method is also an imaging method that enables respiratory-related scans to be performed.

6. Magnetic Resonance (MR)

The invention of the MR imaging method, which received the Nobel Prize in 2003, is a method that has an important place in imaging. Compared with CT, it has advantages such as better soft tissue contrast and theuse of non-ionising radiation. Image in MR method; It is obtained by processing the digital data obtained as a result of the precession of protons in the tissue, using radio frequency (RF) and magnetic field, and converting it into an image. The main components of the MR system are the magnet system with strength in the range of 0.2-3 Tesla, the gradient coils that create the variations of the magnetic field, the radiofrequency system with the transmitter and receiver coils (McRobbie, 2007; Oppelt, 2006). In ordinary MR protocols, images created according to proton density, T1 time and T2 time are obtained (Jenkinson et al., 2007; Villeirs and De Meerleer, 2007).

MR imaging has a superior feature, especially in the differentiation of soft tissues. MR images often play an important role in defining the location and extent of the diseased area. MR imaging also plays an important role in patient radiation therapy planning. In radiotherapy, MR images are fused with CT images to determine the extent of the tumour in the anatomical region. MR imaging has an important place in the workflow in the application of radiation therapy (Dowling et al., 2012; Kapanen et al., 2013; Kerkhof et al., 2010). MR images obtained with contrast agents are used to identify tumour spread and organs, and to determine the treatment planning process. Electron density of images; It is important for estimating the radiation dose that radiation creates in the environment by interacting with substances. The lack of electron density information obtained from MR images may result in a miscalculation of the dose. This is an important reason why MR images are not used in radiotherapy treatment planning.

The information in the MR images is either visually transferred to the CT via some software or directly transferred to the CT by fusion (Jaffray et al., 2007). MR applications are also used to examine the changes in the target volume during radiation therapy and to evaluate the response of the tumour to the treatment after treatment. Today, some studies are carried out to use MR images in radiation treatments. The sample picture is shown in Figure 5. The most comprehensive report on the use of MR in radiotherapy is IPEM report 81 (IPEM, 1999). In addition, IPEM report 80, AAPM report 28, AAPM TG 1 also have important information about MR imaging (AAPM, 1990; IPEM Report 81, 1999; IPEM Report 80, 1999; Price et al., 1990).

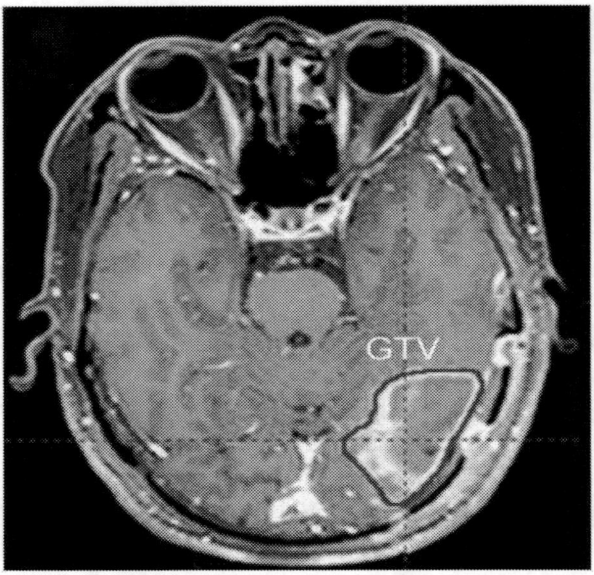

Figure 5. Contour drawn on the MR image.

7. Image Fusion in Radiotherapy

The use of software that combines CT, MR and PET images, which are frequently used in oncological imaging, and allows drawing contours on the image, becomes a basic function for radiation oncology planning, especially in some patient groups. Fusion is the process of displaying different types of images superimposed on a single image. The information combined with different images allows to more accurately determine the regions where the disease has spread and to define the borders of the target region with sharper lines. This greatly contributes to the outcome of the treatment and the preservation of healthy tissues. Most of the treatment planning systems used today have fusion capability. The sample picture is shown in Figure 6. While several fusion algorithms exist, the most commonly used by systems are; point-based, density-based and geometric transformation (Pereira et al., 2014). One of the biggest problems encountered in the fusion process is that the apparatus used in the images are different from each other (table top, head pillow, etc.). This causes anatomical regions to sometimes mismatch when matching images.

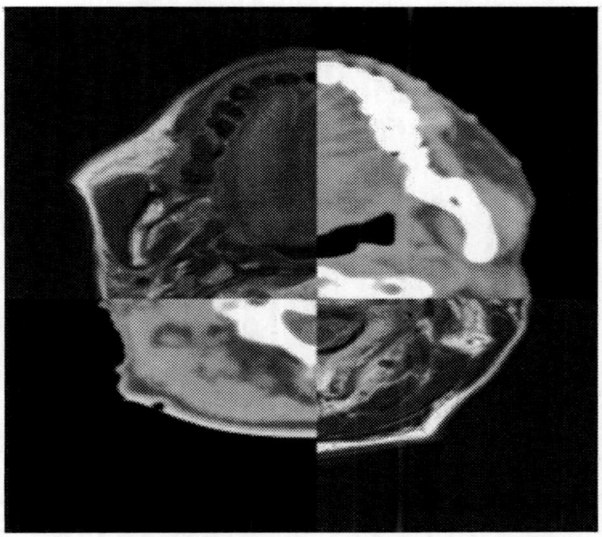

Figure 6. Fusion process of CT and MR images.

8. Portal Imaging

Portal imaging is used to ensure the accuracy of the patient's position before radiation therapy is given. It is used to match the DRR images sent by the TPS and the 2D images taken before the treatment, taking into account the anatomical structures, and to accurately determine the location of the concentric determined in the TPS. Usually, the patient's image is taken from positions where the gantry angle is 0° and 90° (or 270°). When necessary, images can be obtained from the positions of the gantry angle to be used in the treatment. Today, LINAC devices use MV or KV size X-rays for portal imaging. Differences that may occur as a result of portal imaging may be due to misalignment of lasers, misuse of immobilisation tools used on the patient, or incorrect patient positioning. With the development of amorphous silicon type detector systems, there have been significant improvements in image quality. The sample picture is shown in Figure 7. The detector system used by some LINAC devices in portal imaging allows dose measurement to be taken. In this way, some dosimetry operations can be performed comfortably and quickly. In particular, it is very easy to control the quality of the rays used in the IMRT technique with these systems. These quality controls by comparing a 2D dose measurement sometimes need to control the 3D dose measurement as well. This can be seen as a disadvantage of the portal dosimetry system. However, it is not seen as a far technology that the results obtained from the portal dosimeter become 3D with the developing systems.

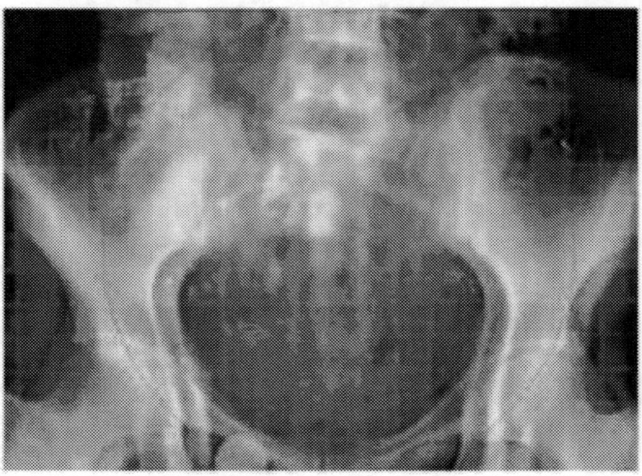

Figure 7. 2-Dimensional (2D) kV image taken for patient setup.

Conclusion

In recent years, developments in imaging have led to some technological innovations in radiotherapy applications. Imaging methods are a rapidly developing field in terms of tumour identification, adaptation and integration into the diagnosis and intervention process. Radiotherapy follows these innovations closely. Advanced imaging methods contribute to radiotherapy in subjects such as better staging, more accurate tumour detection, control of areas that can spread, and more accurate target volume definition. Undoubtedly, the contribution of CT, MR and PET, which are advanced imaging methods, to radiotherapy treatment is very important and it is obvious that it will contribute even more with the developing technology.

References

Atalar B, Özyar E. (2010). Technical Developments and Practice of IGRT (Image Guided Radiotherapy). *Acıbadem Üniversitesi Sağlık Bilimleri Dergisi [Acıbadem University Journal of Health Sciences],* 1, 57-61.

Black QC, Grills IS, Kestin LL, Wong CYO, Wong JW, Martinez AA, and Yan D. (2004). Defining a radiotherapy target with positron emission tomography. *International Journal of Radiation Oncology* Biology* Physics*, 60(4), 1272-1282.

Dowling JA, Lambert J, Parker J, Salvado O, Fripp J, Capp A, Wratten C, Denham JW, Greer PB. (2012). An atlas-based electron density mapping method for magnetic resonance imaging (MRI)-alone treatment planning and adaptive MRI-based prostate radiation therapy. *International Journal of Radiation Oncology* Biology* Physics*, 83(1), e5-e11.

Erdi YE, Mawlawi O, Larson SM, Imbriaco M, Yeung H, Finn R, Humm JL. (1997). Segmentation of lunglesion volume by adaptive positron emission tomography image thresholding. *Cancer*, 80, 2505-2509.

Gayou O, Miften M. (2007). Commissioning and clinicalimplementation of a mega voltage conebeam CT system for treatment localization. *Med Phys*, 34, 3183-3192.

Grosu A-L, Piert M, Weber WA, Jeremic B, Picchio M, Schratzenstaller U, Zimmermann FB, Schwaiger M, Molls M. (2005). Positron emission tomography for radiation treatment planning. *Strahlen Therapie und Onkologie [Radiation Therapy and Oncology]*, 181, 483-499.

Hunter KU, Eisbruch A. (2011). Advances in imaging: target delineation. *Cancer Journal*, 17, 151-154.

IPEM Report 80. (1999). *Quality control in magnetic resonance imaging.* York: IPEM.

IPEM Report 81. (1999). *Physics aspects of quality control in radiotherapy.* York: IPEM.

Jaffray D, Keall P, Mijnheer B, Leach MO, Humm J. (2007). *Imaging in radiotherapy.* Vienna: IAEA.

Jaffray DA, Siewerdsen JH. (2000). Cone-beam computed tomography with a flat-panel imager: Initial performance characterization. *Med Phys*, 27, 1311-1323.

Jenkinson MD, Du Plessis DG, Walker C, Smith TS. (2007). Advanced MRI in the management of adultgliomas. *Br J Neurosurg*, 21, 550-561.

Kapanen M, Collan J, Beule A, Sepp¨al¨a T, Saarilahti K, Tenhunen M. (2013). Commissioning of MRI-only based treatment planning procedure for external beam radiotherapy of prostate. *Magnetic Resonance in Medicine*, 70, 127-135.

Kerkhof EM, Balter JM, Vineberg K, Raaymakers BW. (2010). Treatment plan adaptation for MRI-guided radiotherapy using solely MRI data: A CT-based simulation study. *Physics in Medicine and Biology*, 55, 433-440.

Letourneau D, Keller H, Sharpe MB, Jaffray DA. (2007). Integral test phantom for dosimetric quality assurance of image guided and intensity modulated stereotactic radiotherapy. *Med Phys*, 34, 1842-1849.

Letourneau D, Martinez AA, Lockman D, Yan D, Vargas C, Ivaldi G, Wong J. (2005). Assessment of residual error for online cone-beam CT-guided treatment of prostate cancer patients. *Int J Radiat Oncol Biol Phys*, 62, 1239-1246.

Li T, Schreibmann E, Thorndyke B, Tillman G, Boyer A, Koong A, Goodman K, Xing L. (2005). Radiation dose reduction in 4D computed tomography. *Med Phys*, 32, 3650-3660.

Lu JJ, Brady LW. (2008). *Radiation Oncology, an Evidence-Based Approach.* Verlag Berlin Heidelberg: Springer.

Mak D, Corry J, Lau E, Rischin D, Hicks RJ. (2011). Role of FDG-PET/CT in staging and follow-up of head and neck squamous cell carcinoma. *Quarterly Journal of Nuclear Medicine and Molecular Imaging*, 55, 487-499.

Mao W, Lee L, Xing L. (2008). Design of multi-purpose phantom and automated software analysis tool for quality assurance of on-board kV/MV imaging system. *Med Phys*, 35, 1497-1506.

Mccollough C, Cody D, Edyvean S, Geise R, Gould G. (2008). *The Measurement, Reporting, and Management of Radiation Dose in CT.* American Association of Physicists in Medicine, College Park, MD.

McRobbie DW. (2007). *MRI from Picture to Proton*. Cambridge: Cambridge University Press.

Moseley DJ, White EA, Wiltshire KL, Rosewall T, Sharpe MB, Siewerdsen JH, Bissonnette JP, Gospodarowicz M, Warde P, Catton CN, Jaffray DA. (2007). Comparison of localization performance with implanted fiducial markers and cone-beam computed tomography for online image-guided radiotherapy of the prostate. *Int J Radiat Oncol Biol Phys*, 67, 942-953.

Mutic S, Palta JR, Butker EK, Das IJ, Huq MS, Loo LD, Salter BJ, McCollough CH, Dyk JV. (2003). Quality assurance for computed-tomography simulators and the computed-tomography-simulation process: report of the AAPM Radiation Therapy Committee Task Group No. 66. *Med Phys*, 30, 2762-2792.

Oppelt A. (Ed.). (2006). *Imaging Systems for Medical Diagnostics: Fundamentals, Technical Solutions and Applications for Systems Applying Ionizing Radiation, Nuclear Magnetic Resonance and Ultrasound.* John Wiley & Sons.

Pereira GC, Traughber M, Muzic Jr RF. (2014). The Role of Imaging in Radiation Therapy Planning: Past, Present, and Future. *Bio Med Research International*, 231090.

Pouliot J, Bani-Hashemi A, Chen J, Svatos M, Ghelmansarai F, Mitschke M, Aubin M, Xia P, Morin O, Bucci K, Roach M, Hernandez P, Zheng Z, Hristov D, Verhey L. (2005). Low-dose mega voltage cone-beam CT for radiation therapy. *Int J Radiat Oncol Biol Phys*, 61, 552-560.

Price RR, Axel L, Morgan T, Newman R, Perman W, Schneiders N, Selikson M, Wood M, Thomas SR. (1990). Quality assurance methods and phantoms for magnetic resonance imaging: Report of AAPM nuclear magnetic resonance Task Group No. 1. *Med Phys*, 17, 287-295.

Price RR, Axel L, Morgan T, Newman R, Perman W, Schneiders N, Selikson M, Wood M, Thomas SR. (1990). Quality assurance methods and phantoms for magnetic resonance imaging. *Med Phys*, 17(2), 287-295.

Schlegel W. (2010). If youcan'tseeit, you can miss it: the role of biomedical imaging in radiation oncology. *Radiation Protection Dosimetry*, 139, 321-326.

Van Baardwijk A, Baumert BG, Bosmans G, Van Kroonenburgh M, Stroobants S, Gregoire V, Lambin P, Ruysscher DD. (2006). The current status of FDG-PET in tumour volume definition in radiotherapy treatment planning. *Cancer Treat Rev*, 32, 245-260.

Van den Berge DL, Ridder MD, Storme GA. (2000). Imaging in radiotherapy. *European Journal of Radiology*, 34, 41-48.

Villeirs GM, De Meerleer GO. (2007). Magnetic resonance imaging (MRI) anatomy of the prostate and application of MRI in radiotherapy planning. *Eur J Radiol*, 63, 361-368.

Warburg O. (1956). On the origin of cancer cells. *Science*, 123, 309-314.

White EA, Cho J, Vallis KA, Sharpe MB, Lee G, Blackburn H, Nageeti T, McGibney C, Jaffray DA. (2007). Cone beam computed tomography guidance for setup of patients receiving accelerated partial breast irradiation. *Int J Radiat Oncol Biol Phys*, 68, 547-554.

Xing L, Thorndyke B, Schreibmann E, Yang Y, Li TF, Kim GY, Luxton G, Koong A. (2006). Overview of image-guided radiation therapy. *Med Dosim*, 31, 91-112.

Yoo S, Kim GY, Hammoud R, Elder E, Pawlicki T, Guan H, Fox T, Luxton G, Yin FF, Munro P. (2006). A quality assurance program for the on-boardimagers. *Med Phys*, 33, 4431-4447.

Chapter 5

Target Volume Delineation and Normal Tissue Contouring for Intensity-Modulated Radiation Therapy

Esma Didem Nasuhbeyoglu*
Department of Radiation Oncology, Kahramanmaras Necip Fazil City Hospital, Kahramanmaras,Turkey

Abstract

The radiotherapy (RT) treatment based on bony landmarks historically and the invention of computed tomography (CT) in the 1970s and magnetic resonance imaging (MRI) in the1980s led to the improvement of RT techniques and the application of more precise RT is enabled in terms of modern RT era: 3D conformal RT (3DCRT) and intensity modulated radiation therapy (IMRT). The more the IMRT technique is implemented in clinical practice, the better results for tumour control become possible with less morbidity. On the other hand, the recent precise RT delivery techniques require more attention to target volume delineation and organs at risk (OARs) contouring than historical techniques, because of the sharp dose gradients near the tumour and OARs. The International Commission on Radiation Units and Measurements (ICRU) published the report of ICRU 83 in 2010 that defined the cornerstones for IMRT planning. Thus many guidelines for certain tumour sites were published to improve the clinician's experience and knowledge to minimise variabilities between providers and improve the treatment results. Target volume delineation of IMRT planning is not only affected by the clinician's knowledge but also the technical

---

*Corresponding Author's Email:didemikiz@gmail.com.

In: Frontiers in Intensity-Modulated Radiotherapy Research
Editor: Sibel Karaca
ISBN: 979-8-88697-252-8

capabilities of the clinic and patient-related factors. The patient positioning techniques and definition and/or gating of the tumour motion are challenging issues, especially for tumours affected by internal organ motion (e.g., lung cancer, prostate cancer, gynaecological cancers) to achieve treatment reproducibility in each fraction. Furthermore, it should be taken into account that, even though contouring target volumes in an ideal way is the crucial step of IMRT, it is not adequate to obtain the best treatment results without elaborative RT teamwork.

Keywords: contouring, target volume delineation

1. Introduction

Technological developments in radiation therapy and radiology area led to more precise treatment and improved outcomes of cancer treatment. RT has evolved through 3DCRT to intensity-modulated radiation therapy (IMRT) in recent years. The adaptation of clinical implementations of IMRT in a short time has brought the advantage of increased tumour control results with fewer complications and also patients' quality of life increased.

Although high technology provides technical advantages, it could only turn to accurate results in the hands of medical health care professionals who are well adapted with advanced medical knowledge that turns into medical practice. Contouring is one of the major components of IMRT treatment, accordingly, variations of target volume delineation could result in decreased tumour control and increased toxicity (Abrams et al., 2012; Peters et al., 2010; Ohri et al., 2013).

Therefore, in this chapter, the basic components of target volume definitions (as defined in ICRU 83) (ICRU, 2010) for IMRT planning will be mentioned with demonstrative cases to minimise possible target volume definition errors. In addition, it should be kept in mind that this chapter covers only a small part of the demonstrations and the readers are encouraged to utilise specific guidelines/protocols for detailed information on target volume delineation for each tumour site.

2. ICRU Report 83 Volume Definitions

ICRU published a report of ICRU 83 (ICRU, 2010) in 2010 that aimed to enable recommendations for the basic background of IMRT implementations. The definitions of volumes that were defined in ICRU 83 are as follows:

- Gross tumour volume: GTV
- Clinical target volume: CTV
- Planning target volume: PTV
- Organs at risk: OARs
- Planning organ-at-risk volume: PRV
- Internal target volume: ITV
- Treated volume: TV
- Remaining volume at risk: RVR

In the report, the GTV, the CTV and the OARs are defined as crucial volumes based on anatomy and tumour biology that affected oncological outcomes and side effects, whereas the ITV, the PTV and the PRV are the volumes that are defined to ensure the prescribed dose is delivered to the CTV and the dose constraints of OARs are provided. The TV and the RVR (which are not going to be explained in detail in this chapter) are the concepts about beam arrangements and dose delivery to the body of the patient and are not contoured directly in planning systems. Therefore, the detailed definitions of the GTV, the CTV, the PTV, the ITV and the PRV are going to be covered in this chapter.

2.1. Gross Tumour Volume (GTV)

In ICRU 83 the definition of GTV is 'the gross demonstrable extent and location of the tumour'. GTV contouring is one of the crucial components of IMRT planning. Due to the sharp dose gradient between target volume and normal tissues, GTV delineation must be done with pure attention to avoid possible target missing that could cause inferior oncological outcomes.

The GTV is delineated in computed tomography (CT) images of planning systems and radiological imaging (CT, MRI, a combination of CT and positron emission tomography PET-CT) etc.), physical examination and endoscopic evaluation led determination of tumour extension. Physicians generally prefer to use radiological imaging (CT, MRI, PET-CT, etc.) to describe borders of tumour impeccably, although it should be noted that the spread of tumour with a mucosal path could be defined more precisely with endoscopic or direct (palpation) physical examination procedures (e.g., bladder cancer, head neck cancers, cervical-vaginal-vulva cancer, skin cancer) in addition to radiological procedures.

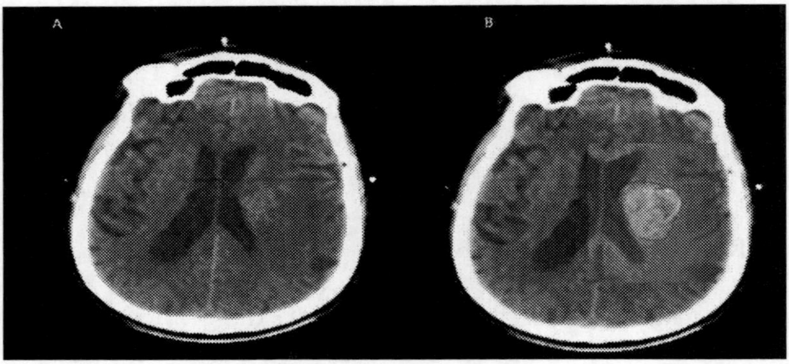

Figure 1. T1 contrast-enhanced MRI image is needed for IMRT planning to delineate GTV in high-grade glioma patients, whereas CT is not adequate to describe borders of tumour and may cause miss the target volume. (A) CT simulation image alone, (B) CT simulation image that is fused with contrast-enhanced axial T1 MRI image and contouring of GTV (red).

The radiological techniques to define the GTV are variable for each tumour site. As demonstrated in Figure 1, for brain tumours MRI sequences are needed to define GTV, whereas PET-CT has a limited role as increased fluorodeoxyglucose (FDG) uptake of normal brain tissue impairs imaging (Cabrera et al., 2016). Lung cancer local-regional target volume delineation could be performed effectively with PET-CT rather than CT and MRI, therefore PET-CT is the crucial imaging for lung cancers (De Ruysscher et al., 2017). In addition, for definitive curative chemo-radiotherapy of cervical cancer for local treatment planning, both MRI (for a detailed assessment of the local spread of the tumor) and PET-CT (especially sensitive and specific for the detection of metastatic pelvic-paraaortic lymph nodes) are required (Chino et al. others, 2020).

To summarise, the definition of GTV for IMRT planning should be improved with advanced imaging techniques (eg, MRI, PET-CT). In order not to miss the target, tumour boundaries must be determined accurately and clinicians must have sufficient radiological imaging knowledge for each tumour type.

2.2. Clinical Target Volume (CTV)

In ICRU 83 the definition of CTV is 'volume of tissue that contains a demonstrable GTV and/or subclinical malignant disease with a certain probability of occurrence considered relevant for therapy'. The potential risk of tumour spread is different for each cancer type. Several published consensus guidelines aimed to standardise CTV delineation.

In this concept, probable subclinical disease infiltration of the malign tumours, such as lymphatic and/or fatty area soft tissue spread, coverage is the main purpose based on clinical experience. In general, the risk of recurrence of 5% to 10% is targeted for CTV contouring, although the consensus regarding what proportion of spread risk to cover is not clear (ICRU, 2010). CTV is not a description for internal motions of the organs (such as respiratory movements, and bladder-rectal filling changes), for that reason delineation of ITV and/or PTV are needed.

The microscopic tumour spread includes the infiltration of the boundary of GTV (e.g., malign cells could easily spread to the soft tissue). However anatomical barriers (e.g., bone cortex, fascia of the muscles) that prevent tumour spread should be considered for CTV delineation. Tumour biology is one of the important factors affecting the spread pattern of tumours and each tumour has different characteristics. For instance, most soft tissue sarcomas tend to infiltrate the muscle compartment without lymphatic metastases, so the CTV of the tumour should cover the related muscle fascia (Wang et al., 2011). On the contrary, the lymphatic area for head and neck cancers, should be delineated for excellent locoregional control (Biau et al., 2019). In addition, perineural invasion risk should be considered for some subtypes of head and neck cancers with different organ localisation (e.g., parotid cancers, lip-buccal mucosa cancers with perinodal spread) (Ko et al., 2014).

Several specific guidelines were published for CTV delineation for each tumour site and the readers are encouraged to utilise special guidelines/protocols to improve their skills in target volume delineation. In addition, some practical resources (demonstrates target volume delineation slice-by-slice for different tumour sites) are recommended for radiation oncologists as follows:

- 'Target Volume Delineation for Conformal and Intensity Modulated Radiation Therapy' (Lee et al., 2014).
- 'econtour.org': The website is useful for radiation oncologists who need to reach main consensus guidelines/ protocols and contoured demonstrative cases.

2.3. Internal Target Volume

The ITV is an optional volume to delineate the PTV. The ITV was defined in ICRU Report 62 (ICRU, 1999) as 'the CTV plus a margin considering uncertainties in size, shape, and position of the CTV within the patient'. The motion of the tumour due to physiological activity of the patient's internal organs (e.g., respiratory changes, heartbeat, bladder filling and rectal filling) may cause missing the target volume while using IMRT techniques. The IMRT technique aids to deliver the dose-escalation for tumours and sparing normal tissues with sharpening dose decreases near the target volume; however, organ motion is a challenging issue to keep the target in the right position, especially for thoracic, intraabdominal and pelvic tumours.

Lung cancer irradiation is one of the challenging areas of tumour motion due to respiratory changes. Because breath control systems require special equipment and/or fiducial implementation (which needs extra implementation and time- consuming), 4DCT simulation is the practical method for treatment planning of lung cancer in daily clinical routine. Although there are many breath control systems (breath-hold techniques, tracking, gating) the recent EORTC report for lung cancer RT recommends two common delineation methods to cover the respiratory tumour motion changes: internal target volume (ITV) concept and mid-ventilation/mid-position concept (De Ruysscher et al., 2017). The movement of the tumour during all phases of respiration or maximum intensity projection (MIP) is contoured in images that are created with 4DCT, thus the probability of target missing is minimised with this technique. The MIP dataset presents the tumour in the highest intensity along the viewing ray of each pixel of volumetric data with the advantage of reasonable correct estimation of tumour motion in less time (Ezhil et al., 2009). However, while contouring the tumours located near the high-density anatomical structures (e.g., chest wall, mediastinum and diaphragm) with the MIP dataset, the extensions of the tumour may be overestimated or underestimated (Bradley et al., 2006; Park et al., 2009).

Contouring of early-stage small-sized lung cancer on MIP images is feasible and takes less time (Underberg et al., 2005). Contouring of the ITV on MIP images is significantly smaller than in all phases of respiration, especially in tumors close to the chest wall, diaphragm, and mediastinum, and completely covers the tumour. (Tibdewal et al., 2021).

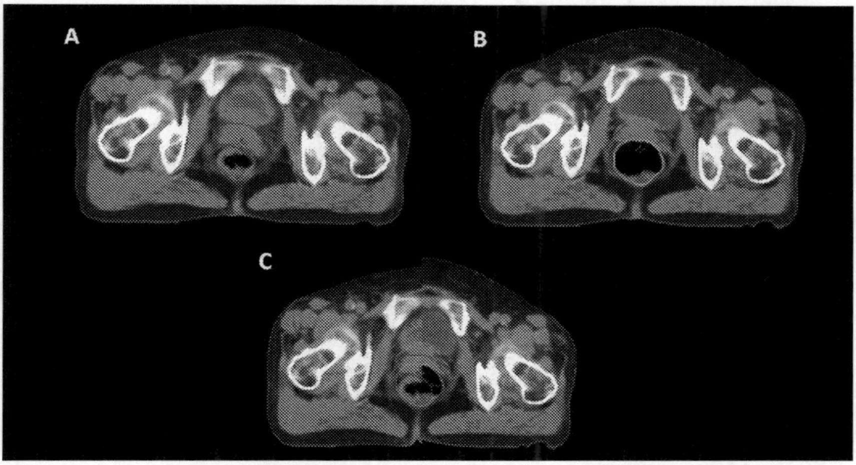

Figure 2. The effect of rectal filling on the movement of the uterine cervix is shown in different images of multiple CT simulations which were performed for individualised ITV delineation: empty rectum (A) and rectum filled with gas (B) are fused according to bony anatomy (C) and rectal filling with gas causes movement of GTV *(green)* to the anterior direction.

Gynaecological cancers are one of the areas in which the ITV concept is needed not to miss the target due to organ mobility such as rectal and bladder filling. The uterus mobility is mainly related to bladder filling, whereas both rectal and bladder filling changes the position of the vaginal apex and the mobility of the cervix and the lower part of the vagina are linked to variations in the filling of the rectum (Mahantshetty et al., 2022). In Figure 2. the movement of the uterine cervix due to rectal filling is demonstrated.

Bondar et al. showed that the movement of vascular structures in contact with lymph node areas is affected by bladder fullness, whereas rectal filling has little impact (Bondar et al., 2011). Bladder repletion also has an impact on the doses received by the small intestine (as the bladder volume increases, the dose that the intestine is exposed to decreases) (Georg et al., 2006). It should be noted that the bladder volume tends to decrease during the RT treatment (due to acute cystitis induced by RT), especially postoperatively (Beadle et al.,

2009). To minimise all the uncertainties that are discussed above, clinics should have protocols for bladder and rectal filling.

Curative intent radio-chemotherapy of locally advanced cervical cancer with IMRT technique is challenging because of the high mobility of the target area and may result in a geographical miss and decreased patient outcome. The EMBRACE-II study protocol (Tanderup et al., 2015), published for definitive radio chemotherapy for cervical cancer with IMRT and MRI-based brachytherapy, provides an acceptable bladder filling protocol as follows: the patient is asked to empty the bladder one hour before the simulation imaging and each radiotherapy fraction, then water intake of 300- 500 mL is applied orally to the patient and the patient is asked not to void before the treatment with the comfortably full bladder. In addition, the rectum should be empty during the simulation and RT fractions. The diameter of the rectum should be kept under 4 cm in any direction, if gas or filling is detected during treatment the patient is asked to empty the stools or deflate with a catheter or offered to delay the treatment simulation to another day. Special diets to reduce the mobility of the intestine are ineffective and not recommended.

EMBRACE-II defined three methods of image-guided RT (IGRT), which of two could be implemented in practice more commonly, to delineate ITV for IMRT:

1. Basic IGRT: CTV to ITV margin is standard and daily online verification for matching verification is required (kilovoltage (kV), cone beam CT (CBCT) image) and CBCT may be performed daily to determine the movement of the uterus and the target volume. The recommended margins are as follows: 10 mm posterior-anterior, 10 mm superior-inferior, and 5 mm lateral. If the tumour location is the upper part of the uterus an extra 5mm expansion should be applied isotropically to the uterus body. It should be kept in mind that in the condition of an empty rectum, the target volume might move to 10-15 mm in the posterior-inferior direction, also the same condition is possible for an empty bladder that the target will move to 10-15 mm in the anterior-inferior direction.
2. Intermediate IGRT: Margins to CTV to ITV is created with multiple simulation scanning and individualised by fusing the images of different imaging series of the patient with a comfortably full bladder and empty bladder and the margin is adapted according to these fused images. For patients with the low motion of the target, the margin of

CTV to ITV expansion can be smaller, whereas the target with high mobility needs larger expansion than standard margins.

3. Advanced IGRT: This method is based on individual plans and one of the appropriate library plans is selected according to the target position in daily CBCT.

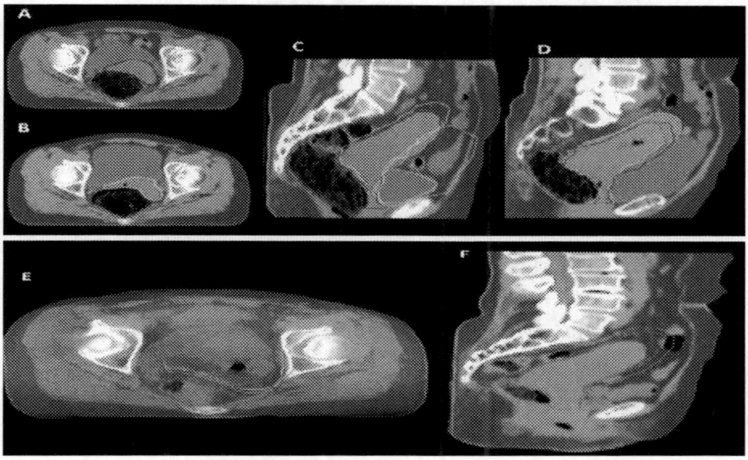

Figure 3. Multiple CT simulation scans with empty (A, GTV in dark blue) and full (B, GTV in white) bladders were fused according to bony anatomy to delineate individual ITV (F, contoured in light blue). It could be noticed that rectal filling was captured as nearly the same volume (rectal diameter was approximately 5 cm) in both full and empty bladder simulation scans (A and B). Even though the bladder volume changed apparently (C), the movement of GTV was not as much as expected (GTV (white) location in the full bladder (yellow) and GTV (dark blue) location in the empty bladder (light green) could be seen). During the treatment, the diameter of the rectum was detected as less than 4 cm on daily CBCT (E) and the new location of GTV with an empty rectum was contoured in purple (D), (E), (F). The new location of GTV (purple, (D)) changed dramatically when bony landmark fusion was evaluated on a simulation scan that had been performed with the full rectum (contoured GTV in simulation with full rectum-empty bladder is dark blue and full rectum-full bladder is white (D)). In the picture (F), individualised ITV (light blue) and PTV (orange) were shown, and the PTV was not cover the new GTV location with an empty rectum. It was noticed that at least 2 cm in a posterior direction from ITV to PTV margin was adequate to cover the target motion. Also, different margins from ITV to PTV in posterior directions are shown (E) to demonstrate the movement range of GTV (GTV was captured in CBCT in the condition of the empty rectum (purple)): 5 mm (orange), 10 mm (yellow), 15 mm (green), 20 mm (red). As a result, despite recommended ITV to PTV margin being 5-15 mm in EMBRACE protocol, it was not adequate to cover tumour movement and for each patient, individualised target motion monitoring should be performed carefully with CBCT during the RT.

The intermediate IGRT with individualised ITV planning is recommended in the EMBRACE II study with daily position verification methods. However, individualised ITV may not be adequate to cover all the potential variations of tumour position. In Figure 3 it is demonstrated that even if individualised ITV contouring is performed in empty and full bladder CT simulation scans, the condition of rectal filling should be considered in both CT scans whether the rectum is full or not. If the same condition of the rectum (filled or empty) is detected in both CT simulation scans, dramatic changes in the target position may not be captured in adequate variations and may cause missing the target unless appropriate margins are given. Furthermore, it should be kept in mind that pelvic organ movements are variable from patient to patient and the ITV margin recommendations in guidelines may not fully cover_the possible target motions. For that reason, during the RT treatment, the position of the target should be carefully checked for each patient on daily CBCT imaging and re-planning should be performed if the localisation of the tumour position is outside the target area.

In a recent prospective study on organ motion effects of radical radio-chemotherapy for cervical cancer, the investigators used bladder filling protocol (CT scan was performed after 45 minutes of 1000 ml water intake orally) for supine position simulation and no empty bladder simulation CT scan was performed for individualised ITV delineation (Mahantshetty et al., 2022). The study reported that the mobility of the cervical region is about 5-6 mm and < 10 mm margin is adequate for coverage of cervical motion, whereas uterine motion was defined as larger and anisotropically. The study suggests CTV to ITV margin for cervix is 10 mm isotropically and for uterus-fundus it is 10-15 mm in superior-inferior, 10-15 mm in laterally, 10-15 mm in posterior and 15-20 mm in anterior (even though strict bladder and rectal filling protocols were applied in study) directions. In high-volume clinics, where individualised ITV (two CT simulation scans with an empty and a full bladder) implementation is not possible, the clinicians may take into account the recommendations of that study in their clinical practice.

As discussed above internal tumour motion is an important point that should be considered while performing IMRT planning and adequate margins should be given from CTV to ITV or directly tumour motion should be analysed by special simulation techniques (e.g., 4DCT simulation, a fusion of multiple CT simulation for pelvic patients such as with full and empty bladder) to keep the target inside the RT field.

2.4. Planning Target Volume

The PTV is a geometrical definition that expansion is given to the target volume (GTV/CTV) to reduce systematic and random uncertainties so that the prescribed dose could be delivered to the main target volume (GTV/CTV) with acceptable probability. The tumour location (target volume could be affected by internal organ motions) and setup uncertainties are considered to create PTV volume and also PTV margin should be calculated for each clinic according to the patient positioning methods and linear accelerator parameters (ICRU, 2010).

Even though GTV and CTV are delineated independently, the PTV depends on the irradiation technique and the prescribed dose of PTV is evaluated and reported according to ICRU 83 (ICRU, 2010). Although in early ICRU reports (ICRU, 1999; ICRU, 2004; ICRU, 2007) compromising of PTV margin was recommended, if PTV encroaches on the OARs, it is not suggested in ICRU 83 report to shrink the margin of PTV anymore. Developments in treatment planning systems enable dose sparing of the OARs with priority rules in optimisation and subdivisions of PTV for overlapping OARs area could be evaluated and accordingly the possibility of under dosage calculation of CTV is avoided. However, the dose reporting should be done for the whole PTV.

The uncertainties and variations that affect CTV coverage could be categorised as (1) internal variations (size, position, and shape of CTV) and (2) external variations (patient and beam positioning). Therefore, an adequate margin should be added to CTV to minimise the probability of coverage missing.

The internal motion of patients (due to rectal filling, bladder filling, and movements of breathing) could be minimised by using protocols (e.g., bowel preparations) and special equipment (e.g., Breath-hold systems, checking bladder filling with ultrasound). Using special equipment gives the advantage of minimising CTV to PTV margin and enables lower OARs dose without compromising target volume coverage. In addition, the application of the equipment could be time-consuming and also brings extra charge; using special equipment is not possible for each clinic (especially in clinics with high patient volumes). External variations could be minimised by using immobilisation devices (e.g., thermoplastic mask, vacuum bed) and daily onboard digital portal imaging (e.g., kV, CBCT imaging).

In Figure 4 the contouring of adjuvant treatment for cholangiocellular cancer patients is illustrated. The illustration demonstrated the importance of using special devices for IMRT planning, especially in patients with the risk of missing the target due to internal motion of breathing (e.g., extrahepatic cancer, intrahepatic cancer, oesophageal cancer, lung cancer) and enlarged PTV margins are needed to cover the uncertainty of internal motion.

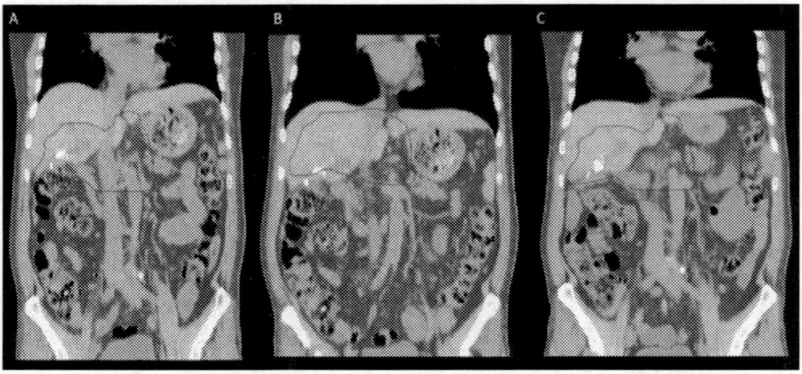

Figure 4. Effect of breathing to target volume *(red)* position changes in intrahepatic cholangiocellular cancer patient. Focusing on the surgical clips (that is included in the target volume) could help to consider the target missing unless adequate CTV to PTV margin is given (>1cm). However, dose constraints for liver and kidney could not be achieved and a lower CTV to PTV margin (5mm) was needed for more normal tissue sparing. Fused images with bone structures to spontaneous breathing (C) on the expiration (A) and inspiration (B) CT images are illustrated and it is shown that CTV to PTV *(red)* margin (5mm) is not adequate to cover the target volume without breath control systems.

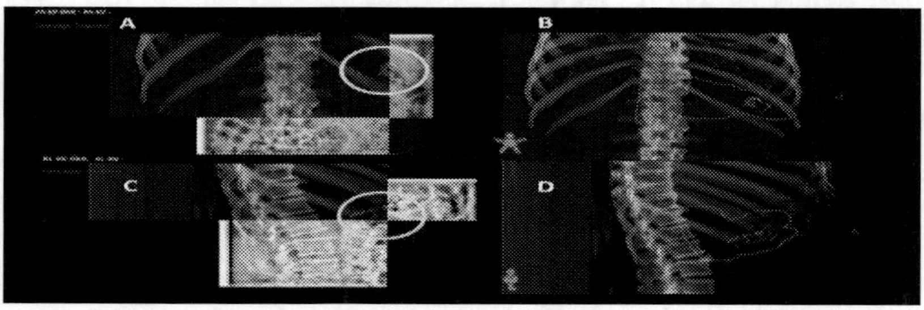

Figure 5. After re-simulation with breath-hold technique in a patient with intrahepatic cholangiocellulary cancer, expansion of 5 mm CTV to PTV margin became reliable for target motion coverage, and was confirmed in daily digital portal imaging. (A) Posterior-anterior (PA) kV image matching, (B) reference image of PA, (C) lateral kV image matching, (D) reference image of lateral and matching of surgical clips is demonstrated in *the yellow* circle and PTV is shown in *the orange* line.

As seen in Figure 4. the movement of the target volume with inspiration and expiration was more than 1 cm and the limits of OARs constraints were exceeded by applying the CTV to PTV margin >1cm (also ITV concept resulted in a large volume). Re-simulation was performed with the breath-hold system and the expansion of a 5 mm margin was applied from CTV to PTV, and the dose limits of OARs were achieved with adequate PTV coverage. The accuracy and reproducibility of the target volume position were confirmed by the breath-hold technique in setup and daily kV imaging (Figure 5).

To summarise, the PTV margin is affected by internal and external factors, and minimisation of these uncertainties is needed for optimal IMRT planning. Stabilising both patient position and internal organ motion is the crucial step for IMRT, accordingly to achieve the ideal treatment results; CTV to PTV margin should cover all the uncertainties. Furthermore, the PTV margin should be calculated according to the facilities of each clinic.

2.5. Organs at Risk

Normal tissue out of the target volume is defined as OARs. However, the importance of sparing the normal tissue is variable according to each tumour site. For example, remaining muscle tissue (the risk of tumour spread is not expected) around the target volume should be spared in RT soft tissue sarcoma to prevent oedema and fibrosis that may have a major impact on treatment morbidity. On the other hand for prostate cancer, the pelvic muscles are not considered OARs and the dose delivery is not affected by the muscle tissue sparing.

The tissue organisation is important (serial or parallel) for the delineation of OARs. For parallel organs (e.g., liver, lung) the volume assessment is crucial and the organ should be delineated completely. In contrast, for the rectum (as a serial-like organ and tubular type anatomy) the wall or the surface contouring (as a rectal wall) is recommended rather than the full organ contouring (ICRU, 2010).

It should be considered that dose-volume constraints data was derived from conventional fractionation (from 1.8 to 2 Gy per fraction) and the tolerance of absorbed doses should be re-evaluated in the concept of simultaneous integrated boost technique (SIB).

2.6. Planning Organ at Risk Volume

To compensate for the uncertainties and variations in the position of the OARs during the RT, the PRV concept is needed (as in the case with PTV). For serial organs (e.g., spinal cord) PRV is more relevant than parallel (e.g., parotid gland, lung) organs.

If the overlap of PTV and PRV occurs, it is recommended that the margins should not be compromised and subdivisions of the overlapped regions should be spared with optimisation priority rules. It is also recommended that the absorbed dose should be reported in the full PRV (ICRU, 2010). OARs to PRV margin should be calculated based on systematic and random uncertainties, as for the PTV.

Conclusion

Target volume delineation is the crucial step of IMRT planning and the specific guidelines/protocols of each tumour type should be followed for detailed information on IMRT implementations. Achieving the best tumour control result with decreased toxicity is affected by multiple factors: the physician's perspective (the knowledge and experience), patient-related uncertainties (e.g., internal organ motions), and technical capabilities (e.g., 4DCT simulation, breath-hold technique, immobilisation devices optimisation system, daily imaging technique). It should be noted that the harmonisation of all these factors in an ideal way in the hands of the RT team (physician, physicist, and radiotherapist) could be turned into optimal results for cancer treatment.

References

Abrams, R. A., Winter, K. A., Regine, W. F., Safran, H., Hoffman, J. P., Lustig, R., Konski, A. A., Benson, A. B., Macdonald, J. S., Rich, T. A. and Willett, C. G. (2012). "Failure to Adhere to Protocol Specified Radiation Therapy Guidelines Was Associated with Decreased Survival in RTOG 9704 - A Phase III Trial of Adjuvant Chemotherapy and Chemoradiotherapy for Patients with Resected Adenocarcinoma of the Pancreas." *International Journal of Radiation Oncology Biology Physics* 82 (2): 809–16.

Beadle, B. M., Jhingran, A., Salehpour, M., Sam, M., Iyer, R. B. and Eifel, P. J. (2009). "Cervix Regression and Motion During the Course of External Beam Chemoradiation for Cervical Cancer." *International Journal of Radiation Oncology Biology Physics* 73 (1): 235–41.

Biau, J., Lapeyre, M., Troussier, I., Budach, W., Giralt, J., Grau, C. and Kazmierska, J., Langendijk, J. A., Ozsahin, M., O'Sullivan, B., Bourhis, J. and Grégoire, V. (2019). "Selection of Lymph Node Target Volumes for Definitive Head and Neck Radiation Therapy: A 2019 Update." *Radiotherapy and Oncology* 134: 1–9.

Bondar, L., Hoogeman, M., Mens, J. W., Dhawtal, G., Pree, I. D., Ahmad, R., Quint, S. and Heijmen, B. (2011). "Toward an Individualized Target Motion Management for IMRT of Cervical Cancer Based on Model-Predicted Cervix-Uterus Shape and Position." *Radiotherapy and Oncology* 99 (2): 240–45.

Bradley, J. D., Nofal, A. N., El Naqa, I. M., Lu, W., Liu, J., Hubenschmidt, J., Low, D. A., Drzymala, R.E. and Khullar, D. (2006). "Comparison of Helical, Maximum Intensity Projection (MIP), and Averaged Intensity (AI) 4D CT Imaging for Stereotactic Body Radiation Therapy (SBRT) Planning in Lung Cancer." *Radiotherapy and Oncology : Journal of the European Society for Therapeutic Radiology and Oncology* 81 (3): 264–68.

Cabrera, A. R., Kirkpatrick, J. P., Fiveash, J. B., Shih, H. A., Koay, E. J., Lutz, S., Petit, J., Chao, S. T., Brown, P. D., Vogelbaum, M., Reardon, D. A., Chakravarti, A., Wen, P. Y. and Chang, E. (2016). "Radiation Therapy for Glioblastoma: Executive Summary of an American Society for Radiation Oncology Evidence-Based Clinical Practice Guideline." *Practical Radiation Oncology* 6 (4): 217–25.

Chino, J., Annunziata, C. M., Beriwal, S., Bradfield, L., Erickson, B. A., Fields, E. C., Fitch, K. J., Harkenrider, M. M., Holschneider, C. H., Kamrava, M., Leung, E., Lin, L. L., Mayadev, J. S., Morcos, M., Nwachukwu, C., Petereit, D. and Viswanathan, A. N. (2020). "Radiation Therapy for Cervical Cancer: Executive Summary of an ASTRO Clinical Practice Guideline." *Practical Radiation Oncology* 10 (4): 220–34.

Ezhil, M., Vedam, S., Balter, P., Choi, B., Mirkovic, D., Starkschall, G. and Chang., J. Y. (2009). "Determination of Patient-Specific Internal Gross Tumor Volumes for Lung Cancer Using Four-Dimensional Computed Tomography." *Radiation Oncology* 4: 1–14.

Georg, P., Georg, D., Hillbrand, M., Kirisits, C. and Pötter, R. (2006). "Factors Influencing Bowel Sparing in Intensity Modulated Whole Pelvic Radiotherapy for Gynaecological Malignancies." *Radiotherapy and Oncology* 80 (1): 19–26.

ICRU 1999. (1999). "ICRU Report 62: Prescribing, Recording and Reporting Photon Beam Therapy (Supplement to ICRU Report 50)." *Journal of the ICRU* os-32 (1).

ICRU 2004. (2004). "Prescribing, Recording, and Reporting Electron Beam Therapy. ICRU Report 71." *Journal of the ICRU* 4 (1).

ICRU 2007. (2007). "International Commission on Radiation Units and Measurements. Prescribing, Recording and Reporting Proton-Beam Therapy. ICRU Report 78." *Journal of the ICRU* 7 (2).

ICRU 2010. (2010). "4. Definition of Volumes." *Journal of the ICRU* 10 (1): 41–53. https://doi.org/10.1093/jicru/ndq009.

Ko, H. C., Gupta, V., Mourad, W. F., Hu, K. S., Harrison, L. S., Som, P. M. and Bakst, R. L. (2014). "A Contouring Guide for Head and Neck Cancers with Perineural Invasion." *Practical Radiation Oncology* 4 (6): E247–58.

Lee, N., Riaz, N., Kohutek, Z. and Unger, K. (2014). Target Volume Delineation for Conformal and Intensity-Modulated Radiation Therapy. *Radiation Oncology*. Vol. 39.

Mahantshetty, U., Naga, P., Nachankar, A., Ghadi, Y., Dheera, A., Scaria, L., Epili, D., Chopra, S., Lavanya, G. and Shrivastava, S. (2022). "Set-Up Errors, Organ Motion, Tumour Regression and Its Implications on Internal Target Volume–Planning Target Volume During Cervical Cancer Radiotherapy: Results From a Prospective Study." *Clinical Oncology* 34 (3): 189–97.

Ohri, N., Shen, X., Dicker, A. P., Doyle, L. A., Harrison, S. A. and Showalter, T. A. (2013). "Radiotherapy Protocol Deviations and Clinical Outcomes: A Meta-Analysis of Cooperative Group Clinical Trials." *Journal of the National Cancer Institute* 105 (6): 387–93.

Park, K., Huang, L., Gagne, H. and Papiez, L. (2009). "Do Maximum Intensity Projection Images Truly Capture Tumor Motion?" *International Journal of Radiation Oncology Biology Physics* 73 (2): 618–25.

Peters, L. J., O'Sullivan, B., Giralt, J., Fitzgerald, T. J., Trotti, A., Bernier, J., Bourhis, J., Yuen, K., Fisher, R. and Rischin, D. (2010). "Critical Impact of Radiotherapy Protocol Compliance and Quality in the Treatment of Advanced Head and Neck Cancer: Results from TROG 02.02." *Journal of Clinical Oncology* 28 (18): 2996–3001.

Ruysscher, D. D., Faivre-Finn, C., Moeller, D., Nestle, U., Hurkmans, C. W., Péchoux, C. L., Belderbos, J., Guckenberger, M. and Senan, S. (2017). "European Organization for Research and Treatment of Cancer (EORTC) Recommendations for Planning and Delivery of High-Dose, High Precision Radiotherapy for Lung Cancer." *Radiotherapy and Oncology* 124 (1): 1–10.

Tanderup, K., Pötter, R., Lindegaard, J., Kirisits, C., Juergenliemk-Schulz, I., Leeuw, A. D., Fortin, I., Kirchheiner, K. Georg, D., Nout, R., Seppenwoolde, Y., Dörr, W., Liederer, T. Tan, L.T. (2015). "EMBRACE-II Protocol." *EMBRACE II Study Protocol v.1.0*, 0–132.

Tibdewal, A., Bushra, S., Mummudi, N., Kinhikar, R., Ghadi, Y. and Agrawal, J. (2021). "Is Maximum Intensity Projection an Optimal Approach for Internal Target Volume Delineation in Lung Cancer?" *Journal of Medical Physics* 46 (2): 59–65.

Underberg, R. W.M., Lagerwaard, F.J., Slotman, B. J., Cuijpers, J. P. and Senan, S. (2005). "Use of Maximum Intensity Projections (MIP) for Target Volume Generation in 4DCT Scans for Lung Cancer." *International Journal of Radiation Oncology Biology Physics* 63 (1): 253–60.

Wang, D., Bosch, W., Roberge, D., Finkelstein, S. E., Petersen, I., Haddock, M.,. Chen, Y. L. E., Saito, N. G., Kirsch, D. G., Hitchcock, Y. J., Wolfson, A. H. and DeLaney, T. F. (2011). "RTOG Sarcoma Radiation Oncologists Reach Consensus on Gross Tumor Volume and Clinical Target Volume on Computed Tomographic Images for Preoperative Radiotherapy of Primary Soft Tissue Sarcoma of Extremity in Radiation Therapy Oncology Group Studies." *International Journal of Radiation Oncology, Biology, Physics* 81 (4): e525–28.

Chapter 6

Algorithms for IMRT in Treatment Plans

Mehmet Ertugrul Erturk[*]
Department of Radiation Oncology, Neolife Medical Centre, Istanbul, Turkey

Abstract

Today, the intensity-modulated radiotherapy (IMRT) option is the default for every linear accelerator (linac) and treatment planning system (TPS). Many researchers have done numerous investigations to develop or improve the components of IMRT for four decades. As part of these studies, they also did various researches on optimisation to find a successful method that solves the inverse problem of IMRT. While early investigations were about to demonstrate the superiority of inverse planning to forward planning via analytic solutions, the succeeding studies on inverse planning utilised sophisticated techniques of optimisation to improve IMRT. In this chapter, a brief introduction to the terminology of the inverse planning algorithms is given. The concept of constraints is explained by classifying it into two groups, which are dosimetric constraints and biological constraints. The optimisation methods used in inverse planning are also classified into two groups named deterministic and stochastic techniques. As there are many optimisation methods used in published research, the most common and successful optimisation techniques are explained. Moreover, an introduction to robust optimisation and direct aperture optimisation is given.

Keywords: inverse planning, IMRT, optimisation algorithms

---

[*]Corresponding Author's Email: mehmet.erturk@mnt.com.tr.

In: Frontiers in Intensity-Modulated Radiotherapy Research
Editor: Sibel Karaca
ISBN: 979-8-88697-252-8

1. Introduction

Before IMRT, three-dimensional conformal radiotherapy (3DCRT) was the default treatment technique to achieve conformal dose distribution. The treatment plan is made straightforwardly in 3DCRT planning. In 3DCRT, the planner is defining gantry angles, collimator angles, jaw openings, field shapes, and beam weights. After the definition of these plan parameters, the dose in the body is calculated with a treatment planning system (TPS). Dose distribution, tumour coverage, and dose-volume histogram (DVH) constraints are used in the evaluation of the plan. If the coverage constraints for target or DVH constraints for organ at risk (OAR) are violated the planner should redo the plan. The treatment is delivered after obtaining a successful plan that does not violate the constraints. In most cases, the 3DCRT planning process is repeated in a loop until achieving a deliverable plan if the planner is not an experienced person. The schematic diagram of 3DCRT was given in Figure 1.

Many patients have been successfully treated with 3DCRT. Unfortunately, sometimes the desired plan cannot be achieved, as a consequence, the plan requires some modifications which can be resulted in a decrease in tumour control probability (TCP), or the plan was delivered by accepting the increase in normal tissue complication probability (NTCP). IMRT was born out of the need for more conformal dose distribution. However, at the beginning of the studies on IMRT, the calculation capacity of computers was limited, and it took more than two decades for IMRT to become one of the standard techniques in radiotherapy.

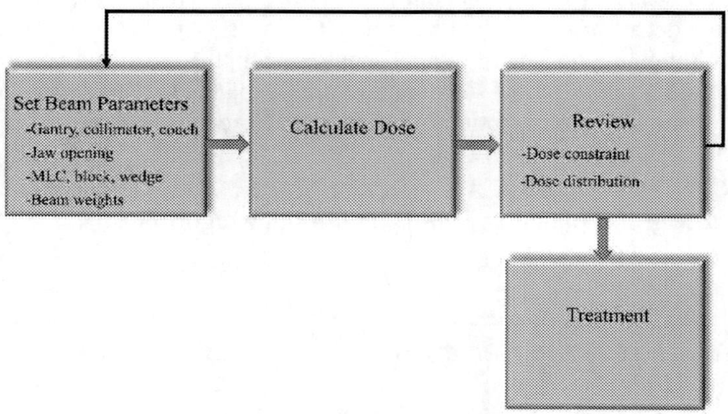

Figure 1. Schematic workflow diagram of 3DCRT.

It was demonstrated by researchers that more conformal dose distributions could be achieved with the modulation of beam fluence. Beam modulation is possible in 3DCRT, but limited. For example, beam modulation can be done with a wedge filter or with a limited number of subfields. Thus, limited conformity can be obtained with straightforward planning. Brahme et al. demonstrated that with the inverse planning techniques, desired modulation of intensities could be achieved (Brahme et al., 1982).

The development of intensity-modulated radiotherapy (IMRT) has been parallel with the development of computers and computing technologies. Although in many applications of engineering, biomedical science, and medical physics the necessity for optimisation was known, it was difficult to implement in real-life problems due to lack of computational power. With the development of computational techniques and beam shaping devices like multileaf collimators, a boost occurred in the field of IMRT research. These researches have an outcome of making IMRT popular worldwide. Today, IMRT is the common treatment technique for most tumour types.

2. Inverse Planning

As an advanced form of 3D-CRT, IMRT also has a similar workflow to 3D-CRT. The number of beams and beam parameters are defined by the users (such as gantry angle, collimator angle, and coach angle). Contrary to 3D-CRT, the user defines objectives, which can be a dosimetric or biological constraint. The inverse planning algorithm tries to find feasible intensity maps that satisfy the constraints for each beam with deterministic or stochastic optimisation methods. The optimisation process produces non-uniform intensity maps; however, only uniform intensity maps can be delivered by linacs. Therefore, the converting algorithm, which is known as the leaf sequencing algorithm, is required to convert the optimum intensity map to a deliverable beam. Details of leaf sequencing algorithms are given in the next chapter. Data is lost during the conversion of optimised fluence to actual fluence, and the direct aperture optimisation method was developed to overcome this problem. Moreover, the expected dose distribution calculated in the optimisation stage and the final dose distribution calculated with fine dose calculation algorithms will be different. In this circumstance, some modern TPSs use the dose distribution calculated with the fine algorithm in optimisation. Finally, if the plan satisfies the desired conditions the treatment is delivered. A schematic diagram of IMRT optimisation is given in Figure 2.

The concept of inverse planning can be understood more easily if the calculation of dose at an arbitrary point is explained. Dose at an arbitrary point *r* can be defined as in Eq. 1 (Boyer and Mok, 1985).

$$D(r) = \int_{V'} \Phi(r')k(r - r').dV' \tag{1}$$

Where D(r) is the dose at point r, Φ(r') is the photon fluence distribution, k (r-r') is the dose spread from point r' to r, and dV' is the volume element. The parameters of the dose spread function depend on the physical properties of the incident beam and the medium of interactions. Therefore, k is varying with energy and medium. The fluence, which is also known as the intensity map, is the number of photons that incident the unit area (Eq. 2). The shape of the fluence is constant (uniform fluence) and depended on the linear accelerator (linac) head design. The objective of inverse planning is to find an intensity map that satisfies the desired constraints for target and OAR. In inverse treatment planning, Φ is the unknown, and the objective is to find the feasible intensity maps for all beams that minimally violated the planning criteria.

$$Fluence = \frac{number\ of\ photons}{unit\ area} \tag{2}$$

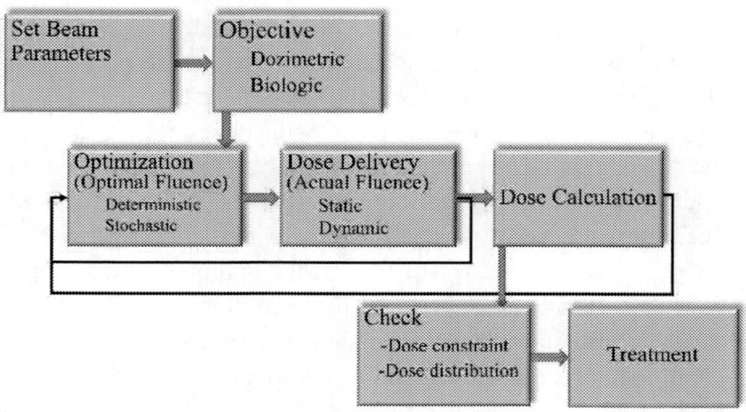

Figure 2. Schematic diagram of IMRT.

Figure 3. Beam-eye view formed by 64 square voxel/beamlet.

The imaginary lines passing through vertically and horizontally form a grid structure, as shown in Figure 3. The squares in this grid structure are the beamlets (bixel) and they are area elements. In 3D-CRT, the intensity of each beamlet is spatially identical, as the fluence is uniform. Contrary, with variable beamlet intensities, a better dose sculpting can be done, and dose distribution would become more conformal. An intensity map with different beamlet weights can be created with inverse planning. As a result, in IMRT, each beam has a non-uniform fluence. In 1982, Brahme et al. raised a similar question and published the solution. It is broadly accepted that the idea of IMRT in radiotherapy was introduced in this article (Brahme et al., 1982). Furthermore, Brahme made various contributions to IMRT such as the invention of the multi-leaf collimator (MLC) (Brahme, 1987).

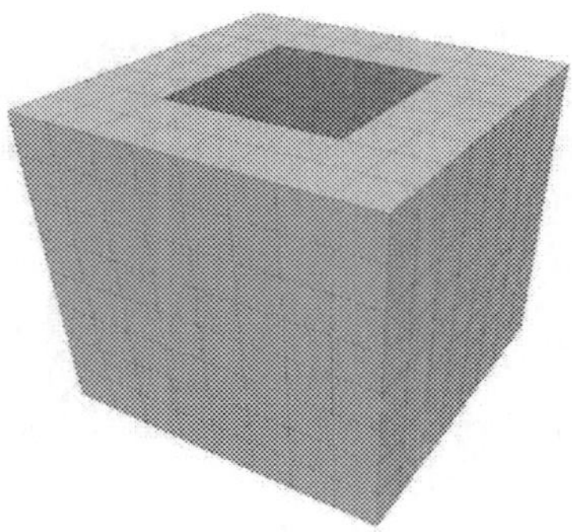

Figure 4. A cube of 512 voxels. The blue small cubes are voxels and the green squares are the projection of beamlets on a virtual phantom.

Like the bixel in 2D, a voxel is an imaginary volume element formed in three-dimensional (3D) grid space, as shown in Figure 4. Therefore, the number of photons passing through each beamlet forms the intensity map, and the convolution of the intensity map with dose spread function over volume for all voxels is dose.

2.1. Objective Function

Inverse planning aims to create a non-uniform intensity map by varying the weight of the beamlet to achieve desired conformity. The change in the beamlet weight results from the change in the dose in the volume. To quantify the effect of the change in dose positively or negatively the objective function is used. For example, let Dp be the maximum allowable point dose of tissue, and a change in the weight of a beamlet can result in exceeding the allowed dose at a point in the tissue. In this case, the value of the cost increases. The set of expected or allowed dose values or intervals are the constraints such as Dp in this example. The difference between constraint and calculated dose value is the objective function, which has to be optimised. The purpose of optimisation is to minimise the objective function. Eq. 3 is the general form of optimisation.

$$\min_{x} \; f(x) \tag{3}$$

In IMRT, a set of constraints is required to express the optimisation algorithm what is desired conformity to the tissue, and the intended dose to the target. Without surprise, the constraints used for plan evaluation in 3D-CRT are being utilised as an objective function in inverse planning. The types of constraints used in IMRT can be classified as DVH (dosimetric) based objectives and biological objectives.

2.1.1. Dosimetric Based Objectives

Dosimetric-based or DVH-based objectives are the most common objectives still used as the cost function in inverse planning. The maximum and minimum dose to the target, V20 volume of lung, etc. are samples of DVH-based constraints. Moreover, DVH-based plan evaluation is still the primary method for IMRT, volumetric modulated arc therapy (VMAT), and other conformal techniques, and numerous studies and many reports were published on DVH-based constraints. In the dosimetric-based objective, the intended dose for the target is usually defined with the maximum and minimum dose constraints, as well as the allowed dose for critical tissues is defined with the maximum and mean dose constraints.

Let a voxel that belongs to a critical structure has a maximum dose constraint Dmax and the calculated dose for this point is Di, j, k. The objective is to keep the calculated dose for points i, j, and k below the constrained dose. However, if Di, j, k is greater than Dmax the value of the cost function should increase. The relationship between constraint and dose is given in Eq. 4.

$$Cost \propto \begin{cases} (D_{max} - D_{i,j,k}), D_{i,j,k} > D_{max} \\ 0, D_{i,j,k} \leq D_{max} \end{cases} \tag{4}$$

Generally, a quadratic objective function, a weight factor, and a Heaviside function are used in inverse planning. The weight factor, which is also known as importance, priority, or penalty, could be a linear or nonlinear function, and it is used to express the relative importance of constraints to each other. Under this circumstance, a cost function can be defined as in Eq. 5. The cost function given in Eq. 5 aims to keep the dose at a point below the prescribed dose.

$$Cost = \sum_i \sum_j \sum_k w_{i,j,k}(D_{max} - D_{i,j,k})^2 H(D_{max} - D_{i,j,k}) \tag{5}$$

Where w is the weight factor for the critical tissue and H (D_p-$D_{i,j,k}$) is the Heaviside function as given in Eq. 6.

$$H = \begin{cases} 1 \; for \; D_{i,j,k} > D_{max} \\ 0 \; for \; D_{i,j,k} < D_{max} \end{cases} \tag{6}$$

To describe the intended dose to the target, usually, a minimum dose (D_{min}) and a maximum dose (D_{max}) are set (Eq. 7).

$$Cost = \sum_i \sum_j \sum_k u_{i,j,k}(D_{max} - D_{i,j,k})^2 H(D_{max} - D_{i,j,k}) + \\ w_{i,j,k}(D_{min} - D_{i,j,k})^2 H(D_{min} - D_{i,j,k}) \tag{7}$$

Where u and w are the weight factors and the Heaviside functions are given in Eq. 8. and Eq. 9.

$$H = \begin{cases} 1\ for\ D_{i,j,k} > D_{max} \\ 0\ for\ D_{i,j,k} < D_{max} \end{cases} \quad (8)$$

$$H = \begin{cases} 1\ for\ D_{min} > D_{i,j,k} \\ 0\ for\ D_{min} < D_{i,j,k} \end{cases} \quad (9)$$

Finally, the total cost is the sum of the cost values of tissues and targets. In IMRT, the cost function quantifies whole variables that affect the objective in a single value.

2.1.2. Biological Objectives

Dosimetric constraints indicate the response of the tumour or tissue to the dose for a single or a couple of volume percentages. The data of DVH constraints have been obtained from the correlation of tumour control or toxicity of tissue. However, the dosimetric constraints depend on the treatment technique. For example, in tangential breast irradiation, the V5 volume of the lung is inherently smaller than the V5 volume of the lung in breast IMRT. V5 dose is not a constraint in the evaluation of tangential breast irradiation. Contrary to tangential irradiation in IMRT, the V5 volume can be high enough to cause grade 3 toxicity. Thus, doses absorbed by different volume ratios of an organ may have the same complication probabilities. For example, the probability of grade 3 toxicity for an organ could be the same for Vx or Vy. More than this, the side effect probability could be a function of these two variables P (Vx, Vy). Hence, by adding a biological model to the optimisation, the effect of dose trade-off between different volume ratios becomes predictable. Contrary to indirect characteristics of physical optimisation, the biological objective is treatment outcome-oriented. On the other hand, biological models are limited to the baseline dataset, and if any variation of the dose in the structure is beyond these datasets, some math is required to predict this clinically obscure situation (AAPM Task Group 166, 2012). Thus, during the evaluation of the plan and the definition of constraints at optimisation, more attention must be paid.

Several dose-response models were studied for normal tissue and tumour such as equivalent uniform dose (EUD), generalised equivalent uniform dose (gEUD), linear-quadratic model, tumour control probability (TCP) model, uncomplicated tumour control probability (UTCP), normal tissue complication model (NTCP). One of the most common biological objectives used as a biological constraint is a generalised equivalent uniform dose (gEUD) given in Eq. 10 (AAPM Task Group 166, 2012).

$$gEUD = (\sum_i v_i D_i^a)^{1/a} \quad (10)$$

Where i denotes the element number or fraction of the organ, v is the volume, D is the dose and a is the biological parameter.

2.2. Optimisation Algorithms

The optimisation problem of an analytic function, which includes a couple of variables, can be solved by setting the first derivative of the function to zero. Contrary, some optimisation problems include dozens or thousands of variables and constraints. In such cases, to reach global minima or maxima, some numerical methods known as optimisation methods are needed. Furthermore, in most problems, it's impossible to obtain a global solution without brute computational force, but brute techniques usually spend enormous time which is not adaptable to the IMRT case to achieve a solution. Therefore, obtaining a solution that reaches sufficiently close to the global result is the purpose of an optimisation calculation in IMRT. Furthermore, the constraints used in IMRT aim for the acceptable plan, not the optimal one. From this point of view, due to the trade-offs between constraints, inverse treatment planning is a multi-criteria optimisation (MCO).

There are numerous attempts with different optimisation algorithms to minimise the objective functions, but most of them are not more than unsuccessful trials. Although analytic solutions were used in the early stage of the investigation of inverse planning (Brahme, 1988), the problem of inverse planning can be solved via numerical methods. The optimisation techniques can be categorised into two groups, which are deterministic methods and stochastic methods (Bortfeld, 1999). However, in various cases, the optimisation techniques were used together to search for feasibility.

2.2.1. Deterministic Algorithms

Deterministic methods assume changes in a variable depend on definite rules instead of probability. Therefore, there is no random step in the optimisation. Hence, the result will always be the same for the particular input, as the algorithm performs the same calculation at each time. The best-known deterministic algorithm is the gradient technique.

2.2.1.1. Gradient Method

The gradient method, also known as steepest descent, is one of the deterministic methods to solve optimisation problems. The gradient method in IMRT was first implemented by Bortfeld et al. (Bortfeld et al., 1990). Let f be the objective function wanted to minimise, and depending on variables x_1, x_2, …, x_n. In the first step, an initial guess f^0 is calculated for the arbitrary variables. Then, the gradient of function (∇f) at the initial arbitrary point is used to search for the next values of the variables. This iteration goes on until it satisfies $\nabla f = 0$. The point “a”, which satisfies $\nabla f = 0$, is the stationary point and could be maximum or minimum (Eq. 11).

$$\nabla f = \frac{df(a)}{dx_1} + \cdots + \frac{df(a)}{dx_n} = 0 \quad (11)$$

If the second derivative at the point “a” is negative, then the point “a” is maximum and if the second derivative is positive, the point “a” is minimum. The advantage of this method is its speed and simplicity. It must be noted that a stationary point doesn’t always satisfy the minimum it could be a saddle point, so the point must be checked with the Hessian operator. Although this method is fast, it has a probability to trap the local minimum.

2.2.1.2. Conjugate-Gradient Method

Conjugate-gradient method is an iterative technique that improves the steepest descending method with successive gradient search directions. This method yields a lower cost relative to the steepest descent method. Spirou and Chui used the conjugate gradient method to optimise beam weights in inverse planning (Spirou and Chui, 1998).

2.2.1.3. Linear Programming

It is also known as linear optimisation, and became popular after 1947, although some researchers had pointed out its potential before (Dantzig, 1982). Linear programming is a type of constrained optimisation technique that deals with linear inequalities and linear objective functions. Inverse planning in radiotherapy is difficult to approximate as a linear system. This method fails if it finds non-negative beamlets. Convery and Rosenbloom used Linear programming to generate the IMRT field with collimators (Convery and Rosenbloom, 1992). Dose weight, position, and orientation of each beam of Cyberknife were determined with linear programming (Tombropoulos et al., 1998).

The simplex method is one of the most successful methods used in linear optimisation, and it was introduced by Dantzig in 1947 (Dantzig, 1982). The simplex method optimises the cost function f(x) (Eq. 12).

$$f(x) = c_1x_1 + \cdots + c_mx_m \tag{12}$$

Where c_1 to c_n are the coefficients of variables x_1 to x_n, and f(x) subject to constraints (Eq. 13)

$$a_{11}x_1 + \cdots + a_{1m}x_m = b_1$$

$$a_{n1}x_1 + \cdots + a_{nm}x_m = b_n \tag{13}$$

$$x_i \geq 0$$

Where a_{11} to a_{nm} are the coefficients, and the constraints can be defined as AX=b. Thus, a matrix called simplex tableau (T) is formed as in Eq. 14

$$T = \begin{bmatrix} 1 & c^T & 0 \\ 0 & A & b \end{bmatrix} \tag{14}$$

The optimum values of the variable are obtained after some algebraic operation on the tableau.

2.2.2. Stochastic Algorithms

Stochastic algorithms are global optimisation methods that seek the absolute maximum/minimum of the objective function. Stochastic algorithms use random variables in optimisation, and the main advantage of generating random variables is escaping from the local minimum. For example (Figure 5), in gradient methods, if the starting point is at the left side of the hump, such as x_1, the solution will converge to x_3, which is a local minimum. However, if the starting point is selected on the right-hand side of the hump, such as x_4, the solution will converge to x_6, which is the global minimum. In stochastic optimisation, passing through x_3 to x_4 or x_5 is possible, so it may be not trapped at the local minimum. As a consequence, due to the search for a global minimum, the stochastic algorithms spend extra time, which makes them relatively slow to gradient methods. Also, the starting point, or in other words initial guess, is affecting the result in gradient methods, but this effect is limited by stochastic methods.

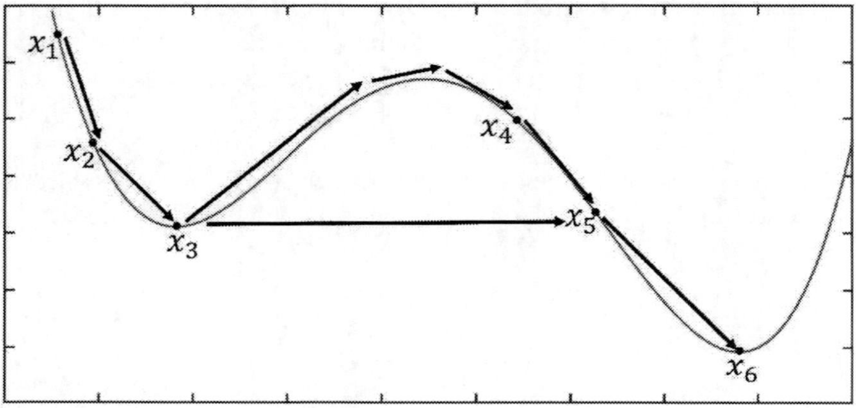

Figure 5. Comparison of the gradient methods and stochastic methods on one-dimensional optimisation problem.

2.2.2.1. Simulated Annealing

The simulated annealing method, which takes its name from a metallurgical process, is a global optimisation method, developed by Kirkpatric, Gellat, and Vecchi in 1983 (Kirkpatrick et al., 1983). Webb implemented the simulated annealing method to optimise beamlet weights (Webb, 1989). Although there were complaints of slowness in the early years, the enhancement of the method and increase in the computer processing power made this slowness insignificant. In 1995, Carol published about the use of simulated annealing in the optimisation of beam sequences in rotational therapy (Carol, 1995). Shepard et al. utilised this algorithm to optimisation of direct apertures, which is a milestone method in the delivery of the beam (Shepard et al., 2002).

Let the cost value at the nth step of iteration be c^n, and a beamlet value is changed in the $(n + 1)^{th}$ step of the iteration. In that case, if the cost function in the new step is smaller than the cost value of the previous step ($\Delta c = c^{n+1} - c^n < 0$) then the new value for the beamlet is accepted. However, if the difference ($\Delta c = c^{n+1} - c^n > 0$) is positive, in that case, the new beamlet value is accepted or rejected according to the Boltzmann distribution. The probability of acceptance decreases with the increase of the magnitude of the Δc and the iteration step number.

2.2.2.2. Genetic Algorithms

The genetic algorithm, which is a non-gradient method, is a member of the stochastic algorithms. It uses evolutionary biology and mechanisms such as mutation, crossover, etc. for optimisation. The genetic algorithm works well with many local optima. Ezzell published a report about the implementation of genetic algorithms in radiotherapy and compared the genetic algorithm with simulated annealing (Ezzell, 1996). It was also utilised to optimise segment shape, weights, and the selection of beam angles (Cotrutz and Xing, 2003; Li et al., 2004).

2.3. Dose Computation for Optimisation

The purpose of inverse planning is to achieve a suitable intensity map (fluence) distribution that satisfies the objectives and constraints. The response of a change in the intensity map must be known to find the cost (penalty) value. Therefore, it should be known how the change in the variable during the iteration affects the dose distribution. Thus, a dose calculation algorithm must be used in optimisation. Moreover, lots of iteration is performed in the optimisation. However, the dose calculation algorithm in the optimisation cannot be the algorithm used in the final dose calculation due to the nature of the problem. The final dose calculation algorithms require relatively more computation time, which makes them useless for optimisation. Hence, the dose computation algorithm used at optimisation must be a simplified algorithm that calculates the dose at a point relatively in a short time, but with acceptable accuracy. The algorithms used for dose calculation during optimisation can be called coarse algorithms and the algorithm used during final dose calculation can be named fine dose algorithms.

Brahme, Roos, and Lax used an exponential to calculate the dose distribution in their pioneering study as given in Eq. 15 (Brahme et al., 1982).

$$d(x,y) = d(x)e^{-\mu_p z} \tag{15}$$

Where μ_p is the attenuation coefficient, d(x) is the dose along the x-axis and z can be considered as depth. Dose build-up was ignored in Eq. 15, however, Brahme used Eq. 16, which was not disregarding dose build-up (A Brahme 1988), in the paper on algebraic inverse problems.

$$d(z) \propto (e^{-\mu_p z} - v e^{-\mu_e z}) D_0 \tag{16}$$

Where μ_p and μ_e are the attenuation coefficients, and v is the build-up factor. More sophisticated dose computation algorithms such as pencil kernel and point kernel were introduced, with the increase of high horsepower computers (Jeleń et al., 2005; Papanikolaou et al., 1993).

2.4. Direct Aperture Optimisation

There are two tasks in inverse planning which are the evaluation of the fluence and conversion of this fluence to a deliverable field. The optimal fluence map is calculated by an optimisation algorithm, and this map is needed to be converted to a map called the actual fluence map, which could be delivered by linac. Leaf sequencing algorithms are the algorithm that converts the non-uniform fluence of the IMRT beam to a deliverable uniform beam. Leaf sequencing algorithms can create these deliverable beams with static or moving MLCs. The details of leaf sequencing algorithms and delivery types are discussed in the upcoming chapter.

In the leaf sequencing algorithms, linac and MLC parameters are used particularly to convert the maps. The conversion of the optimal fluence to the deliverable fluence results in a loss in dose distribution. To overcome this problem, a method was proposed by Shepard et al. to omit the leaf-sequencing algorithm for segmental IMRT by using MLC parameters in optimisation. In this model, the number of apertures was also a constraint, and the proposed model tried to directly optimise the weight and aperture shapes (Shepard et al., 2002). Although some previous studies had attempted to eliminate the leaf sequence algorithm, global optimisation was first introduced to the elimination of leaf sequencing in Shepard's algorithm. The simulated annealing method was used for optimisation. Changes in aperture size are accepted or rejected according to the rules of simulated annealing if the new position of MLCs does not violate the MLC constraints. In the direct aperture optimisation, N apertures in a direction create a 2^N-1 intensity level, which makes the model effective.

In 2003, Earl et al. published an article on the optimisation of leaf positions and weights with direct aperture optimisation to IMAT (Earl et al.,

2003). Moreover, direct aperture optimisation was utilised to optimise the leaf speed, dose rate, and gantry rotation speed in VMAT optimisation (Otto, 2008). The physically impossible conditions such as overlapping of MLCs and negative beam weights were rejected during optimisation. The proposed model for VMAT was using a progressive approach to increase leaf and gantry position samplings from coarse to fine. In the progressive approach, the sampling interval of variables starts with a larger step size, then after a couple of iterations, the step size decreases and becomes finer.

2.5. Robust Optimisation

Robust optimisation is an optimisation technique that can be applied if the accuracy of the available data is in doubt or if the future value of the data is concerned and this value is uncertain. The motivation for robust planning is the uncertainties in radiotherapy. Inter-fraction organ motion in pelvic tumours or intra-fraction organ motion in lung tumours, as well as delineation of the planning target volume (PTV), limitation of imaging, and setup error can be given as examples of these uncertainties. The ultimate goal of robust optimisation is to add these uncertainties into the optimisation process and minimise the outcome of the worst case. Unkelbach et al. published a review on robust optimisation in 2018 and explained the details of this conceptual approach in radiotherapy (Unkelbach et al., 2018).

Conclusion

The first paper about IMRT was published four decades ago, and IMRT became an option for treatment over the last two decades in many countries. IMRT is the most preferred treatment method currently. Numerous studies are showing that IMRT provides better conformity in most tumour sites than 3D-CRT. With IMRT being such an effective method, there are studies conducted by researchers in parallel with technological developments. In the past, many studies have been carried out both in software and hardware, which enable the development of inverse planning. Inverse planning has been studied with different optimisation techniques using deterministic methods and sometimes both methods. Moreover, many studies have been made on how to use dosimetric and biological objectives. The invention of the MLC and the leaf motion calculation or direct aperture optimisation research on how to use this invention are part of this success. Undoubtedly, some studies did not meet expectations, such as genetic algorithms. Although genetic algorithms were promoted in Bortsfeld's visionary review, they found a place for themselves in a limited area (Bortfeld, 1999). IMRT has not only benefited from development but also tends to new developments. IGRT methods have been improved to ensure the correct positioning of the steep dose gradient of IMRT in the patient. The flattening filter-free (FFF) x-ray energies have become available as an option through inverse planning. Today, there are studies in different disciplines of science, such as artificial intelligence applications, that can directly affect IMRT. As stated previously, there are still some ongoing studies such as robust planning and biological constraint-based optimisation. In addition, with the application programming interfaces (API) provided by some TPS vendors or open source software such as MATRAD (Wieser et al., 2017) anyone can be a part of these researches. It is a fact that IMRT and related methods will go further than they have today, and thus more successful treatments will be delivered.

References

AAPM Task Group 166, Therapy Physics Committee. (2012). *The Use and QA of Biologically Related Models for Treatment Planning Report of AAPM Task Group 166*. New York.

Bortfeld, T., Bürkelbach, J., Boesecke, R., & Schlegel, W. (1990). Methods of image reconstruction from projections applied to conformation radiotherapy. *Physics in Medicine & Biology*, *35*(10), 1423.

Bortfeld, T. (1999, January). Optimized planning using physical objectives and constraints. In *Seminars in radiation oncology* (Vol. 9, No. 1, pp. 20-34). WB Saunders.

Boyer, A., & Mok, E. (1985). A photon dose distribution model employing convolution calculations. *Medical physics*, *12*(2), 169-177.

Brahme, A., Roos, J. E., & Lax, I. (1982). Solution of an integral equation encountered in rotation therapy. *Physics in Medicine & Biology*, *27*(10), 1221.

Brahme, A. (1987). "*Multi Leaf Collimator*." Google Patents, no. 19.

Brahme, A. (1988). Optimization of stationary and moving beam radiation therapy techniques. *Radiotherapy and Oncology*, *12*(2), 129-140.

Carol, M. P. (1995). Peacock™: A system for planning and rotational delivery of intensity-modulated fields. *International Journal of Imaging Systems and Technology*, *6*(1), 56-61.

Convery, D. J., & Rosenbloom, M. E. (1992). The generation of intensity-modulated fields for conformal radiotherapy by dynamic collimation. *Physics in medicine & biology*, *37*(6), 1359.

Cotrutz, C., & Xing, L. (2003). Segment-based dose optimization using a genetic algorithm. *Physics in Medicine & Biology*, *48*(18), 2987.

Dantzig, G. B. (1982). Reminiscences about the Origins of Linear Programming. *Operations Research Letters*, 1 (2): 43–48.

Earl, M. A., Shepard, D. M., Naqvi, S., Li, X. A., & Yu, C. X. (2003). Inverse planning for intensity-modulated arc therapy using direct aperture optimization. *Physics in Medicine & Biology*, *48*(8), 1075.

Ezzell, G. A. (1996). Genetic and geometric optimization of three-dimensional radiation therapy treatment planning. *Medical Physics*, *23*(3), 293-305.

Jeleń, U., Söhn, M., & Alber, M. (2005). A finite size pencil beam for IMRT dose optimization. *Physics in Medicine & Biology*, *50*(8), 1747.

Kirkpatrick, S., Gelatt Jr, C. D., & Vecchi, M. P. (1983). Optimization by simulated annealing. *science*, *220*(4598), 671-680.

Li, Y., Yao, J., & Yao, D. (2004). Automatic beam angle selection in IMRT planning using genetic algorithm. *Physics in Medicine & Biology*, *49*(10), 1915.

Otto, K. (2008). Volumetric modulated arc therapy: IMRT in a single gantry arc. *Medical physics*, *35*(1), 310-317.

Papanikolaou, N., Mackie, T. R., Meger-Wells, C., Gehring, M., & Reckwerdt, P. (1993). Investigation of the convolution method for polyenergetic spectra. *Medical physics*, *20*(5), 1327-1336.

Shepard, D. M., Earl, M. A., Li, X. A., Naqvi, S., & Yu, C. (2002). Direct aperture optimization: a turnkey solution for step-and-shoot IMRT. *Medical physics*, *29*(6), 1007-1018.

Spirou, S. V., & Chui, C. S. (1998). A gradient inverse planning algorithm with dose-volume constraints. *Medical physics*, *25*(3), 321-333.

Tombropoulos, R., Latombe, J. C., & Adler, J. R. (1998). Inverse treatment planning for the CyberKnife. In *Radiosurgery 1997* (Vol. 2, pp. 236-250). Karger Publishers.

Unkelbach, J., Alber, M., Bangert, M., Bokrantz, R., Chan, T. C., Deasy, J. O., ... & Xu, H. (2018). Robust radiotherapy planning. *Physics in Medicine & Biology*, *63*(22), 22TR02.

Webb, S. (1989). Optimisation of conformal radiotherapy dose distribution by simulated annealing. *Physics in Medicine & Biology*, *34*(10), 1349.

Wieser, H. P., Cisternas, E., Wahl, N., Ulrich, S., Stadler, A., Mescher, H., ... & Bangert, M. (2017). Development of the open-source dose calculation and optimization toolkit matRad. *Medical physics*, *44*(6), 2556-2568.

Chapter 7

Delivery Methods of IMRT

Cemile Ceylan[1,2,*]

[1]Radiation Oncology, Istanbul Oncology Hospital, Istanbul, Turkey
[2]Department of Medical Physics, Yeditepe University, Istanbul, Turkey

Abstract

Intensity-modulated radiation therapy (IMRT) is a more sophisticated form of external beam radiotherapy that modulates the intensity of each beam by splitting it into numerous beamlets. The beams are modulated by the IMRT delivery techniques to the required intensity maps generated by the inverse planning. The individual beamlets' intensities are optimised independently concerning achieving the desired dose distribution by inverse planning algorithms, which are made applicable by MLC movements on linacs with leaves. Initially, the cast metal compensator was used to modify the density of beams, but this method was quite cumbersome due to the requirement for uniquely shaped blocks in each segment, and it was challenging to acquire a homogeneous dose distribution, particularly in concave-shaped PTVs. Additionally, to the ideas of inverse planning and optimisation, the methodologies for delivering IMRT are considered to be the second cornerstone of IMRT. The current state of IMRT technology is that it is a mature radiotherapy technology and it is not the method in which nonuniform beam intensities are generated only by metal compensators, which can only modify binary intensity and are therefore unsuitable for complicated intensity patterns. With the development of MLC as a replacement for cast blocks to perform desired field shaping, IMRT was accepted as an advanced type of external beam radiotherapy and quickly took its place in clinical applications. To deliver an extremely conformal dose to one or more

[*]Corresponding Author's Email: cemile.ceylan@istanbulonko.com.

In: Frontiers in Intensity-Modulated Radiotherapy Research
Editor: Sibel Karaca
ISBN: 979-8-88697-252-8

targets calculated by inverse optimisation approaches, MLCs have become an essential component of all types of IMRT delivery methods, including static and dynamic IMRT, rotational fan, and cone beam delivery systems, and more recently, robotic arm linacs. Even though the first IMRT applications were performed using the binary MIMiC, which was an add-on to the linac heads, linear accelerator-based IMRT treatment delivery systems including step-and-shoot MLC, dynamic MLC (sliding window), IMAT, and VMAT have been developed since then, computer-controlled MLCs became commercially available. Currently, the majority of radiotherapy applications, including SRS or SRT, are successfully performed on patients using these delivery methods. Besides these IMRT delivery techniques, non-C-arm linac designs, including the Cyberknife and Helical Tomotherapy tools, have been constructed and are accessible today. This chapter will address contemporary IMRT delivery approaches in clinical settings with a concentration on MLC-based IMRT delivery methods, from a physicist's perspective, briefly covering commissioning and quality assurance issues related to these delivery methods.

Keywords: IMRT delivery, sliding window, step and shoot, tomotherapy VMAT

1. Introduction

Typically, the outcome of an inverse treatment plan is optimum photon-fluence distributions for each given beam angle or gantry rotation (Alber et al., 2001). As discussed in previous chapters, the optimum treatment plan is not immediately available for delivery. The issue in Intensity Modulated Radiation Therapy (IMRT) treatment planning that begins after the generation of the fluence map is to design prescribed dose distribution that can be administered to the patient effectively and precisely while still achieving the designated treatment aims (Bortfeld, 2006; Webb, 2003). A leaf sequencing algorithm must be utilised to convert each acquired optimum intensity pattern into a sequence of applicable field geometries. The leaf sequencing process considers the limits factored by the multileaf collimator. Finally, the IMRT delivery approaches modulate the beams according to the required intensity maps created by the inverse planning of the IMRT plan. There are primarily three strategies used in clinical practice for the delivery of nonuniform fields. Intensity modulators, binary beam modulators, and multileaf collimators were used to modulate the beam intensities (IMRT-CWG, 2001; Webb, 2003a; 2003b, 2005).

For a long period, cast metal compensators have been used to increase dose uniformity on target volumes (Chang et al., 2004; Opp et al., 2011), but their use is inconvenient because each patient requires a unique tissue compensator, and changing compensators throughout therapy to accomplish varied intensity modulation from varied directions of incidence is inefficient. The abilities of computer control and multileaf collimator (MLC) systems have enabled the realisation of complex plans. Metal compensators were unable to successfully deliver IMRT plans with the recently established inverse approach. Therefore, it was found that multileaf collimators, which were designed to shape the area to be irradiated, are the appropriate device for this purpose (Chang et al., 2000).

As previously mentioned, IMRT can be given through a variety of techniques, some of which include MLC-generated field-shaping in combination with modulating intensities of each beam direction. Two distinct dose delivery strategies are distinguished using the MLC computer-control system: (a) the "step-and-shoot" and (b) the "dynamic" dose administration approaches (Galvin, 2006). The static delivery of IMRT, step-and-shoot (SS), and sliding window (SW) deliver dose from various and restricted gantry angles. For SW, the beam is retained while the multileaf collimators "paint" a continuous fluence pattern across the treated area at different leaf speeds. In comparison, SS modulates the MLC to a series of distinguishable aperture patterns and only beams on while the leaves are stable in every location. The SS approach requires a intensity pattern with multiple discrete stages, which will be utilised subsequently to generate segment forms (Galvin et al., 1993; Xia and Verhey, 1998).

A newer technique, the most advanced and sophisticated of these modes is the form of rotational IMRT which can be delivered the dose via the conventional C-arm linear accelerators (linac) concept with the gantry rotation around the patient for a half or complete rotation at a persistent or varying dose rate. This approach is initially named intensity-modulated arc therapy (IMAT) and this approach was initially referred to as intensity-modulated arc therapy (IMAT) and then called volumetric-modulated arc therapy (VMAT) (Yu et al., 1995; Otto, 2008).

In the beginning, the majority of scientific research focused on IMRT performed on conventional cone beam C-arm linacs featuring with MLCs, which is the mainstream IMRT equipment used today. In contrast, the first commercially accessible IMRT delivery technology for patient treatment was used as supplementary equipment called a binary Multileaf Intensity Modulating Collimator (MIMiC), which allowed conventional linear accelerators to administer serial fan beam tomotherapy (Carol et al., 1995). The MIMiC multileaf collimator is a slice design collimator that is installed on the gantry of a linac as the third part of the collimator and operates in place of the linac collimator system. Arc rotation is used to administer the dose across a narrow slice of the patient. Bilateral leaf pairs of the MIMiC can be switched open and closed on a binary system to generate beamlets of varied intensity (Saw et al., 2001).

Mackie et al. (1999) conceived the idea of rotational irradiation of IMRT in 1993, where the couch and gantry are continuously moving, similar to a helical CT scanner. Helical tomotherapy became commercially available in 2002 and is currently available using dedicated machines that deliver fan beams in a helical (spiral) pattern with replaced the MIMiC. The treatment unit is comprised of a mega-voltage linear accelerator waveguide that is positioned on a Computed Tomography (CT) gantry and has a number of CT detector rows that have been fitted as in a conventional CT, to supply megavoltage CT imaging during the delivery of IMRT. The gantry and couch movements of the Tomotherapy are comparable to those of a single-slice spiral CT. A binary MLC device comparable to the NOMOS MIMiC was applied for beam collimation to define opening geometry and intensity modulation throughout therapy delivery. The intensity of the radiation beam can be modulated by altering the leaf opening timing and gantry velocity, as well as by rotating the treatment couch, similar to a helical CT scanner (Beavis, 2004).

The most recent third class of clinical IMRT delivery systems consists of specialised robotic approaches that do not easily fit into the other delivery techniques. The high-precision stereotactic radiation termed the CyberKnife treatment system is based on a linear accelerator that is combined with a robotic arm and has a 6-MV photon energy linear accelerator installed on a robotic system that travels around the patient across predetermined, non-isocentric pathways (or trajectories) around the patient (Adler et al., 1997).

Early in this century, Magnetic Resonance-guided radiotherapy (MRgRT) has recently been available in clinical settings. The concept of hybrid systems for MRgRT, which combine MR scanners with linac (MRLinac), was initially presented and has recently been introduced into clinical practice (Raaymakers et al., 2017). Currently, two alternative systems are available to use external radiotherapy, including radiosurgery applications equipped with onboard magnetic resonance imaging (MRI) for patient alignment, and are capable of delivering IMRT in a step-and-shoot method (Lagendijk et al., 2014; Mutic and Dempsey, 2014).

As emphasised above, while various delivery methods have been utilised in the establishment of IMRT, MLC-based techniques methods have been considered to be a forerunner in terms of relevance and usefulness in contemporary therapeutic applications. Simultaneously with the advancements in image-guided radiotherapy (IGRT), MLC-based delivery techniques are now reaching unprecedented levels of accuracy, which in turn is also increasing the success rate of administered radiotherapy. The understanding of the physical features, capabilities and inherent inaccuracies associated with MLC-based delivery systems enables the medical physicist to implement these approaches effectively and accurately in the clinic.

The physical characteristics and the core principles and procedures for administering fluence patterns as an outcome of inverse planning encompassing MLCs-based innovative IMRT delivery techniques including tomotherapy, conventional linear accelerators modulated by MLCs, robotic linear accelerators, and MR Linac equipped with MLC will be discussed in the context and their methods of IMRT dose delivery will be described in detail.

2. Historical Background of the IMRT Delivery Techniques

IMRT is a recently introduced advanced and crucial component of external beam irradiation for the treatment of malignant and non-malignant disorders in many radiotherapy departments. This is because of the capability of IMRT to shape the high-dose volume the surrounding the potentially irregular area being treated, which could be utilised to construct highly uniform dose volumes, resulting in enhanced tumour control probability (TCP) without allowing unintended irradiation effect on healthy tissues and a reduced risk of normal tissue complication probability (NTCP) (Nutting, 2003).

In principle, IMRT delivery methods use intensity-modulated beams created by a combination of a large number of small beams called *beamlets or segments* shaped by dynamic multileaf collimator (MLC) motion or static MLC fields rather than non-modulated-uniform intensity beams across each field to achieve a highly conform the pattern of the intended dose as a proportion of the geometry of volume to be irradiated and anatomical location of the nearby organs-at-risk (OARs) (Bortfeld et al., 1994; Boyer et al., 2000; Keller-Reichenbecher et al., 1999; Spirou and Chui, 1994; Webb, 1998). The shape and weight of the beam intensity at a certain gantry angle are defined in IMRT by the merging of segments, each with a different density adjusted with an optimisation technique to produce an aimed dose to the target. The process of IMRT planning and delivery due to having a great number of beams of differing doses, dimensions, or forms, and alignments to conform irregularly shaped target volumes by prescription dose could be described as more complex compared to three-dimensional conformal radiotherapy (3DCRT). With the development of the MLC beam shaping system and the assistance of computer-assisted sophisticated plan optimisation techniques of treatment planning systems (TPS) to create the intensity map to customise the dose distribution as a requirement of a planning target volume (PTV), IMRT has become a useful and important component of the routine treatment modality of delivery for conventionally fractionated radiotherapy as well as for radiosurgery applications (ICRU Report 83, 2010).

Historically, Brahme et al. defined the fundamental and mathematical concept of IMRT in 1982, and Bortfeld et al. described a clinical implementation of IMRT in 1990. Webb (1989) and Bortfeld et al. (1990) introduced simulated-annealing inverse planning for IMRT to be integrated into TPSs in the same years to solve the optimisation problem of reducing the discrepancy between the prescribed and delivered doses. Currently, the majority of IMRT planning is conducted through an inverse optimisation approach with various algorithms on TPS taking into consideration stated dose constraints for the delineated target volumes and organs at risk and beam numbers with different gantry angles. The intensity modulation of the beams is calculated using an iterative approach and various algorithms to achieve the desired dose distribution which is physically and technically can be delivered by several different modes (Ezzel et al., 2003). At the beginning of IMRT research and adoption into clinical practice, it was unclear how to shape the intensity of the beam with a non-uniform dose using either a linac equipped with commercially available MLCs or a linac without MLCs. Until the development of computer-controlled MLC-based delivery methods, beam compensators with varying thicknesses have been used for each different field, with the homogeneity of the beam thus modulated after the beam passes through the different thicknesses of the compensators (Chang et al., 2004; Helyer et al., 1995). The disadvantage is that separate filters must be built for each beam and each patient treated (Chang et al., 2000). Additionally, the filters must be changed manually during the radiation therapy between intensity-modulated radiation fields belonging to the different gantry angles, precluding the use of time-saving automatic setups. Although Popple and

Rosen (2000) introduced a novel technique for delivering multiple-field IMRT utilising a compensator, IMRT with the newly developed inverse planning approach to create a complex intensity map couldn't be delivered efficiently with binary intensity modulated beams formed by metal compensators. The concept of the modern, commercial MLC patent was first articulated by Brahme and was realised by Scanditronics in 1984. In the 1990s, cone beam IMRT was developed by combining conventional linacs equipped with computer-controlled MLCs and various delivery methods to generate beam intensity patterns.

On the other hand, as a result of research into IMRT applications in linacs without MLCs by Mackie and Paul Reckwerdt (1992), the first clinical implementation of commercialized IMRT based on MLC, known as serial tomotherapy, by NOMOS in 1992 (Mackie et al., 1993). Subsequently, the first IMRT device clinically accessible (Peacock, NOMOS Corp.) as a serial tomotherapy IMRT principle became accessible and employed with a special binary Multileaf Intensity Modulating Collimator (MIMiC) as an add-on tool for a standard linear accelerator (linac) for arc delivery. This was a binary (open/closed) slit fan-beam system that was controlled by a computer while the gantry was rotating. The MIMiC modulated the intensity of linac rotating around the patient to treat slice by slice utilising a fan beam in the approach of early CT scanner design. Helical Tomotherapy was developed in the 1990s by the same group and the history of this first commercially available system for planning and execution of IMRT was published by Mackie, 2006. Treatments are provided using a linac that rotates around the patient and a binary collimator (Nomos MIMiC), similar to serial tomotherapy treatment delivery. During radiotherapy, MLCs turn segments on and off as the patient is moved longitudinally across the machine. Whereas serial tomotherapy uses discontinuous table intervals between each axial gantry rotation to produce numerous fan beams, helical tomotherapy uses helical CT-type movements with uninterrupted synchronised gantry and table motion. The timetables for the IMRT delivery procedure were listed in Table 1.

Simultaneously, as innovations on the linac side addressed technological concerns, the question of how to invert non-uniform intensity patterns into clinical settings for inverse optimisation problems in planning algorithms began to be addressed independently by several groups. Brahme et al. (1982) provided a possible answer to an integral equation encountered in rotational treatment and formulated the IMRT plan as an inverse problem in their publication, which is widely regarded as the cornerstone IMRT paper. Researchers Brahme et al. (1982) and Cormack et al. (1987) demonstrated that the utilisation of nonhomogeneous beam intensities allows for the administration of dose distributions that adapt to the desired shape in terms of the treating volume while simultaneously conserving any adjacent organs at the risk due to the radiation dose distribution. Steve Webb (1989) presented a paper in which he described the inverse approach of IMRT as an optimisation issue and proposed the optimisation technique of 'simulated annealing, which is used to minimise an objective function or 'cost function'. The solution provided by Webb has been accepted as a milestone in modern IMRT planning.

Convery and Rosenbloom (1992) invented a system in essence still in use in clinical IMRT as a dynamic delivery today wherein the leaf pairs of an MLC shift in a single direction ‘sweep motion’ at a changeable speed while the beam is on. They developed an algorithm for calculating leaf trajectories that produce arbitrary intensity profiles with the minimal possibility of beam-on time. Bortfield et al. (1990) also constructed a solution for an optimisation approach to the inverse planning problem with gradient descent methods. In summary, in the late 1980s and early 1990s, numerical IMRT optimisation algorithms were developed to obtain optimal intensity profiles as desired. These algorithms iteratively explore spaces of physically realisable (without negative fluence) IMRT delivery sequences in order to find dose distributions that are the closest match to physically unachievable ideal distributions.

Nearly four decades have elapsed since IMRT was "invented" (Brahme et al., 1982) and the development in technology and planning approaches to enable it has prepared the foundation for the rapid development of IMRT delivery possibilities, making it a routine treatment modality in clinical applications today. IMRT technology now available enables the treatment of patients in a variety of modalities, including tomotherapy, segmented or "step and shoot" (SS), and dynamic "sliding window" (SW), using linear accelerators equipped with different types of MLC. The shapes and weights of individual segments are different and depend on the prescribed dose and dose gradient, as well as the technical characteristics of the MLC design regarding delivery methods.

As will be addressed later in this chapter, MLC-based IMRT delivery systems are well-establish however, they are limited by a number of physical restrictions that must be overcome. The MLC leaf width limits the dosimetric spatial resolution that interleaf leakage and tongue-and-groove effects impair dosimetric precision, and the degree of leaf motion restricts the maximum field size that can be provided. Thus, different types of MLCs have been designed and constructed to decrease transmission, sharpen the penumbra, and increase speed and positioning accuracy during IMRT delivery. Due to the mechanical and physical restrictions of MLCs, IMRT delivery methods including sliding window and step and shoot have prolonged treatment times and exposed an enhancement volume of normal structures to low radiation doses. To overcome these limitations of MLCs, Yu et al. (1995) and Otto et al. (2008) suggested an MLC-based IMRT technique that adds collimator rotation and so gives more flexibility in producing leaf sequences for the intended intensity pattern. A cone beam alternative to tomotherapy was proposed by Yu et al. (1995) called intensity-modulated arc therapy (IMAT), which incorporates gantry motion, MLC leaves/diaphragms, and dose rate modulation during delivery to produce a cone beam alternative while preventing the junction problems associated with slice-based tomotherapy and utilising a standard linear accelerator that is capable of performing IMRT.

VMAT is a novel concept in rotational IMRT that employs a traditional C-arm linear accelerator with synchronised MLC leaves and gantry rotations in combination with a traditional C-arm linear accelerator (arc movements). By employing a number of arcs based on the anatomical site to be treated, these approaches could attain comparable dosimetric achievement to fixed-gantry IMRT delivery approaches (Yu and Tang, 2011). Additionally, VMAT therapies have the potential to drastically minimise the amount of time and monitor units necessary for a patient's irradiation.

MLC technology was recently released for clinical application in 2015 with the Cyberknife system, which is the first commercial MLC to be installed on a robotic radiotherapy machine (McGuinness et al., 2015). Non-isocentric, non-coplanar delivery of the radiation beams shaped by different radius size cones and dynamic collimators that enable variable field size during treatment delivery were used in this device until 2014. The new MLC system, dubbed InCiseTM, consists of 41 leaf pairs and enables fields to be dynamically sculpted to match the contour of the tumour. A considerable number of beams incident with a circular cone at various directions and with sizes less than the target projection were necessary to completely cover an irregularly shaped target, resulting in a prolonged treatment course. Although the dosimetric benefits and clinical indications of the technology are still being evaluated, the investigations by Fürweger et al., (2016) and Calusi et al., (2020) stated that the recent implementation of MLCs in the Cyberknife system could give the possibility to treat larger tumours and minimise irradiation duration and the overall amount of monitor units these characteristics make this MLCs the preferred option for stereotactic body therapy (SBRT) of large body lesions.

Table 1. Timeline and specifications of IMRT delivery modalities

Procedure	Realised/First Clinical Usage	Specification of Technology
Custom Block Compensators	1930s/1930s	Simple metallic absorbers (compensators) of variable thickness with limited modulation
Static IMRT Step and Shoot Delivery	1991/1997	Multiple MLC shapes per field with fixed gantry
Dynamic IMRT Sliding Window Delivery	1994/1995	Multiple moving MLC leaves shapes per field with fixed gantry
MIMiC Tomotherapy	1992/1994	A mechanical binary intensity modulator-Slice by slice rotational delivery with the coach movement
Helical Tomotherapy	1993/2002	Multiple moving MLC leaves during gantry rotation with coach increment
CyberKnife Circle Collimator	1994/1994	Cone beam delivery with robotic gantry movement
IMAT	1995/2001	Rotational delivery with a cone beam of homogeneous intensity per arc.
VMAT	2007/2007	Delivery with variable dose rate, gantry speed with dynamic MLC shape per cone beam
MRIdian (Co^{60} Source)	2012/2014	Step and Shoot IMRT delivery
CyberKnife MLC Based Delivery	2015/2015	MLC based delivery with robotic gantry movement
MR LINAC IMRT	2009/2017	Fixed-beam with Step and Shoot IMRT delivery
MR LINAC VMAT	2021	Dynamic MLC shapes with multi-arc cones at fixed gantry speeds

The point we have reached in recent years in the historical process of IMRT delivery methods is the combination of a low-field (0.35T) or a high-field (1.5T) magnetic resonance (MR) scanner with a conventional linac called MR Linac has been clinically introduced for MR-guided radiotherapy (MRgRT) (Raaymakers et al., 2017). Before the newly published work by Kontaxis and colleagues in 2021, the commercially available MR Linacs were restricted to only supporting fixed-gantry step-and-shoot IMRT delivery They demonstrated that the delivery of dynamic arc therapy similar to the VMAT approach on the 1.5 T Unity MR Linac was successfully applied for prostate treatments (Lagendijk et al., 2014; Mutic and Dempsey, 2014).

Consequently, the various innovative delivery methods of IMRT are now commercially available, and the variations in the dose distributions administered to the patients using these types of innovative IMRT delivery methods are intended to improve the efficiency of radiotherapy.

3. Leaf Sequencing Algorithms

IMRT optimisation algorithms as discussed previous chapter iteratively search for the optimum solution to create an intensity map depending on dose constraints of tumour volumes and OARs and as well as their geometry. *Fluence map optimisation* is a term that refers to the process of determining the optimal intensity map given the defined dose constraints using an inverse planning optimisation algorithm (Suss et al., 2007; Webb 2000; Webb 2003b). Assuming that IMRT treatment planning optimisation consists of four steps, namely:

1. Definition of dose constraints for target volumes, OARs, and beam directions
2. Fluence (intensity) map optimisation
3. Leaf sequencing
4. Final dose calculation

The procedure for turning fluence distributions into the corresponding shape of the radiation field obtained by the motion patterns of leaves is called *leaf sequencing*. A software component distinct from intensity map optimisation governs the motion of the MLC throughout delivery by translating the ideal intensity patterns into a series of leaf sequence information (Kamath et al., 2003). The leaf sequencing step in the major of treatment planning systems utilises two approaches during the optimisation circuit to calculate the leaf sequences based on the optimal fluence map (Cameron et al., 2005). The fact is that the desired set of intensity patterns resulting from the inverse IMRT optimisation algorithm may not be ideal regarding defined dose constraints or even clinically deliverable (Saw et al., 2001). For IMRT delivery using an MLC, a fluence map must be converted into leaf sequence data that guides the MLC's directions during radiation delivery. Depending on the specific TPS inverse algorithm employed, optimisation may generate continuous 2D intensity profiles required by sliding window sequencing to generate dynamic segments, or discrete 2D intensity matrices required by static sequencing algorithm to generate segments delivered via step and shoot delivery technique with respect to predetermined spatial resolution size and intensity level increment (Xia et al., 2010). The fluence map will be delivered via the leaf sequence file produced after the sequencing optimisation as shown in Figure 1 should be as near as possible to the intensity map created by the inverse process to achieve desired dose distribution while considering the dosimetric specifications of the treatment machine and MLCs.

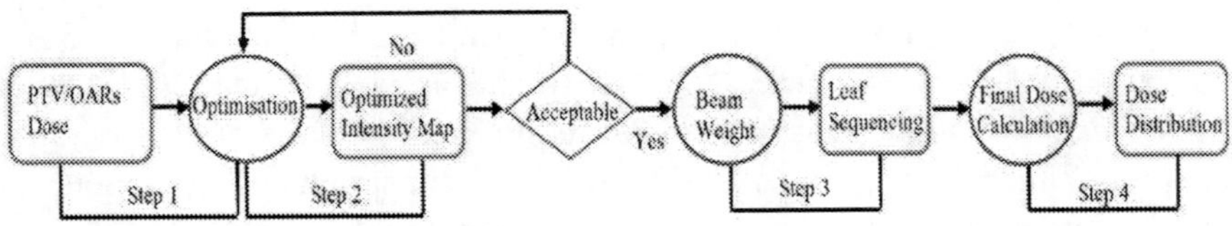

Figure 1. Flowchart of inverse planning IMRT.

Numerous physical and mathematical issues influence the degree to which MLC leaf sequences successfully approximate the specified fluence maps. In most cases, the resulting dose distribution is compromised and mostly degraded after the sequencing process due to considering minimising the number of subfields or segments without compromising the coverage of the target by the intended dose level. It also needs to be considered for physical restriction of the collimator and the need to minimise dosimetric issues including the tongue-and-groove effect and the leaf transmission (van Santvoort, 1996; Wu, 2007). To obtain deliverable and precise dose distribution, the relationship between inverse planning optimisation techniques and sequencing must take into account the MLC leaf width and speed when optimising the intensity map. Figures 2(a) and (b) demonstrate the fluence map outcomes following inverse planning optimisation, which is step1, and sequencer optimisation, which is step 2, respectively, whereas (c) illustrates the level of degradation between the two distributions as a result of MLC restrictions. As an illustration of a sequencing optimisation outcome for VMAT delivery to the lung, which is depicted in Figure 3, while the homogeneity and conformity of the planning target volume (PTV) may decrease as a result of segmentation, the dose distribution remains acceptable and deliverable. It will be appropriate to explain briefly the optimising algorithms that will construct the leaf sequencing pattern for the delivery methods of IMRT in the part of the present chapter. The essential features of the inverse planning approach used to generate an optimal intensity map can be found in the previous chapter written by Erturk, which covers most of the useful details. Physical limitations of the collimator and the necessity to minimise dosimetric concerns including the tongue-and-groove effect and leaf transmission must also be considered (van Santvoort, 1996; Wu, 2007).

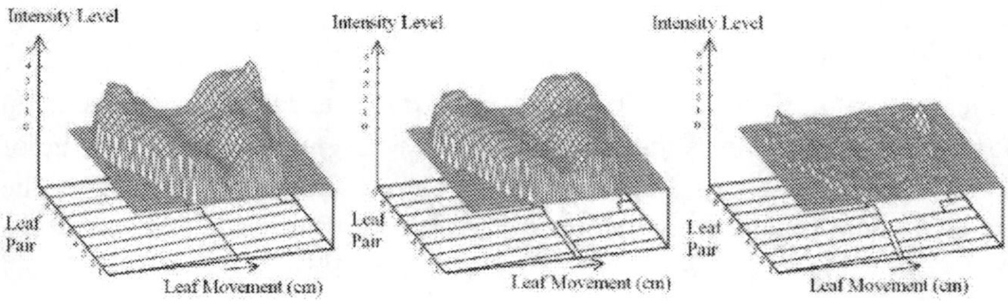

Figure 2. (a) Fluence map as the outcome of the inverse planning optimisation. The resolution of the map is generally defined by the leaf increment size through the movement direction(X) of the MLC. (b) The outcome of the leaf sequencer optimisation which discrete the fluence map into the beamlets with the resolution defined by MLC leaf width and step increment size. (c) The difference between two fluence maps.

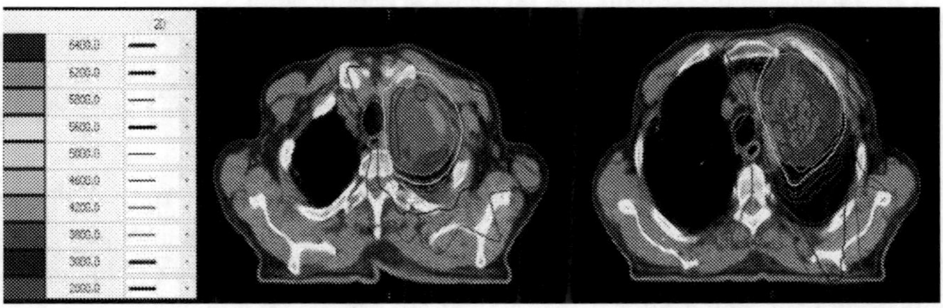

Figure 3. The dose distribution of before and after leaf sequencing algorithm for VMAT plan of a lung case.

Leaf sequencing is the inverse problem that does not have a unique solution (Bortfeld, 1994). However, since the numerous distinct leaf motion sequences could produce the desired pattern of intensity, a robust leaf sequencing technique is required which has a considerable effect on the overall accuracy of IMRT application, to find a set of MLC segments that deliver an optimised fluence map to deliver the nonuniform field in the systematically shortest delivery time, as well as accurately and precisely (Convery et al., 1995). Several algorithms have been developed in order to produce a leaf sequence with an efficient solution, which includes both the monitor units and the number of segments being kept to a minimum (Bortfeld et al., 1994; Convery and Rosenbloom, 1992; Dirkx et al., 1998; Langer et al.,

2001; Ma et al., 1998; Xia and Verhey, 1998). One of the two well-described approaches for leaf sequencing described by Bortfeld (1994), yielded a solution with decreasing monitor units (MU) per segment although it may result in more segments than requires. The other approach defined by Xia (1998) yielded a solution by reducing the number of segments but resulting in an increased number of MU. Therefore, more comprehensive leaf sequencing approaches must decrease the number of overall segments and MU value of them without adversely affecting the dose conformity tuning with the homogeneity of intensity distributions, the degrees of intensity levels, and the positional resolution of the intensity map with consideration of the mechanical limitations of MLC, such as the tongue-and-groove effect and the leaf transmission (Langer et al., 2001, Croock et al., 2002). Briefly, the following two well-known leaf sequencing approaches are generally utilised in IMRT delivery, which are:

(i) Beamlet-based optimisation

- Static Multileaf Collimation (SMLC) Sequencing
- Sliding Window (Dynamic Multileaf Collimation, (DMLC)) Sequencing

(ii) Direct Apertured-based optimisation

In the fourth step of the inverse optimisation process, it is essential to ensure that the finalised "deliverable" plan remains satisfactory by using the second dose calculation. Following segmentation, a final dose calculation is required considering a full scatter calculation. The dose calculation algorithm is employed to compute the absorbed dose by delineated targets and structures using the segmented intensity in the final step of the process.

The leaf sequencing resulted in shorter treatment times, which are related to leaf sequences with fewer movements and MU, which are preferred in clinical settings among the multiple valid leaf sequences. The result of the sequencing could be evaluated with two important measures of sequence efficiency, which are the total MU value and the number of segments. The sequences describe the segments with different leaf positions as a function of the beam MU. Generally, the generated IMRT fields as a result of the sequencing optimisation are inefficient with respect to MU. MU effectiveness could be described as the ratio of dose provided with an IMRT beam to the MU given by it at a certain location in the patient. The projected width of an individual MLC leaf determines the width of the beamlet. Each beamlet in a nonbinary MLC is variable in length, depending on the dose that must be delivered as well as the dose gradient that should be achieved, and on the technical parameters of the MLC device (Sharpe et al., 2000; Suss, 2007). Increased MUs and the number of segments have a detrimental effect on treatment delivery by increasing machine leakage, increasing the risk of secondary malignancy, and prolonged the treatment time of each fraction, resulting in inaccuracy in patient positioning (Mohan et al., 2006).

3.1. Beamlet-Based Optimisation

According to the principle of IMRT, the low-intensity beams that pass through high-risk organs (OARs) and the high-intensity beams that pass through the target volume are used in combination with each other. As a result, IMRT mainly relies on the synergistic effects of beamlets of the specific gantry angle beams formed by the sequencing algorithm as an optimum solution by utilising MLC specifications and dose constraints to achieve improved target volume coverage by prescription dose line and/or conserving of organs OARs. A typical method for solving the inverse problem is to create an optimum leaf sequence set either for step and shoot or dynamic delivery, which will be expressed in later sections that a beamlet-based technique is utilised for IMRT optimisation challenges. The beamlet-based sequencing approach is widely accepted as a second step in the inverse planning optimisation process in which the segment forms and weights are optimised instantaneously. The following fluence map optimisation according to the dose constraints of the desired plan the beamlet-based sequencing begins as shown in the flowchart of the inverse planning process in Figure 1, and is referred to as a 'two-step solution' for achieving a clinically acceptable and deliverable IMRT plan.

The process of beamlet-based sequencing begins with the segmentation of the field into a grid of beamlets where the fluence map discretises the two-dimensional (2D) grid areas into quadratic elements called "bixels" or "beamlet" which can be explained as the smallest beam element typically with 0.5x0.5 cm or smaller by assigning different intensity levels covering the respective beamlet shape, and then the weights (doses) of the beamlets are optimally determined (Coselmon et al., 2005). Thus, an intensity function is specified for each gantry angle to represent the amount of radiation delivered at each bixel. To define and optimise the desired intensity (weight) of each bixel labeled with w (θ, i, j) which can be expressed in 2D with (i, j) and identified by an intensity matrix, that is a positive integer $m \times n$ matrix at the gantry with an angle of θ, the formula in equation (1) should be solved by the inverse algorithm iteratively. Each voxel in the area to be irradiated (in the delineated structure) is identified by a three-dimensional (3D) coordinate system with the coordinates (x, y, z), and the desired dose D (x, y, z) is delivered by the beamlet (p, q) presented in Equality (1) and is calculated using the superposition principle as represented in Equality (1):

$$D(x,z,y) = \sum_{(\theta,i,j)} w(\theta,i,j).\, d_{(\theta,i,j)}(x,y,z) \quad (1)$$

$d_{(\theta, i, j)}$ (x, y, z) element of the formula is the dose given to voxel (x, y, z) by beamlet (i, j) from gantry angle θ. This calculation should be done by assuming *mxn* number of beamlets with a vast number of variable shapes for each defined gantry angle of beams and prescribed intended constraints of the PTVs and OARs (Rocha et al., 2012).

3.1.1. Static Leaf Sequencing

Static leaf sequencer transforms fluence weight profiles into static MLC field shapes will be delivered. The objective of the translation is to reduce the disparity between the original fluence weight profile and the resultant profile. It also operates a number of field shape restrictions and MLC design constraints. In addition, the algorithm attempts to generate the smallest number of apertures with shapes as regular as possible. Due to the reduced leaf travel, accurate dose calculation and quick delivery have become possible. Static leaf sequencing algorithms require the discrete map of the intensity distribution generated by the dose optimisation algorithms into the beamlets in order to deliver intensity-modulated beams via MLC settings, which are obtained by concatenating a series of variously shaped uniform fields resulting from various leaf position combinations to produce the corresponding intensity map. As previously stated, a collection of bixels with the same intensity in relation to the MU value is referred to as a "segment." These segments are shaped by various MLC positioning variations. Each segment consists of small beamlets that will be shaped by the MLC. The sequencer algorithm's purpose is to acquire those segments in order to deliver IMRT. Some sequencers utilise integers to represent equidistant fluence levels, while others employ clustering approaches to select levels with the least amount of approximation error (Ahnesjö et al., 2006). Typically, the discretised map into the regular grid described above section (3.1) has a resolution set by the width of the MLCs and an intensity level of discretisation defined by the user. If the intensity level of 5 is used, the grey value of the inverse optimisation's resultant intensity map is separated into five levels of intensity. As shown in Figure 4, for each row of the intensity matrix that has been discretised into intensity levels, a pair of leaves, a left leaf, and an opposing leaf can be changed in the manner in which the row is assigned. While Figure 4 (a) illustrates the positioning of the MLC and the patient geometry, Figures 4 (b) and (c) illustrate the profile as a continuous function of the optimal intensity map generated by inverse optimisation and the corresponding discretised profile used as an input function for sequencing algorithms, respectively. The discretised profiles can be used either the SMLC to create segments or the DMLC methods to derive leaf trajectory, depending on the selected delivery method. As illustrated in Figure 4b, the continuous intensity profile generated by inverse optimisation is first discretised into the equal distance part (Δx), which is equal to the distance between consecutive points on the x-axis where the leaves move uni-directionally; this results in the determination of the intensity values $I(x)$ corresponding to those coordinates on the x-axis that correspond to the desired intensity values after segmentation. In this manner, $I(x_i)$ which is related to MU denotes the intended intensity profile at the x_i location.

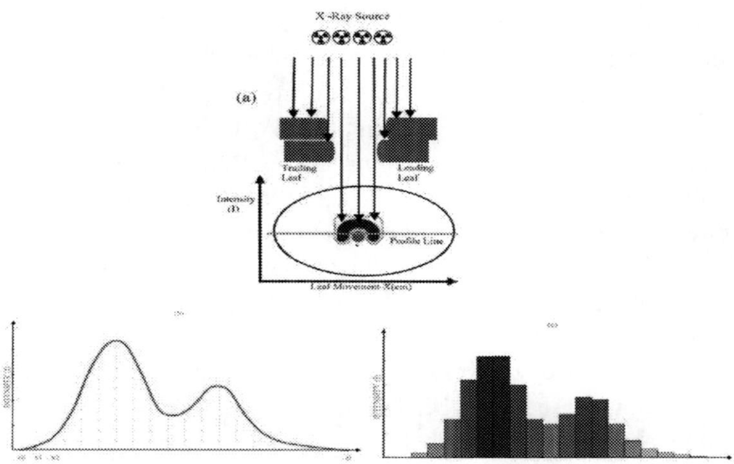

Figure 4. (a) Geometry of the beam, MLCs, and patient during the IMRT delivery. (b) Optimised fluence map using the inverse approach. (c)he discretised fluence map to be used as an input to sequencing algorithms. The intensity levels are depicted using a greyscale scale, with the darkest colour representing the greatest intensity level with the highest MU value.

The intensity level indicates the degree of complexity of the segment shape, which determines also leaf travelling and the number of segments to be established. The primary concern with static leaf sequencing is the prolonged treatment duration associated with the presence of numerous segments. The beam is switched off between segments while the MLC are changing their locations to create the next segment, which is another factor that contributes to the treatment's length being prolonged. As a result of the static leaf sequencing algorithm, the various segments with varying shapes created by static MLCs are realised by the "step and shoot" delivery technique wherein the radiation is switched off while the MLCs are shifting (Galvin et al., 1993). In the static mode, the entire therapy comprises the irradiation and the intervals between the irradiation and the moving of the leaves. The total irradiation time, which is related to the amount of MU per segment, and the total treatment time, which is related to the number of segments generated by the static sequencing, are the two important considerations of the static sequencing algorithm. Numerous algorithms have been developed with the primary aim of generating such a segmentation by grouping or smoothing the intensity distributions focused on addressing two concerns of the static algorithm, namely minimising the overall number of monitor units and number of segments (Galvin et al., 1993; Xia and Verney, 1998). Consequently, there are many different sequencing approaches to create static segments for step and shoot delivery of intensity-modulated fields. However, with the current delivery systems and improved MLC constraints such as leaf width, maximum speed, and the minimal gap between opposing leaves and also interdigitation abilities, the smallest number of subfields would yield the shortest treatment time (Medeiros et al., 2020). Significant improvements had been developed to the MLC sequencing algorithms in order to avoid spending time in MLC movement, improve the quality of beam delivery, and decrease the overall treatment time.

On the other hand, delivery-related effects of MLC such as leakage, tongue and groove design, and head scatter variations result in a decrease in plan quality and delivery efficiency, as the leaf sequencing procedure is frequently performed beyond the scope of inverse planning optimisation cycle, particularly in the beamlet-based sequencing algorithm (Arnfield et al., 2001). The consequent reduction in plan quality will become more noticeable in cases when the fluence map has a strong gradient, and its realisation will demand the inclusion of more MU. Figure 5 illustrates the optimal intensity dose distribution obtained from (a, b) inverse optimisation while maintaining the same MLC and intensity parameters for the pelvis region, as well as segmented dose distributions and differences obtained using static (c) and dynamic sequencing (d), respectively. Due to the goal of keeping the number of apertures low, there is a greater disparity between the targeted fluence map and the actual fluence map, resulting in a disagreement that does not typically arise with dynamic (sliding window) delivery (Xia et al., 2007).

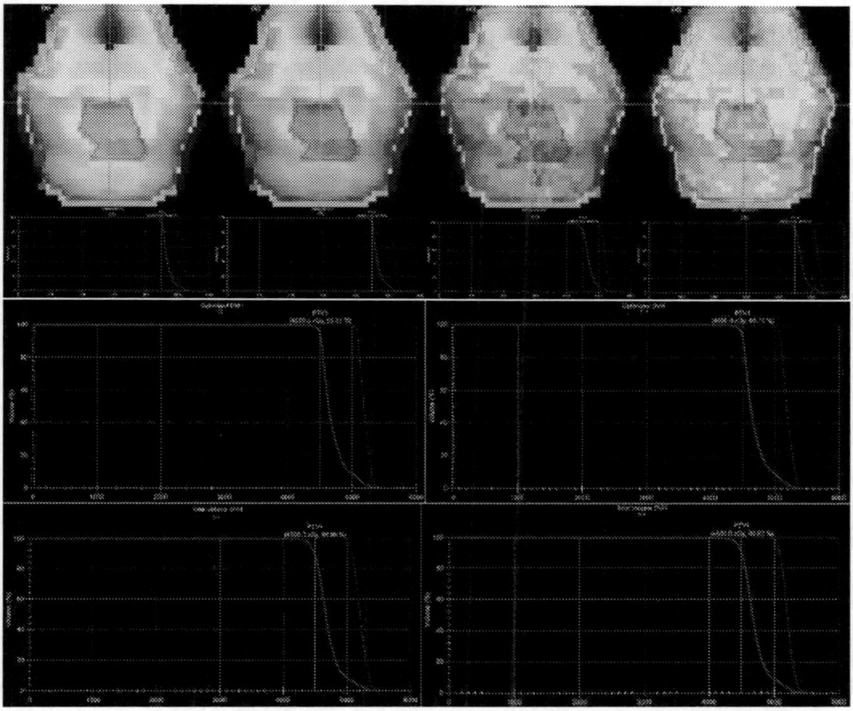

Figure 5. A diagram of the human body. The optimal intensity maps produced by inverse optimisation with selection SMLC and DMLC sequencing, as well as the corresponding Dose-Volume Histograms (DVHs), are depicted in (a) and (b). The calculated dose distribution following the sequencing of step and shoot and dynamic delivery with corresponding DVHs, in (c) and (d).

3.1.2. Sliding Window (Dynamic Leaf) Sequencing

In contrast to static leaf sequencing techniques, dynamic leaf sequencing algorithms have been developed to transform the required fluence distribution generated by an IMRT optimisation algorithm into leaf trajectories, i.e., unidirectional leaf motion sequences as a function of MUs (Bortfeld et al., 1994b; Convery and Rosenbloom, 1992; Kallman et al., 1988; Spirou and Chui, 1994, Stein et al., 1994). The most significant distinction between the dynamic and step and shoot delivery techniques is that the leaf sequence for Static SMLC defines a finite set of static segments, whereas the leaf sequence for DMLC defines trajectories of opposite pairs of leaves. When using step and shoot delivery, the radiation is turned off when the leaves move, however in dynamic mode, the radiation is kept on throughout the treatment, and modulation is accomplished by altering the velocity of the leaf motion. This opportunity results in a more efficient approach, but also adds to the complexity of the problem. The leaf speed and acceleration must be taken into account by the sliding window sequencer algorithm for dynamic delivery to occur. In comparison to the static segmentation problem, some theory on the optimal method of segmentation has been developed using sliding window sequencing, a condition in which the leaves only travel in a unidirectional with varied leaf spacing and leaf speed or the dose rate to modulate the intensity map without compromising the optimum intensity map obtained via inverse optimisation. Thus, this approach becomes the more flexible method compared to step and shoot delivery.

The leaf trajectories must provide an accurate intensity profile by employing either a stepwise constant fluence profile of radiation intensity, similar to that used in step-and-shoot, or a smooth continuous intensity pattern (Svensson et al., 1994) in relation to the desired profile (Ma et al., 1998). The intensity pattern can be generated by altering either the leaf speed or the dose rate, with the segmentation process being more customisable than step and shot delivery.

As illustrated in Figure 5, the length of the modulating beam can be fixed in dynamic mode using a single pair of leaves. Then, with the radiation turned on, a modulation would be formed by actively sweeping the opposite leaf pair. The "trailing jaw" pursues the "leading jaw" during the beam on time, and the positions of the leading leaf or trailing leaf as a function of time are determined by the central quantities, which are leaf trajectories. Thus, the geometry of the segment is retrieved using a specified intensity level, and MUs are calculated simultaneously. This is a well-known and frequently used technique referred to as a "sliding window," wherein the leaf pairs are moving in a uni-direction with varied leaf spacing in order to modulate the fluence. There are additional bidirectional algorithms, such as the close-in method, in which the leaves are moving toward one another, although this strategy is unlikely to find practical application due to its inefficiency compared to the sliding window (Kamath et al., 2004). As a result of the uni-direction sliding window sequencing technique, the positions of the leading and trailing leaves are determined as a function of time (in this case, MU), in accordance with the intensity value to be created at any given position of the profile where the leading leaf exposes at that point or where the trailing leaf shields. When designing the leaf trajectories, it is important to ensure that at least one of the trailing or leading leaves travels at maximum leaf speed while the other travels at a reduced velocity in order to modulate the beam as desired. According to the assumption that the leading leaf is moving forward at its maximum velocity while the trailing leaf is moving forward with lower velocity, as a result, the gap between the leading and trailing leaves will expand and increase the beam on time for all new locations previously under the leading leaves. In contrast, when the trailing leaf closes in at maximum speed toward a slower leading leaf, a descending gradient is created. Figure 6 depicts a schematic illustration of the irradiation process of the sliding window method, adapted from Cho's (2018) review article. Figures 6(a) and 6(b) demonstrate the generation of leaf trajectories for the unidirectional sweep approach. The dashed lines reflect the movement pattern of a leaf pair (x-axis) as a function of beam-on time (y-axis), which is proportional to the intended intensity I (x), whereas the solid line shows the intended intensity profile that will be delivered to the patient trough below this leaf pair. The independent motion of the right and left parallel leaf pairs of MLC leaves in unidirectional donation with R and L, respectively, would result in a two-dimensional intensity in terms of the profile pattern of the optimal profile achieved through the inverse planning stage.

The profiles of the MLC leaf trajectories $t_R(x)$ and $t_L(x)$, respectively, are derived directly from the required fluence profile I(x), taking into account the constant dose rate of the machine. At every point x, the difference $t_R(x)$-$t_L(x)$ equals the intended treatment time to create the intended density. Finally, inverting $t_R(x)$ and $t_L(x)$ yields the leaf motion patterns $x_R(t)$ and $x_L(t)$, which are then assigned to each leaf.

The higher MLC leakage could be regarded as a drawback of DMLC and should be taken into account while applying dynamic mode delivery. Typically, the backup jaws remain motionless during the sequence, and the MLC covers a large amount of the field in a number of MUs. Calculations must account for leakage and beam hardening caused by the MLC characteristics (Kim et al., 2001).

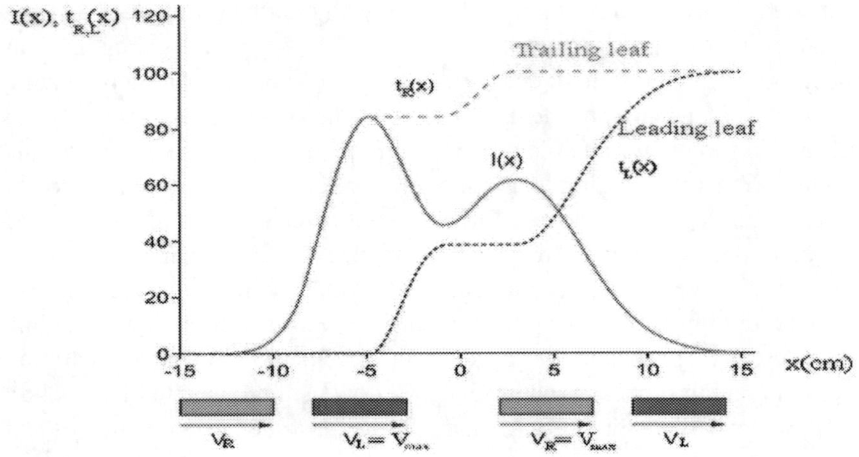

Figure 6. (a) Trailing and leading leaf trajectories as a function of position x, t1(x), and t2(x), as defined by the intensity profile I(x). To produce a rising part of the I(x) profile, the leading leaf moves at the maximum permitted speed, V_{max}, while the trailing leaf X_R slows down proportionally to the rate of intensity increased (b). In contrast to (a), to create a decreased I(x) value at the profile, while the trailing leaf X_L moves at the permitted maximum speed Vmax and the leading leaf X_R slows in accordance with the falling intensity rate. Graphs adapted from Cho B. (2018) with accepting terms stated with Open Access article distributed under the terms of the Creative Commons Attribution Non-Commercial License.

3.2. Direct Apertured-Based Optimisation

The idealised optimal fluence maps derived through inverse optimisation frequently differ from the fluence maps acquired using the previously discussed MLC sequencing algorithms. In contrast to two-step approach with beamlet based sequencing, the direct aperture-based optimisation (DAO) concept was introduced by Shepard et al. (2002) skipping the sequencing step to minimise the difference between the optimised fluence map and segmented fluence maps, as the optimisation already includes a set of deliverable segments, with each optimisation step taking MLC delivery constraints into account. Thus, direct aperture-based optimisation is accepted as an alternative method to the beamlet-based approach for determining the MLC shape of the segments, which results in a generally smaller potential MU (Van Asselen et al., 2006).

Following a few initial iterations, the shape of the segments in DAO is defined, the apertures are found, and the dose distributions for all fields are calculated. A large number of selected apertures are sampled and evaluated to determine whether adding the new aperture improves the plan, called aperture, is determined directly at the start with fluence map optimising using a set of criteria that tends to follow the anatomic contours seen in the beam's-eye view for each beam angle. By comparison of both sequencing algorithms, the DAO also leads to photon plans that can be delivered more efficiently, as fewer segments and fewer MU are necessary to deliver the treatment (Yu et al., 2006). However, not all available planning systems provide a DAO method. The shapes and weights of the beamlets are optimised concurrently with the fluence map optimisation process in this sequencer solution. Therefore, the optimised treatment plan does not require leaf sequencing and the plan is available for delivery after the optimisation. Direct aperture optimisation using a simulated annealing optimisation approach to optimise the MLC leaf positions and segment weights was initially used for step-and-shoot IMRT and was then utilised to solve intensity-modulated arc therapy (IMAT) optimisation problems in a highly robust and reliable manner to overcome gantry rotation and MLC leaf motion combination (Cameron et al., 2005). Before optimisation, DAO requires the segment number for each beam angle, the minimum size and weight of each segment, the dosage limitations on the structures, and the beam energies and angles. The segments are selected depending on a few initial iterations, and the dose distribution is then determined for all fields. A large number of potential segments are sampled and accepted or rejected based on whether the plan is enhanced by the addition of the new segment (Ahunbay et al., 2007). However, the DAO concept was initially applied to IMRT sequencing, which led to the development of intensity modulated arc treatment, which was subsequently introduced by Yu et al. (1995).

4. MLC Based IMRT Delivery Techniques

MLC-based IMRT is one of the most common and current methods of IMRT delivery which can be either a step-and-shoot or sliding window application using the conventional MLC which is an essential component of linacs. The approaches used in the delivery of IMRT can be divided into two basic categories. One method is referred to as "fan-beam delivery," and it involves the use of a rotating gantry to deliver IMRT in either a sequential or spiral form of tomotherapy. The radiation beam is collimated with binary MLC to generate a narrow-slit beam, and the intensity of the beam is modulated as the gantry rotates around the patient during treatment. IMRT delivery utilising a "fixed gantry" approach is the other type of IMRT delivery. Figure 7 categorised the various IMRT delivery methods currently available. Fixed-gantry IMRT accepted as a conventional MLC-based IMRT also referred to as "fixed field" IMRT, is capable of producing highly conformal radiotherapy dose distributions with a few fixed-gantry angle beams delivered by standard clinical linacs and modulated by conventional multileaf collimators operating in either dynamic or step-and-shoot modes. In addition to the IMRT delivery methods described above, innovative and enhanced IMRT delivery methods that are combined with IGRT technologies, which were developed in the early 2000s as a result of extensive scientific research, primarily using static or dynamic IMRT approaches, can be accepted as additional methods of IMRT delivery.

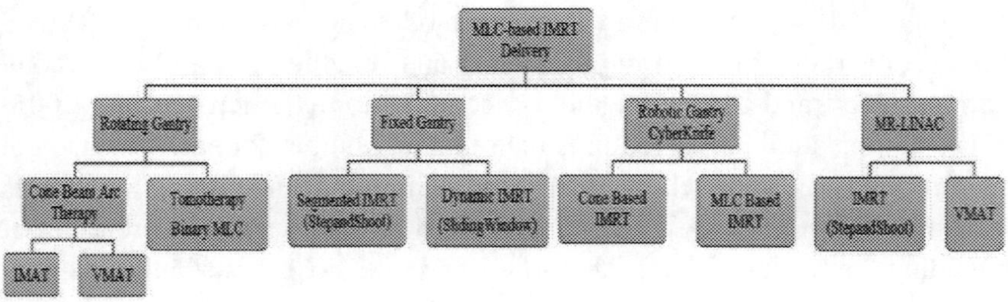

Figure 7. Diagram of the MLC-based delivery methods and available treatment modalities.

As listed below, six different delivery systems are routinely employed by the majority of clinics for either conventional fractional external radiotherapy or SBRT/SRS applications. These techniques modulated beam delivery methods are either step-and-shoot or dynamic delivery, but their implementations differ. Since the first four modalities are widely acknowledged as the primary means of delivering IMRT therapy, these methods will be discussed in detail in the following subsections:

- SMLC (Step and shoot) technique
- DMLC (Sliding window) technique
- Tomotherapy; Serial and helical
- Intensity-Modulated and Volumetric Arc Therapy; IMAT/VMAT

- Robotic Delivery; Cyberknife
- MR Linac

4.1. Static MLC (Step and Shoot) Delivery

SMLC, sometimes referred to as the step-and-shoot delivery method, is one of the IMRT delivery modalities with a wide variety of clinical uses in the majority of clinics. With the SMLC method on the linac, the delivery of those segments is accomplished in such a way that each IM field is delivered in a sequence of IM fields known as "steps," in which the leaves move to their respective designated positions while the beam is turned off, and IM fields known as "shoots," in which the leaves remain stationary while the beam is turned on. As described in chapter 3.1.1, SMLC necessitates that the intended profile be approximated by discrete levels of intensity resulting from the static sequencing method, which consists of merging variously shaped segments and the corresponding MU value for each segment. The number of segments acquired by the sequencing method for a given intensity pattern is dependent on the intensity pattern's complexity and the segmentation algorithm utilised (Sun et al., 2004). Most of the time, the segmentation process will inevitably result in a degradation in the dose distribution due to spatial resolution, the number of intensity levels used in the approximation, and the physical limitations of the MLC. The higher the level of intensity, the more intricate the intensity pattern, and the higher the number of segments needed to achieve the required dose distribution that may require prolonged treatment time for irregularly shaped beams.

On the other hand, the SMLC method is more similar to treatment with the combination of numerous static fields similar to 3DCRT fields, and as a result, quality control of those fields can be verified more easily. Compared to SMLC quality assurance, DMLC quality assurance is more complicated. In SMLC, only the leaf position must be verified, whereas, in DMLC, both the leaf position and speed must be verified (Chui et al., 2001).

4.2. Dynamic MLC (Sliding Window) Delivery

DMLC-based IMRT is a kind of fixed gantry IMRT that employs an infinite number of constantly altering MLC shapes in addition to an infinite number of predefined small incremental doses. In the DMLC method, the leaves move continuously at variable speeds while the beam is on. Within the limits given by the MLC design, the sequence of alternating "step" and "shot" segments in the SMLC method or the various speeds of leaf motion in the DMLC method can be appropriately constructed to irradiate practically any desired intensity profile. The main advantage of using a DMLC is that the continuous leaf motion enables the delivered intensity to closely match the optimal fluence calculated by the inverse optimisation algorithm, accurately preserving both the spatial and intensity resolutions.

Figure 7 demonstrates that an SMLC technique MIMiCs a traditional multi-segmented treatment and necessitates approximating the intensity profile into discrete intensity levels, resulting in a decreased resolution. However, while the delivery of DMLC is generally considered to be faster than that of the step-and-shoot technique, calculations are more challenged because the discretisation of the beams into well-defined beamlets is not as straightforward as it is for the step-and-shoot technique as explained by the sequencing algorithm section of this chapter.

4.3. Rotating Gantry Delivery: Tomotherapy

Previous scientific investigations focused on the application of IMRT to conventional cone beam C-arm linear accelerators with multileaf collimators (MLC), which is considered to be the mainstream IMRT technique. However, the first commercially available rotational IMRT delivery technology for clinical use was achieved through the use of tomotherapy in combination with add-on equipment to the linac called the MIMiC, which was commercialised by NOMOS and allowed standard linear accelerators to deliver serial, fan-beam tomotherapy. A binary collimator is mounted to the head of a typical 6-MV linear accelerator in serial tomotherapy. A binary collimator is mounted to the head of a typical 6-MV linear accelerator in serial tomotherapy. The collimator consists of two banks of 20 MLC leaves and the width of each leaf is 1 cm at the isocentre that are pneumatically positioned either within or outside the fan beam generated by the linear accelerator. The fan beam is modified by intermittently positioning the MLC within the radiation field. The fan beam's width can be opened to 2 or 4 cm at the isocentre, and the patient must be irradiated with many consecutive arcs when the PTV length exceeds the beamwidth of the fan (Elith et al., 2011). The uncertainty of intersections between fields as the couch when treating such large tumours and the absence of an imaging system in serial tomotherapy inspired the creation of helical tomotherapy, in which the machine moves in a helical manner to avoid junctions (Mallick et al., 2020).

Tomotherapy is now also offered through dedicated machines and a planning software system for helical tomotherapy became commercially available through Tomotherapy Inc. in collaboration with the University of Wisconsin (Beavis, 2004; Mackie et al., 1993; Welsh et al., 2002). Helical Tomotherapy is an IMRT delivery method integrated with IGRT employing fan beam megavoltage computed tomography (MVCT) technology. The design of Tomotherapy machine is similar to that of a helical computed tomography scanner with a linac in place of the diagnostic x-ray tube. In helical tomotherapy, modulated beams are administered using a dynamic field shaping technique without interruption with continuous helical motion, which decreases the problem of junctions when treating broad fields of serial delivery. While the patient is being transported along the gantry of the tomotherapy on a treatment couch, the linac rotates continuously (Mackie et al., 1999). A computer-controlled binary MLC with two sets of interlaced leaves modifies the radiation beam continuously throughout the rotation in tomotherapy to irradiate the tumour slice by slice, similar to the dynamic delivery of IMRT. The binary MLC similarly consists of numerous leaf pairs, but each leaf pair has just two possible states: open or closed also in synchrony with the beam rotation and couch translation to produce a 3-D intensity-modulated beam. The current generation of tomotherapy systems has a conical secondary collimator followed by binary MLC, which is a MIMiC-adopted technology with considerable enhancements to beam modulation speed and width. The maximum fan-beam field size of 5x40 cm can be reached by continually opening and closing movable jaws and employing 64 interleaved leaves with a nominal width of 6.25 mm at the isocentre.

As stated previously, one of the most significant benefits of helical tomotherapy delivery is the elimination of field junctions and dose gaps, especially for complicated and lengthy target volumes. Tomotherapy delivers a more uniform dose distribution than other IMRT delivery systems in clinical treatments such as craniospinal irradiation due to this feature (Sun et al., 2019). In addition, with the ability of the binary MLC to generate a very small field in helical treatment delivery, in comparison with other delivery techniques, better sparing of healthy tissue can be achieved while the target volume is covered uniformly by the prescribed dose. Consequently, this may result in prolonged treatment durations (Kraus et al., 2020).

4.4. VMAT: Volumetric Modulated Arc Therapy

VMAT is a method of delivering IMRT that refers to radiotherapy treatments in which, as opposed to the original IMAT technique, the gantry continuously rotates around the patient, varying the MLC leaf, the gantry rotation speed, and the dose rate over the specified arc range. Therefore, the delivery constraints comprise the allowed limits of all variable parameters, including dose rate, gantry rotation speed, and position of MLCs (Craft et al., 2018). Due to this feature, VMAT has the potential to achieve excellent dose conformity and sparing of normal tissue, while concurrently decreasing the number of MUs and the delivery times relative to other established IMRT delivery approaches. VMAT differs from existing techniques such as rotational IMRT or IMAT in that it delivers dose to the entire volume rather than slice by slice.

The delivery constraints comprise the allowed limits of all variable parameters, including dose rate, gantry rotation speed, and position of MLCs. The MLC aperture shape is determined during the treatment planning process as a function of discrete gantry angle position. Also, the dose or MU to be delivered for each MLC aperture is determined during this stage and this defines a treatment plan which becomes an invariant for the delivery.

VMAT can be delivered using a conventional linac equipped with a conventional MLC, resulting in an effectively intensity-modulated field with a high degree of complex modulation. It has been the most often utilised delivery technique in recent years because of its ability to significantly reduce overall treatment time in most clinical applications when compared to SMLC and DMLC (Yu et al., 2011). While it is categorised as rotational IMRT, the optimisation processes for planning and segmentation of VMAT are more complex than SMLC and DMLC, due to the need to account for the constraints of both the leaves and the gantry (Rangaraj et al., 2010). Therefore, algorithm development for VMAT planning has been scarce and the ability to deliver VMAT on traditional linacs has been delayed in part due to a scarcity of treatment planning systems (TPSs) that are capable of providing VMAT treatment plans. Many treatment planning studies have shown that it is possible to develop VMAT plans for various treatment sites that are comparable in quality to those for SMLC and DMLC but significantly shorter treatment time, which is extremely beneficial in clinical application due to treatment accuracy. The majority of VMAT planning algorithms adapt already published IMRT planning methods to the VMAT optimisation and segmentation that most of the VMAT planning (Palma et al., 2010, Papp et al., 2014). During the treatment planning phase, the shape of the MLC for each segment is defined as a function of the position of the discrete gantry angles, which is accomplished by utilising a sequencing algorithm.

Yu (1995) proposed IMAT, in which the intended dose distribution was provided via dynamic arcs approximated by a sequence of static beams with optimum leaf positions. Due to the large number of segments emerging from sequencing, precautions must be taken to assure that the resultant leaf sequence control points are relevant to the plan's delivery. Earl et al. (2003) suggested direct aperture optimisation (DAO) as an alternative to the traditional IMRT sequencing phase for producing IMAT plans, optimising both leaf positioning and beam weights concurrently. However, VMAT algorithms differ in the component most of the commercial implementations use DAO methods as a sequencer algorithm. In this category is RapidArc (Varian), which adopts a global stochastic optimisation approach to DAO rather than relying on intensity map optimisation or sequencing approaches to achieve results. SmartArc (Philips) and Monaco (Elekta) both use a local gradient-based optimisation approach to DAO, and they both employ intensity map optimisation and arc sequencing methods to acquire a starting point for DAO before moving on to the next step. Unkelbach et al. 2015 published a report addressing the physicist's perspective on VMAT planning, sequencing, and delivery formulation, in which readers can find additional information regarding the planning, sequencing, and delivery formulation of VMAT, as well as additional discussion about advantages and limitations of the approaches of VMAT optimisation. In accordance with the classification in this report, the three components of VMAT planning are as follows, with the majority of them being similar to IMRT delivery as described in the preceding portion of this chapter:

1. Optimisation of fluence map: Optimisation of fluence profiles at discrete incident beam angles is carried out in a similar approach as the IMRT fluence map optimisation algorithm is carried out.
2. Arc Sequencing: In the arc sequencing step, in which fluence maps are turned into apertures, are used. When compared to fixed field IMRT planning using the two-step approach described above, this process is relatively similar; however, additional restrictions on the shape of the apertures are placed in VMAT planning in order to allow for efficient radiation delivery during the treatment. For example, it is needed that neighbouring apertures should be similar to allow for efficient delivery and promote dose calculation accuracy. In the first step, after fluence map optimisation, the resulted fluence is divided

into a relatively large number of equispaced beam angles. In the second step, an arc sequencing method is used to convert the flexible mask optimization (FMO) solution into deliverable arcs.

3. Shaping apertures with direct aperture-based optimisation (DAO): An aperture collection, typically one aperture per two-arc-sector, characterises a VMAT plan when using a DAO approach to VMAT. Once this is accomplished, DAO approaches are used to optimise the shape and intensity of each aperture.

The published study demonstrates (Nagarajan et al., 2020; Yin et al., 2012) that the VMAT method of IMRT delivery has the clinical advantage of providing improved conformality when compared to the usage of a limited number of gantry locations such as SMLC or DMLC delivery. VMAT can also deliver single or multiple arc delivery, coplanar or non-coplanar delivery, as well as collimator rotation, hence increasing the number of degrees of freedom and allowing for a more conformal plan to be achieved.

Conclusion

Radiation therapy is strongly reliant on a variety of critical technologies, including imaging, treatment planning, and administration of radiation therapy treatments. These technologies are pushing each other aiming to improve the treatment precision and ultimately improve cure. The IMRT planning and delivery technique offer many degrees of freedom to shape dose distributions for photon beam irradiation. The delivery of the resulting treatment plan using MLCs is performed either in the step-and-shoot or sliding window technique via different treatment machines such as conventional linac, Tomotherapy, Cyberknife, and recently MR Linac.

References

Adler Jr, J. R., Chang, S. D., Murphy, M. J., Doty, J., Geis, P., & Hancock, S. L. (1997). The Cyberknife: A frameless robotic system for radiosurgery. *Stereotactic and Functional Neurosurgery*, 69: 124–128.

Ahnesjö, A., Hårdemark, B., Isacsson, U., & Montelius, A. (2006). The IMRT information process-mastering the degrees of freedom in external beam therapy. *Physics in medicine and biology*, 51(13), R381–R402.

Ahunbay, E. E., Chen, G. P., Thatcher, S., Jursinic, P. A., White, J., Albano, K., & Li, X. A. (2007). Direct aperture optimization–based intensity-modulated radiotherapy for whole breast irradiation. *International Journal of Radiation Oncology Biology Physics*, *67*(4), 1248-1258.

Alber, M., & Nüsslin, F. (2001). Optimization of intensity modulated radiotherapy under constraints for static and dynamic MLC delivery. *Physics in Medicine & Biology*, *46*(12), 3229.

Arnfield, M. R., Wu, Q., Tong, S., & Mohan, R. (2001). Dosimetric validation for multileaf collimator-based intensity-modulated radiotherapy: a review. *Medical Dosimetry*, *26*(2), 179-188.

Beavis, A. W. (2004). Is tomotherapy the future of IMRT? *The British journal of radiology*, *77*(916), 285-295.

Bentzen, S. M. (2005). Radiation therapy: intensity modulated, image guided, biologically optimized and evidence based. *Radiotherapy and Oncology*, *77*(3), 227-230.

Bortfeld, T., Bürkelbach, J., Boesecke, R., & Schlegel, W. (1990). Methods of image reconstruction from projections applied to conformation radiotherapy. *Physics in Medicine & Biology*, *35*(10), 1423.

Bortfeld, T. R., Kahler, D. L., Waldron, T. J., & Boyer, A. L. (1994). X-ray field compensation with multileaf collimators. *International Journal of Radiation Oncology Biology Physics*, *28*(3), 723-730.

Bortfeld, T. (2006). IMRT: a review and preview. *Physics in Medicine & Biology*, *51*(13), R363.

Boyer, A., Xing, L., Luxton, G., Chen, Y., & Ma, C. (2000). IMRT by dynamic MLC. In *The Use of Computers in Radiation Therapy* (pp. 160-163). Springer, Berlin, Heidelberg.

Brahme, A., Roos, J. E., & Lax, I. (1982). Solution of an integral equation encountered in rotation therapy. *Physics in Medicine & Biology*, *27*(10), 1221.

Brahme, A. (1987). Multi leaf collimator (US Patent No. 4,672,212). Washington, DC: US Patent and Trademark Office.

Calusi, S., Doro, R., Di Cataldo, V., Cipressi, S., Francolini, G., Bonucci, I., ... & Masi, L. (2020). Performance assessment of a new optimization system for robotic SBRT MLC-based plans. *Physica Medica*, *71*, 31-38.

Cameron, C. (2005). Sweeping-window arc therapy: an implementation of rotational IMRT with automatic beam-weight calculation. *Physics in Medicine & Biology*, *50*(18), 4317.

Carol, M. P. (1995). Peacock™: A system for planning and rotational delivery of intensity-modulated fields. *International Journal of Imaging Systems and Technology*, *6*(1), 56-61.

Chang, S. X., Cullip, T. J., Deschesne, K. M., Miller, E. P., & Rosenman, J. G. (2004). Compensators: an alternative IMRT delivery technique. *Journal of Applied Clinical Medical Physics*, *5*(3), 15-36.

Chang, S. X., Cullip, T. J., & Deschesne, K. M. (2000). Intensity modulation delivery techniques: "Step & shoot" MLC auto-sequence versus the use of a modulator. *Medical physics*, *27*(5), 948-959.

Cho, B. (2018). Intensity-modulated radiation therapy: a review with a physics perspective. *Radiation oncology journal*, *36*(1), 1.

Chui, C. S., Chan, M. F., Yorke, E., Spirou, S., & Ling, C. C. (2001). Delivery of intensity-modulated radiation therapy with a conventional multileaf collimator: comparison of dynamic and segmental methods. *Medical physics,* 28(12), 2441–2449.

Convery, D. J., & Rosenbloom, M. E. (1992). The generation of intensity-modulated fields for conformal radiotherapy by dynamic collimation. *Physics in medicine & biology*, *37*(6), 1359.

Convery, D. J., & Rosenbloom, M. E. (1995). Treatment delivery accuracy in intensity-modulated conformal radiotherapy. *Physics in Medicine & Biology*, *40*(6), 979.

Coselmon, M. M., Moran, J. M., Radawski, J. D., & Fraass, B. A. (2005). Improving IMRT delivery efficiency using intensity limits during inverse planning. *Medical physics*, *32*(5), 1234-1245.

Cormack, A. M., & Cormack, R. A. (1987). A problem in rotation therapy with X-rays: dose distributions with an axis of symmetry. *International Journal of Radiation Oncology Biology Physics*, *13*(12), 1921-1925.

Craft, D., & Halabi, T. (2018). Sliding window IMRT and VMAT optimization. *Decision Analytics and Optimization in Disease Prevention and Treatment*, 307.

Crooks, S. M., McAven, L. F., Robinson, D. F., & Xing, L. (2002). Minimizing delivery time and monitor units in static IMRT by leaf-sequencing. *Physics in medicine and biology*, *47*(17), 3105–3116.

Dirkx, M. L., Heijmen, B. J., & van Santvoort, J. P. (1998). Leaf trajectory calculation for dynamic multileaf collimation to realize optimized fluence profiles. *Physics in medicine and biology*, 43(5), 1171–1184.

Earl, M. A., Shepard, D. M., Naqvi, S., Li, X. A., & Yu, C. X. (2003). Inverse planning for intensity-modulated arc therapy using direct aperture optimization. *Physics in medicine and biology*, 48(8), 1075–1089.

Elith, C., Dempsey, S. E., Findlay, N., & Warren-Forward, H. M. (2011). An Introduction to the Intensity-modulated Radiation Therapy (IMRT) Techniques, Tomotherapy, and VMAT. *Journal of Medical Imaging and Radiation Sciences*, 42(1), 37–43.

Ezzell, G. A., Galvin, J. M., Low, D., Palta, J. R., Rosen, I., Sharpe, M. B., Xia, P., Xiao, Y., Xing, L., & Yu, C. X. (2003). Guidance document on delivery, treatment planning, and clinical implementation of IMRT: Report of the IMRT subcommittee of the AAPM radiation therapy committee. *Medical Physics*, 30: 2089–2115.

Fürweger, C., Prins, P., Coskan, H., & Heijmen, B. J. (2016). Characteristics and performance of the first commercial multileaf collimator for a robotic radiosurgery system. *Medical Physics*, *43*(5), 2063-2071.

Galvin, J. M., Chen, X. G., & Smith, R. M. (1993). Combining multileaf fields to modulate fluence distributions. *International Journal of Radiation Oncology Biology Physics*, *27*(3), 697-705.

Galvin, J. M., Smith, A. R., & Lally, B. (1993). Characterization of a multileaf collimator system. *International Journal of Radiation Oncology Biology Physics*, *25*(2), 181-192.

Galvin, J. M. (2006, October). Alternative methods for intensity-modulated radiation therapy inverse planning and dose delivery. In *Seminars in Radiation Oncology* (Vol. 16, No. 4, pp. 218-223). WB Saunders.

Helyer, S. J., & Heisig, S. (1995). Multileaf collimation versus conventional shielding blocks: a time and motion study of beam shaping in radiotherapy. *Radiotherapy and Oncology*, *37*(1), 61-64.

ICRU. (2010). ICRU Report 83: prescribing, recording, and reporting photon-beam intensity-modulated radiation therapy (IMRT). *J ICRU*, 10(1):1–106.

IMRT-CWG. (2001). Intensity-modulated radiotherapy: current status and issues of interest. *Int. J. Radiat. Oncol. Biol. Phys.,* 51: 880–914.

Kamath, S., Sahni, S., Li, J., Palta, J., & Ranka, S. (2003). Leaf sequencing algorithms for segmented multileaf collimation. *Physics in medicine and biology*, 48(3), 307–324.

Keller-Reichenbecher, M. A., Bortfeld, T., Levegrün, S., Stein, J., Preiser, K., & Schlegel, W. (1999). Intensity modulation with the "step and shoot" technique using a commercial MLC: A planning study. *International Journal of Radiation Oncology Biology Physics*, *45*(5), 1315-1324.

Kim, J. O., Siebers, J. V., Keall, P. J., Arnfield, M. R., & Mohan, R. (2001). A Monte Carlo study of radiation transport through multileaf collimators. *Medical Physics,* 28(12), 2497–2506.

Kontaxis, C., Woodhead, P. L., Bol, G. H., Lagendijk, J. J. W., & Raaymakers, B. W. (2021). Proof-of-concept delivery of intensity modulated arc therapy on the Elekta Unity 1.5 T MR-linac. *Physics in Medicine & Biology*, *66*(4), 04LT01.

Kraus, K. M., Kampfer, S., Wilkens, J. J., Schüttrumpf, L., & Combs, S. E. (2020). Helical tomotherapy: Comparison of Hi-ART and Radixact clinical patient treatments at the Technical University of Munich. *Scientific Reports*, *10*(1), 1-10.

Lagendijk, J. J., Raaymakers, B. W., & Van Vulpen, M. (2014, July). The magnetic resonance imaging–linac system. In *Seminars in radiation oncology* (Vol. 24, No. 3, pp. 207-209). WB Saunders.

Langer, M., Thai, V., & Papiez, L. (2001). Improved leaf sequencing reduces segments or monitor units needed to deliver IMRT using multileaf collimators. *Medical Physics*, 28(12), 2450–2458.

Nagarajan, M., Banu, R., Sathya, B., Sundaram, T., & Chellapandian, T. P. (2020). Dosimetric Evaluation and Comparison Between Volumetric Modulated Arc Therapy (VMAT) and Intensity Modulated Radiation Therapy (IMRT) Plan in Head and Neck Cancers. *The Gulf journal of oncology*, 1(33), 45–50.

Ma, L., Boyer, A. L., Xing, L., & Ma, C. M. (1998). An optimized leaf-setting algorithm for beam intensity modulation using dynamic multileaf collimators. *Physics in medicine and biology*, 43(6), 1629–1643.

Mackie, T. R., Holmes, T., Swerdloff, S., Reckwerdt, P., Deasy, J. O., Yang, J., Paliwal, B., & Kinsella, T. (1993). Tomotherapy: a new concept for the delivery of dynamic conformal radiotherapy. *Medical physics*, 20(6), 1709–1719.

Mackie, T. R., Balog, J., Ruchala, K., Shepard, D., Aldridge, S., Fitchard, E., Reckwerdt, P., Olivera, G., McNutt, T., & Mehta, M. (1999). Tomotherapy. *Seminars in radiation oncology*, 9(1), 108–117.

Mackie, T. R. (2006). History of tomotherapy. *Physics in Medicine & Biology*, *51*(13), R427.

Mallick, S., Benson, R. (2020). Helical Tomotherapy. In: Mallick, S., Rath, G., Benson, R. (eds.). *Practical Radiation Oncology.* Springer, Singapore.

McGuinness, C. M., Gottschalk, A. R., Lessard, E., Nakamura, J. L., Pinnaduwage, D., Pouliot, J., Sims, C., & Descovich, M. (2015). Investigating the clinical advantages of a robotic linac equipped with a multileaf collimator in the treatment of brain and prostate cancer patients. *Journal of applied clinical medical physics*, 16(5), 284–295.

Medeiros, H., Goldbarg, E., & Goldbarg, M. C. (2020). On the three-objective static unconstrained leaf sequencing in IMRT. *Medical & biological engineering & computing*, 58(9), 2025–2037.

Mohan, R., & Bortfeld, T. (2006). The potential and limitations of IMRT: a physicist's point of view. In *Image-Guided IMRT* (pp. 11-18). Springer, Berlin, Heidelberg.

Mutic S., Dempsey J.F. (2014). The ViewRay system: magnetic resonance-guided and controlled radiotherapy. *Semin Radiat Oncol,* 24: 196–199.

Nutting, C. (2003). Intensity-modulated radiotherapy (IMRT): the most important advance in radiotherapy since the linear accelerator? *Br J Radiol* 76, 673.

Otto, K. (2008). Volumetric modulated arc therapy: IMRT in a single gantry arc. *Medical physics*, *35*(1), 310-317.

Opp, D., Forster, K., & Feygelman, V. (2011). Commissioning compensator-based IMRT on the Pinnacle treatment planning system. *Journal of Applied Clinical Medical Physics*, *12*(2), 310-325.

Palma, D. A., Verbakel, W. F., Otto, K., & Senan, S. (2010). New developments in arc radiation therapy: a review. *Cancer treatment reviews*, *36*(5), 393-399.

Papp, D., & Unkelbach, J. (2014). Direct leaf trajectory optimization for volumetric modulated arc therapy planning with sliding window delivery. *Medical physics*, *41*(1), 011701.

Popple, R., & Rosen, I. (2000). Delivery of multiple IMRT fields using a single physical attenuator. In *The Use of Computers in Radiation Therapy* (pp. 191-193). Springer, Berlin, Heidelberg.

Rangaraj, D., Oddiraju, S., Sun, B., Santanam, L., Yang, D., Goddu, S., & Papiez, L. (2010). Fundamental properties of the delivery of volumetric modulated arc therapy (VMAT) to static patient anatomy. *Medical physics*, *37*(8), 4056-4067.

Raaymakers, B. W., Jürgenliemk-Schulz, I. M., Bol, G. H., Glitzner, M., Kotte, A. N. T. J., Van Asselen, B., ... & Lagendijk, J. J. W. (2017). First patients treated with a 1.5 T MRI-Linac: clinical proof of concept of a high-precision, high-field MRI guided radiotherapy treatment. *Physics in Medicine & Biology*, *62*(23), L41.

Rocha, H., Dias, J. M., Ferreira, B. C., & Lopes, M. C. (2012). Combinatorial optimization for an improved transition from fluence optimization to fluence delivery in IMRT treatment planning. *Optimization*, *61*(8), 969-987.

Saw, C. B., Ayyangar, K. M., Thompson, R. B., Zhen, W., & Enke, C. A. (2001). Commissioning of peacock system for intensity-modulated radiation therapy. *Medical Dosimetry*, *26*(1), 55-64.

Saw, C. B., Siochi, R. A. C., Ayyangar, K. M., Zhen, W., & Enke, C. A. (2001). Leaf sequencing techniques for MLC-based IMRT. *Medical Dosimetry*, *26*(2), 199-204.

Sharpe, M. B., Miller, B. M., Yan, D., & Wong, J. W. (2000). Monitor unit settings for intensity modulated beams delivered using a step-and-shoot approach. *Medical physics*, *27*(12), 2719–2725.

Shepard, D. M., Earl, M. A., Li, X. A., Naqvi, S., & Yu, C. (2002). Direct aperture optimization: a turnkey solution for step-and-shoot IMRT. *Medical physics*, 29(6), 1007–1018.

Spirou, S. V., & Chui, C. S. (1994). Generation of arbitrary intensity profiles by dynamic jaws or multileaf collimators. *Medical Physics*, *21*(7), 1031-1041.

Sun, Y., Liu, G., Chen, W., Chen, T., Liu, P., Zeng, Q., Hong, J., & Wei, R. (2019). Dosimetric comparisons of craniospinal axis irradiation using helical tomotherapy, volume-modulated arc therapy and intensity-modulated radiotherapy for medulloblastoma. *Translational cancer research*, 8(1), 191–202.

Sun, X., Xia, P., & Yu, N. (2004). Effects of the intensity levels and beam map resolutions on static IMRT plans. *Medical physics*, *31*(9), 2402-2411.

Unkelbach, J., Bortfeld, T., Craft, D., Alber, M., Bangert, M., Bokrantz, R., Chen, D., Li, R., Xing, L., Men, C., Nill, S., Papp, D., Romeijn, E., & Salari, E. (2015). Optimization approaches to volumetric modulated arc therapy planning. *Medical physics*, 42(3), 1367–1377.

Webb, S. (1989). Optimisation of conformal radiotherapy dose distribution by simulated annealing. *Physics in Medicine & Biology*, *34*(10), 1349.

Webb, S. (1994). Optimizing the planning of intensity-modulated radiotherapy. *Physics in Medicine & Biology*, *39*(12), 2229.

Webb, S. (1998). Configuration options for intensity-modulated radiation therapy using multiple static fields shaped by a multileaf collimator. *Physics in Medicine & Biology*, *43*(2), 241.

Webb, S. (2000). Advances in three-dimensional conformal radiation therapy physics with intensity modulation. *The Lancet Oncology*, *1*(1), 30-36.

Webb S. (2003a). Historical perspective on IMRT. In: Palta J. R., Mackie T. R., Chen Z. *Intensity-modulated radiation therapy: the state of the art.* Madison, WI: Medical Physics Publishing; 1-23.

Webb, S. (2003b). The physical basis of IMRT and inverse planning. *The British journal of radiology*, *76*(910), 678-689.

Webb, S. (2005). Intensity-modulated radiation therapy (IMRT): a clinical reality for cancer treatment, 'any fool can understand this: The 2004 Silvanus Thompson Memorial Lecture *Br. J. Radiol.* (spec no 2), 78: S64–72.

Welsh, J. S., Patel, R. R., Ritter, M. A., Harari, P. M., Mackie, T. R., & Mehta, M. P. (2002). Helical tomotherapy: an innovative technology and approach to radiation therapy. *Technology in cancer research & treatment*, 1(4), 311–316.

Wu, V. W. (2007). Effects of multileaf collimator parameters on treatment planning of intensity-modulated radiotherapy. *Medical Dosimetry*, *32*(1), 38-43.

Xia, P., & Verhey, L. J. (1998). Multileaf collimator leaf sequencing algorithm for intensity modulated beams with multiple static segments. *Medical Physics*, *25*(8), 1424-1434.

Xia, P., Xing, L., Amols, H. I., and Ling, C. C. (2010). Three-dimensional conformal radiotherapy and intensity modulated radiotherapy. In Hoppe, R. T., Phillips, T. L., Roach, M. (ed). *Leibel And Phillips Textbook of Radiation Oncology* 3th Edition, (pp 170-192), Elsevier Health Sciences.

van Santvoort J. P. C. and Heijmen B. J. M. (1996). Dynamic multileaf collimation without 'tongue-and-groove' underdosage effects. *Phys Med Biol,* 41 2091–105.

van Asselen, B., Schwarz, M., van Vliet-Vroegindeweij, C., Lebesque, J. V., Mijnheer, B. J., & Damen, E. M. (2006). Intensity-modulated radiotherapy of breast cancer using direct aperture optimization. *Radiotherapy and oncology, 79*(2), 162-169.

Yin, L., Wu, H., Gong, J., Geng, J. H., Jiang, F., Shi, A. H., Yu, R., Li, Y. H., Han, S. K., Xu, B., & Zhu, G. Y. (2012). Volumetric-modulated arc therapy vs. c-IMRT in esophageal cancer: a treatment planning comparison. *World journal of gastroenterology*, 18(37), 5266–5275.

Yu, C. X. (1995). Intensity-modulated arc therapy with dynamic multileaf collimation: an alternative to tomotherapy. *Phys. Med. Biol*, 40 1435–49.

Yu, C. X., Li, X. A., Ma, L., Chen, D., Naqvi, S., Shepard, D., Sarfaraz, M., Holmes, T. W., Suntharalingam, M., & Mansfield, C. M. (2002). Clinical implementation of intensity-modulated arc therapy. *International journal of radiation oncology, biology, physics*, 53(2), 453–463.

Yu, C., Shepard, D., Earl, M., Cao, D., Luan, S., Wang, C., & Chen, D. Z. (2006). New developments in intensity modulated radiation therapy. *Technology in cancer research & treatment*, 5(5), 451–464.

Yu, C. X., Tang G. (2011). Intensity-modulated arc therapy: principles, technologies and clinical implementation. *Physics in Medicine & Biology*, 56(5), R31.

Chapter 8

Verification and Geometric Uncertainties in Intensity Modulated Radiotherapy

Nural Ozturk*
Department of Radiation Oncology, Aydın Adnan Menderes University, Faculty of Medicine Aytepe Campus, Aydın, Türkiye

Abstract

In intensity-modulated radiotherapy (IMRT) non-standard field shapes and sizes are intertwined and use contiguous fields with critical organs and planning target volume (PTV) The aim of IMRT is to increase the probability of tumour control by providing the least irradiation of the normal tissues around the PTV while the dose distribution fully covers the PTV volume. Although extremely suitable dose distributions can be obtained with IMRT, the determination of the parameters of the linear accelerator device, beam modeling, treatment planning system software together with the data and information flow of the software algorithms must be correct. It also requires that the calibration of the therapy device be correct and its operation reliable during patient treatment. Error anywhere in the process can lead to serious, irreversible errors in dose distribution and patient treatments. In order to make an accurate IMRT plan, it is necessary to very well determine the error rates that may occur from both the device, the planning and the geometric uncertainties. About 30% of these errors occur during the measurement. Causes of errors in the measurement period; non-optimal measurement techniques in the system, deficiencies or errors in measuring devices, and human errors during application. Errors at the rate of about 50% include erroneous data loading, incorrect and insufficient modeling, and software errors during

---

*Corresponding Author's Email: nural.ozturk@adu.edu.tr.

In: Frontiers in Intensity-Modulated Radiotherapy Research
Editor: Sibel Karaca
ISBN: 979-8-88697-252-8

the beam modeling phase in treatment planning. The complexity of the IMRT plan during implementation is also included in this rate. The remaining about 20% of errors include patient positioning, errors from the multi-leaf collimator (MLC), and geometric error sources, which are defined as the deviation between the intended geometry of the radiotherapy plan and treatment. Total geometric uncertainty consists of small errors that are possible to classify as errors related to setup, organ movement, organ contouring, and technical condition. In this chapter, the points to be considered to plan an accurate IMRT in general and the sources of error will be discussed.

Keywords: errors from MLC, geometric uncertainties, IMRT, out-put errors

1. Introduction

An advanced special form of three-dimensional conformal radiotherapy (3D-CRT) is intensity modulated radiotherapy (IMRT). While 3D-CRT multi-leaf collimators (MLC) are shaped according to the planned target volume (PTV), photon beams with non-uniform photon fluxes, optimised according to PTV, are used throughout the beam fields in IMRT. In the IMRT treatment technique, a large number of small complex and asymmetrical fields with varying densities of radiation, varying along the beam, are used to adapt the dose to the target. Thus, it is possible to give a high and homogeneous dose to the target volume. This ensures that local control is increased and critical organs within the treatment field or near the target receive a minimum dose, thus reducing possible side effects. However, IMRT is a complex process that includes treatment delivery, patient choice, immobilisation, simulation, goal and identification of tissue and dose, planning of treatment and evaluation in addition to patient quality control (Neeley, 2009).

2. Beam Modeling Errors

While wedge filters and compensators are used to create homogeneous dose distribution in 3D therapy (Khan et al., 2014; Menzel, 2010; Palma et al., 2010), MLC is used to generate homogeneous dose distribution in IMRT (Brahme, 1988). They are systems that can move independently and automatically. MLCs are special collimators that are used in 3D-CRT, IMRT, and volumetric-modulated arc therapy (VMAT) in addition to primary and/or secondary collimators, unlike standard radiotherapy (RT). MLC leaves are produced from tungsten alloy, and the physical thickness corresponds to leaf thickness. On the other hand, the leaf width is measured at the centre concentric. The maximum possible field size for a single IMRT treatment field is a function of the number of leaves, the predicted leaf width, and the distance a leaf can pass through the centre of the field (Mukherji, 2018). These collimators:

1. The regular and/or irregular PTV field and target volume of the beam can be shaped according to the beam eye view.
2. MLCs can move fully or partially across the field according to a computer-optimised model. It can also modulate the flux along the beam.
3. Especially, instead of standard wedges, it can act as a beam modifier as a dynamic wedge with planned movements.

The MLC can be mounted on the accelerator head as a tertiary collimator either above the upper secondary collimator jaws assembly or below the lower secondary collimator jaws assembly (Figure 1).

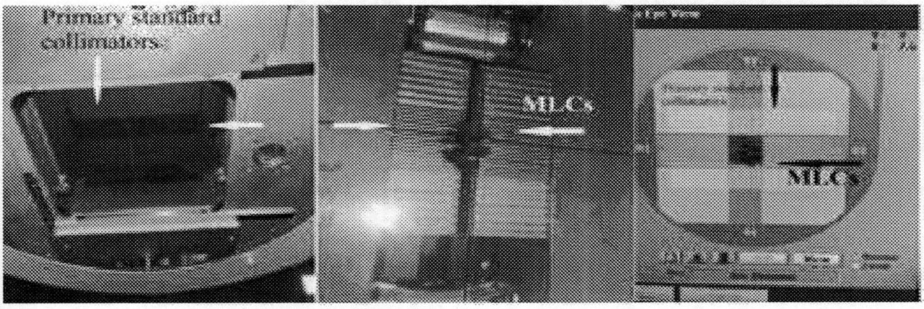

Figure 1. A linear accelerator head with MLC and beams eye view A) Primary standard collimators, B) MLCs, C) Beam Eye View of collimators (Vital BEAM: Varian Medical Systems Palo Alto, CA).

In designs from the three major manufacturing companies, MLCs substitute the upper (Y) jaws additionally with 3 cm thick Y jaws to decrease radiation leakage from the MLC (Elekta) even the lower (Y) jaw replacement. (X) jaws (Siemens) help act as a tertiary collimator and furthermore to conventional X and Y secondary collimators (Varian). Provided that MLCs are below sets of secondary collimators, they are near the patient and geometric penumbra improves, but the result is in a larger device head with a smaller space between the MLC and the patient. On the secondary collimator MLC case, there is no strong geometric penumbra. The MLC design is smaller and lighter with a physical space increment between the accelerator head and the patient (Mukherji, 2018). These structural differences can be sources of error in IMRT.

2.1. The Importance of MLC at IMRT

The basis of IMRT planning is based on the MLC. Computer software provides leaf sequencing, which converts the intensity pattern of the beam generated by inverse planning (IP) into a set that describes the movement of the MLC leaves during the transmission of the beam. There are numerous sequence alternatives for leaf motion-producing density pattern requirements by taking into account the distribution method. Software is useful in minimisation of segment number, monitor units (MUs) total number, motion distance of leaf, and the total delivery time (Bortfeld et al., 1994; Galvin, et al., 1993; Spirou and Chui, 1994; Xia and Verhey, 1998).

During irradiation, these MLCs can be either fixed or dynamic. In the step and shoot technique (Figure 2), where fixed MLCs are used, MLCs cover the organs around the PTV volume and irradiate at determined angles.

In the dynamic IMRT technique, in a fixed isocentre within the scope of PTV, the MLC shapes and dose rate change according to the target volume, while continuously rotating around the field to be treated. Head structures and MLCs of the devices used in IMRT differ according to the device model.

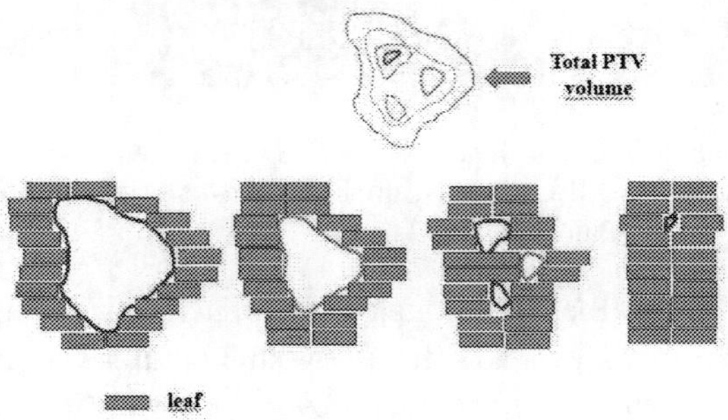

Figure 2. Step and Shoot technique: Irregular-shaped treatment areas, called segments, are irradiated with a specific Monitor Unit (MU) defined for each segment. The beam is switched off until the next segment is turned on. This process is repeated for the calculated angles and segments.

Although it is possible to obtain the desired dose in PTV and to preserve normal tissues with the use of MLCs, isodose distributions at the margins of the field are not certain due to the limited widths of the MLCs. This poses a risk to critical organs located at field edges. The fact that the MLC ends are not fully focused causes a gap between the leaves.

Since dose distribution and critical organ protection are provided by MLC leaf movement in IMRT planning, the slightest error arising from the MLC position will affect many points within the tumour, causing significant hot or cold dose zones to occur, since it is not only at the edge of the field, but also within the treatment field during irradiation. Regarding this, LoSasso et al. (1998) showed in their study that a ±1 mm MLC position error in the sliding window technique could cause a 10% dose error in the 1 cm irradiation zone (LoSasso et al., 1998).

In the sliding window technique (Figure 3), depending on the errors in the leaf positioning, cold and hot dose points may occur in small fields, especially in the regions where the rays are adjacent, as well as cause output changes and profile irregularities.

Since MLC leaves move according to the field size during irradiation in dynamic IMRT, leaf speed, leaf positions and dose rate must be simultaneously controlled very precisely. These hot and cold dosing points may cause undesirable low dose and organ at risk (OAR) overdose in PTV.

Regarding treatments using static MLCs, another study of IMRT stated that spots for static MLC, 13% where adjacent field segments overlap, and 18% MV (Million Volts = MV) photon beams at 6 MV 17%, hot and it is stated that the cold dose is 13% and the average dose in the overlapping regions (approximately per millimeter) is formed (Low et al., 2001).

MLCs focusing only on the Y direction are single MLCs, and focusing on both the x and y axes are dual focus MLCs (Mukherji, 2018). IMRT has significance such that field edge of radiation is planned in accordance with MLC leaf tip nominal position. Each MLC leaf width is slightly smaller on the side of leaf exposed to radiation source than on the side of the radiation source. When MLCs are designed with rounded tips (single focus), they create an offset (gap) between the beam edge defined by the light field and the line that reduces the radiation field by 50%. The design of this offset leaf is between 0.4 mm and 1.1 mm, depending on the beam energy and the distance from the central axis. For this reason, hot spots occur in equidistant positions due to radiation leakage (Ezzell et al., 2003).

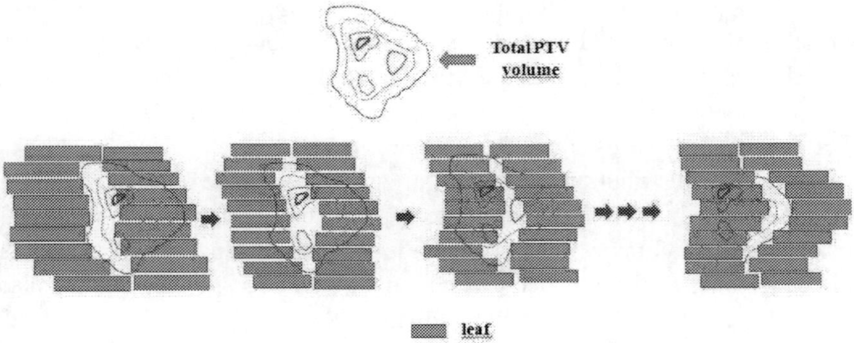

Figure 3. Sliding Window Technique: It is a technique made without interrupting the treatment beam. In this technique, while the Gantry is rotating around a fixed isocentre, the MLCs are positioned by moving them relative to the PTV and irradiated according to the planned MU value.

The effect of rounded end leaf permeability is more effective, especially in sliding window MLC treatments and causes high doses in small fields.

Studies have shown that a photon field approximately 0.5 mm larger than the light field is formed on both sides of a field. This problem can be solved in two ways:

1. Leafs can be calibrated to match the actual photon field,
2. An adjustment in treatment planning can be made to adjust for this difference.

This issue can be understood by a user who can make the necessary justification to correct dose delivery. The penumbra of the device must be defined very well in the planning system. Hardcastle et al., (2007) in their study of Varian Millennium MLC, they found that in cases where the modelling of penumbra was inadequate, leaf leaching could result in an additional absorption dose of 2 Gy to 3 Gy during each treatment period (Hardcastle et al., 2007).

The penumbra part of the leaf tips in the direction of leaf movement should be detected with a suitable high-resolution measurement system such as a film, diode, or small volume ion chamber and modelled accurately in the planning system (Ezzell et al., 2003; Low et al., 2011). In addition to other protectors in the accelerator head, due to radiation leakage through and between the MLC leaves, the targeted dose in PTV can only be achieved, but in the form of a MU higher than desired. This increases the whole-body dose in IMRT applications (Galvin et al., 2004). For this, it is necessary to determine the leaf leakage and permeability of MLC, which is the most important factor affecting IMRT treatment planning. In order to minimise the leakage between two adjacent MLCs, one of the solutions offered by the manufacturers according to each device brand is different tongue and groove designs (Figure 4).

In these designs, the transmissions of the left and right corners of the MLCs are different from each other. In addition, the velocities of two adjacent MLCs are also different from each other (Bayouth et al., 2003; Ezzell et al., 2003; Kung and Chen, 2000; Ling et al., 2008). Due to the tongue and groove effect, dose changes are mentioned in the literature up to 15% in a single field and up to 1.6% in a multi-field treatment (Huq et al., 2002)

In tongue and groove design, if leaves are not properly synchronised with the leaf sorting algorithm, IMRT can cause undesirable blocking and dose reduction in small fields of the treatment field (Que et al., 2004; Nill et al., 2006; Yu, 1998). In their study, Kamath et al. (2004) showed that the tongue and groove effect can cause doses as low as 10-25% in static and dynamic MLC treatment techniques (Kamath et al., 2004). Deng et al. (2001) showed that these dose reductions are significant when the number of beams in the treatment plan is low (<5) (Deng et al., 2001).

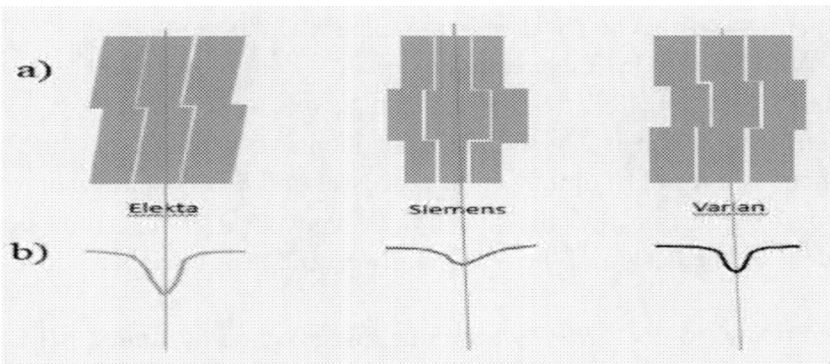

Figure 4. a) Tongue & groove designs in Multi Lief Collimators from different companies b) Dosimetric implications of three different collimator designs.

Yu (1998) study, on the other hand, shows that the tongue and groove effect is significantly reduced with Monte Carlo simulation and the use of an accurate leaf sorting algorithm (Yu, 1998).

IMRT fields consist of many beamlets with dimensions of 0.5 x 0.5 cm^2. The rays have a wide intensity range of values (0-100%), which is the output of complex software steps calculating the ideal radiation intensity for the appropriate dose distribution optimisation achievement for a given target. Another programme transforming the ideal density map is suitable for PTV as the appropriate density map, taking into account the characteristics of the linear accelerator and the MLC. Two methods are commonly used for this type of conversion (Burman et al., 1997; Deng et al., 2001; Kamath et al., 2004; Mott et al., 1999).

In segmental IMRT (also known as step and shut), the MLC shape is fixed during irradiation and only changes when the beam is "off." For dynamic IMRT, leaf positions change while the beam is "on." In both cases, the position of each leaf is continuously monitored. As a function of tracking units, a feedback mechanism is used to ensure that the leaves are in their determined positions (Convery and Webb, 1998; Ezzell et al., 2003; Purdy, 2001; Spirou, 1994).

In static MLC-based IMRT, the targeted intensity model is obtained by manually dividing the beam modulation array into multiple segments or software based on the system used whether forwarding or backward planning.

The total segment number is proportionally related with the field shape, size and treatment complexity. Most of these segments can provide < 5 MU and a significant number < 1 MU. Therefore, the dose/MU should be validated within the range of clinically given values. In addition, field flatness and symmetry should also be checked in the same MU range.

In MLC-based IMRT technique, quality control for MLC plays an important role in IMRT treatment planning and dose delivery, since the treatment fields consist of multiple segments depending on the MLC movement as a result of optimisation processes and leaf positions control the steep dose gradient. Specific quality assurance (QA) tests are heavily dependent on the design of the MLC, and specific tests have been developed for MLC.

According to the IMRT technique used (static-dynamic) MLC leaf velocity (dynamic), leaf position accuracy and repeatability, leaf permeability, round tip leaf permeability, gap, beam stability at low MUs, effects of stopping treatment, etc., specific tests should be carried out (Hansen et al., 1998; LoSasso et al., 1998). Leaf permeability (intra-leaf) is the amount of radiation that passes through the leaf thickness. Leaf permeability can be determined in a given field size by closing the MLCs with the jaws fully open and measuring with a film, water phantom, or small volume ion chamber. Leaf permeability varies according to leaf design and energy but is usually <3%. The average permeability value for treatment planning is accepted as 2%. The factor affecting planning is not only MLC leakage, but device head scattering, leaf travel length, penumbra modelling of MLC and main jaws. In addition, the correct determination of the output factor in small fields, which are frequently used in IMRT, the deep dose values of the off-axis points, the dose profiles and the grid size used in dose calculation (which is the smallest value such as 0.2 mm is recommended). The parameters needed for the planning should be determined with detailed measurements under appropriate conditions and modelled in the existing treatment planning system (Menzel, 2010; Ting et al., 2005).

In order to make an accurate IMRT plan, it is necessary to very well determine the error rates that may occur from both the device, the planning and the geometric uncertainties.

3. Installation Tests at IMRT

Task Group (TG) 53 divides installation tests into three main categories: These are benchmark tests with computer hardware, software functionality and features of the treatment planning system (Fraass et al., 1998). In most cases, these tests will be functional (yes or no), while some tests may be quantitative and based on the manufacturer's tolerances (Low et al., 2005).

Collecting, entering and verifying the data of the linear accelerator required by the planning system for modelling in the treatment planning system (TPS) forms the basis of these tests. In addition, the tests should be performed and documented both at device setup and when software is changed for any reason. The tests required for the IMRT treatment planning system have been reported in detail in the American Association of Physicists in Medicine (AAPM) TG 40, 53, 142, and 430 reports (Fraass et al., 1998; Johnson, 2004; Klein et al., 2009, Kutcher et al., 1994).

3.1. Out-Put Effect in IMRT

Commissioning processes usually start with the collection of basic beam data such as out-put factors, percent deep dose and dose profiles suitable for the treatment fields required by the planning system for beam modelling of each linear accelerator. The beam data should be carefully measured with detectors suitable for different field sizes and measurement techniques (ion chambers, diode, diamond, etc.) in all energies from the smallest field used to the largest field, taking into account the recommendations of the device company. The selection of ion chambers is very important during these measurements (Lee et al., 2002; Martens et al., 2000).

The detector volume effect is the most important parameter invalidating the IMRT plan. If the ion chamber will be used; In 4 x 4 cm^2 and smaller field measurements, small-volume ion chambers should be preferred instead of large-volume ion chambers, because they cause lateral electron balance deficiencies (Hansen et al., 1998; Low et al., 2011). In the studies of Laub et al., (2003), it was reported that the volume effects of ion chambers increase as the treatment field gets larger 0.6 cc farmer type (Lauba and Wong, 2003). Its reading represents an average value, as ion chambers with a large volume, such as ion chambers, will measure a large field during measurement. Small-volume ion chambers with a volume of 0.01 cm^3 have a weak signal-to-noise ratio. This can cause erroneous measurements in IMRT. The recommended ion chamber volume in IMRT modelling measurements is ion chambers with an active volume of ~ 0.1 cm^3. If micro-MLC capable of providing a field size < 5 mm is used then smaller volume micro ion chambers (< 0.01 cm^3) can be used. In addition, it is recommended to use tissue-equivalent detectors in very small fields (Figure 5).

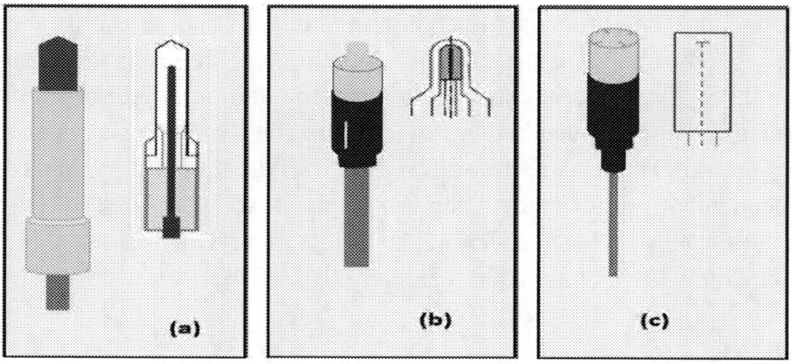

Figure 5. Different types of ion chambers used in commissioning and control of IMRT patient plans. e.g., a) 0,6 cc Farmer type ion chamber b) pinpoint ion chamber c) microdiamond ion chamber.

To obtain reproducible reliable results with an ion chamber, measurements should be made in the dose region with a low dose gradient. This is because small differences in the relative position of the measuring point within the IMRT field cause significant errors in the measured values, no matter how small the measuring volume of the detector. The mean dose and standard deviation can be obtained and compared with the measured values. By detecting the relative deviation (standard deviation divided by the mean value), it can be quantitatively determined whether the measurement point is on the high dose gradient. If the relative deviation exceeds 5%, it may be useful to choose a different measuring point, as small uncertainties in the setup can lead to difficult-to-interpret measurements. It is also important to keep a record of the measurements obtained during commissioning. These records will serve as a basis for patient-specific measurements during treatment. Small variable gaps between leaves create local output variations. A variation of 0.2 mm in the gap width can cause a dose change of ±3% for each dynamic MLC field (tolerance ≤ 0.2 mm). Also, the error in the ion chamber measurements should be within the limits of ±2% at most. Output factors that change rapidly depending on the field size should be modelled within 0.5% uncertainty (Dieterich et al., 2011).

Sharpe et al. (2000) reported that a 2 mm deviation in field size for 6MV photon beams changes the output factor by 2% for a 2 x 2 cm^2 field and 15% for a 1 x 1 cm^2 field (Sharpe et al., 2000). Most of the time, an irradiation consists of many small fields. In order to add them correctly, the penumbra of the fields must be determined very precisely and measured with special care. In order to control the off-axis ratios, the profiles of both symmetrical and asymmetrical fields needed for planning should be measured (Boyer et al., 2001). A detailed and careful commissioning is required. Also, for small MU (<2 MU) output, flatness and symmetry stability should be tested with suitable detectors (diode, diamond, film) and appropriate phantoms. It has been noted that some therapy systems have dosimetric differences within the nominal range of use for clinical treatments in small MU due to the communication delay between the MLC control system and the linear accelerator console. Simple beams modulated with MLC should be created and absolute dose verification should be done with appropriate phantom and dosimetry (Dieterich et al., 2011; Ezzell et al., 2003).

3.2. Treatment Planning System Effect on IMRT

While IMRT can deliver highly matched dose distributions, it requires reliance on treatment planning system software, data and algorithms, information transfer process, and linear accelerator calibration and operation unprecedented in radiation therapy. Errors anywhere in the process can lead to serious errors in dose distribution that can first be detected by clinical consequences. Before continuing, it is important to distinguish commission-level QA from patient-specific QA. In unheterogeneity-corrected TPS, heterogeneity in IMRT affecting some beamlets more than others may result in different localised dose differences (Ezzell et al., 2003).

In lung or head and neck cancers whose tumours are usually located at the air-tissue interfaces, tissue inhomogeneity should be corrected without error, especially when stereotactic radiosurgery treatment using very small and multiple fields is planned. The effects of transient electronic instability in air and increased lateral electron spacing may result in a significant reduction in central axis dose beyond the gap, resulting in a low dose of the tumour. It is especially important when the target is surrounded by low-density tissues such as the lungs. Therefore, dose calculation algorithms that take into account loss of electronic balance and lateral electron scatterings, such as lung tissue interface or tumour margin in a low-density environment, need to be used. It is recommended to use Monte Carlo dose calculation for accurate tissue inhomogeneity corrections (Benedict et al., 2010; Dieterich et al., 2011).

Parameters to consider when calculating the dose for an IMRT plan are as follows.

1. The more complex the density modulation, the more MUs increase,
2. Device suitable MLC structures (factors such as the structure of the tips of the leaves, leaf permeability and leakage rates in the grooves of the MLCs) should be considered correctly in IMRT planning,
3. The overall leaching from MLC leaves may be up to several percent of the total IMRT dose,
4. Calculation of the output factor can be complicated due to the variable field sizes and the effect of collimator scattering during irradiation in IMRT.

Studies have shown that the Monte Carlo (MC) calculations are valid for dose calculation accurately concerning tissue corrections in addition to collimator and leaf scattering effects. It should be known that in the MC calculation method, the computation time is longer than in other algorithms and requires high-speed computers (Wang et al., 1996). In order to calculate heterogeneity corrections in planning systems, an electron-based and/or mass density-based Computed Tomography (CT) density model should be introduced to the system. The user should know which density type the system uses for each dose calculation algorithm and should follow the recommendations set forth in AAPM TG66 and National Council on Radiation Protection and Measurements (NCRP) Report No: 99 for CT quality control (Mutic et al., 2003; Poznanski et al., 1988).

3.3. Data Transfer Issues on IMRT

The compatibility of the treatment planning system and data transfer tests should be tested. After generating an acceptable IMRT plan, intensity profiles for each beam are sent via Digital Imaging and Communications in Medicine (DICOM) to the accelerator, which is electronically equipped with the appropriate hardware and software to provide the planned intensity-modulated beams. The accuracy of the patient's data must be checked. As a result, data transfer compactness over the system (CT simulator, treatment planning, registration and verification, and control of IMRT accelerator) needs to be verified, as in conventional 3DCRT (Kutcher et al., 1994).

4. Sources of Geometric Uncertainty

Geometric errors in IMRT are defined as the difference between the IMRT plan geometry and the actual RT treatment geometry. In IMRT, if technical conditions are adjusted by quality assurance systems, geometric errors include patient fixation and movement deviations of organs around the tumour. Both deviations consist of systematic and random components. In fractional IMRT applications, systematic errors occur if the mean irradiation geometry in the treatment differs from the geometry in the treatment plan. Systematic errors are position errors that are likely to recur throughout the treatment period, most of which occur during the determination of target volumes, and whose magnitude generally does not change much during the entire treatment period. Some causes of systematic errors are summarised in Table 1.

Systematic errors; laser mismatch in CT-Simulator (CT-Sim) and treatment unit, sagging or collapse of table or gantry in CT-Sim and treatment unit, bending of collimator wires determining the centre of the field, errors in Digitally Reconstructed Radiographs (DRR) formation, radiation and light field, the inconsistency between marker movement used for the treatment position can be given as an example. Systematic errors cause a change in dose distribution by acting in the same direction across all fractions of the patient (Mileusnić, 2005; Thomas et al., 2005). Systematic mean errors are denoted by "S." representing the duplicate difference between intended and actual geometry. Considering the geometric uncertainties in radiotherapy, systematic error is examined in two different ways as individual and population.

From the reference, geometry deviation is more or less different during each fraction with total deviation being expressible as systematic fraction-specific error summation. In this case, random errors are fraction-to-fraction variations representing the total error floating component. In general, standard deviations (SDs) is a measure of random errors corresponding to frequency distributions, which are usually denoted by "s" (Mileusnić, 2005). Random errors are errors that result from daily set-up differences that change in magnitude and direction during treatment (Manning et al., 2001). The magnitude and effects of these errors depend on the treatment field depends on the quality of the immobilisation materials used in patient positioning and their correct use (Astreinidou et al., 2005).

The patient's treatment may have a systematic error during the period from the initial positioning of the patient with immobilisation to the application of definitive therapy. Once this error is detected, this error can be fixed. If not corrected, a known discrepancy will occur between intended and actual target coverages. Random errors occur frequently during treatment execution differing between fractions. The total geometric error (external - setup deviations and internal - organ movement) is considerable in treatment planning even though they are not estmatable for each patient (Burnet et al., 2004).

Table 1. Possible sources of systematic error in IMRT

Coordinate errors
Laser calibration errors
Errors in treatment and/or CT table movements
Mechanical calibration errors
Dose measurement parameters from the treatment unit to TPS (Profile, output, collimator scattering factors, MLC modelling etc.) wrong entry
Incorrect drawing of treatment volumes (PTV, CTV, OAR)

4.1. Electronic Portal Imaging Device (EPID)

Both systematic and random errors measured for an individual patient can be evaluated exactly after completion of all treatment fractions. Systematic error can be corrected partially with an on-line and off-line correction procedure measuring before treatment start with the Electronic Portal Imaging Device (EPID). Also, random error can be fixed just by using on-line. On the other hand, geometrical error components are measurable patient treatment group of similar previous treatments using standard deviations. After knowing specific patient group typical values, they can be employed for institutional correction protocols generation and the patient becomes important when defining the PTV (Stroom and Heijmen, 2002).

EPIDs clinical uses are necessary for geometric errors detection and correction during radiotherapy treatment. It is also one of the most practical systems for quality assurance of dose accuracy of IMRT plans as they depend on the therapy device.

In the work of Fielding et al., (2004) 15-segment step and shoot IMRT plans, 1 mm phantom position shifts in a single segment, 2 mm leaf position errors, and 10% dosimetry errors of less than 1% of the total dose were detected. They reported that they could detect it with EPID (Fielding et al., 2004).

QA programme based on portal images reflects overall treatment compliance verification. With Portal View, and it is not possible to reveal errors in patient set-up, field size, positioning and shaping of the MLC. Inconsistencies in the resulting portal images are investigable and correctable under the light of clinical criteria and protocols. Then, when its accuracy is finalised, it must be confirmed electronically by the responsible persons. By using Portal Dose Images (EPI), it is possible to take portal dose images of the patient and confirm the dose to be given to the patient. Chang et al. (2000) reported in their study that an EPID can be used for profile verification and absolute isocentric dose measurement for Internal Mammaria (IM) fields (Chang et al., 2000).

4.2. Reducing Treatment Volume and Organ Identification Errors

The two sources of uncertainty in treatment duration, irradiation and positioning, can be considered separately, but they combine to reduce the overall effectiveness of treatment. Target location ambiguities arise in two ways, but the distinction between the two is often not made. First, there are differences in the position of the patient's bony anatomy with respect to the beam (so-called setup errors), and second, there are differences in the target organ movement within the patient, usually relative to the bony structures (Jaffray et al., 1999; Van Herk et al., 1995).

In order to determine and record the dose and dose levels to be administered, and to express the target volume and the level of dose critical organs receive, it is necessary to define the target and/or critical organs first. Accurate definition of all these volumes is necessary for the treatment planning process in radiotherapy application. Detailed target definitions are available in the International Commission on Radiation Units and Measurements (ICRU) protocols 50 and 62 (Allisye et al., 1999; Lanberg et al., 2016).

According to reports, a margin is added to the Gross Tumour Volume (GTV) to account for subclinical disease and invisible cells, thereby creating a Clinical Target Volume (CTV). An additional margin is then added to account for geometric uncertainties, including patient set-up errors, to create the Planning Target Volume (PTV). Then, by adding the necessary margins as detailed in the protocols, Treated Volume (TV), Irradiated Volume (IV), Organ at Risk (OAR) and Planning Organ at Risk Volume (PRV) should be defined correctly using appropriate anatomy atlases within the framework of the clinical protocol.

OAR is normal tissues such as medulla spinals, lung, heart, kidney, eye, which affect the treatment planning or defined dose by staying within the treatment field and have significant radiation sensitivity.

It should be known that the systematic and random uncertainties of the equipment used in patient positioning during treatment planning and implementation lead to changes in the target volume. Therefore, when determining the planned target volume, the Set-up Margin (SM) should be determined by considering the uncertainties in Table 2.

Table 2. Uncertainties to consider when determining PTV limits

Errors in patient positioning between fractions
Tumour movements varying between fractions
Mechanical uncertainty of equipment, patient immobilisation
Dosimetric uncertainties
Setup errors
Human factor (Uncertainties in tumour volume and OAR shaping)

The actual PTV margin, expressed as a geometric parameter, is determined by taking into account the uncertainties that may arise in the IM and SM. Van Herk et al., (2004) in their study, in which different techniques are examined to determine the necessary margins to reduce geometric uncertainties, he mentions that it is possible to reduce the margin between 2-3.5 mm by using patient-specific immobilisation (Van Herk et al., 2004).

Kanakavelu and Samuel's (2016) study results show that the causes of patient set-up errors in different anatomical reasons are the immobilisation equipment used, the clinical patient set-up protocol, the geometric accuracy of the IMRT treatment device, and the room lasers, CT sim and image guide are related (Kanakavelu and Samuel, 2016).

Furthermore, unavoidable geometric uncertainties from visceral movement may result in a lower Conformity Index (CI), a decrease in the Probability of Tumour Control (TCP), and an increase in the Probability of Normal Tissue Complications (NTCP) during treatment. The CI of the IMRT plan is largely dependent on the steep dose gradients between the PTV and the organ at risk. Geometric uncertainties reduce planned dose gradients and result in a less steep or "fuzzy" dose gradient. With a good CT imaging protocol, it is possible to reduce the effect of organ movement to some extent. A relatively simple way of influencing the movement of certain organs is to control physiology habits (urine and stool passage) and adjust to treatment timing (Mileusnić, 2005).

For treatment validation, CT scan imaging provides accurate detection of geometric variations such as uncertainties in patient position, concentric localisation, changes in the patient's outer contour such as organ movement, weight loss, or tumour shrinkage. It can also be used to generate three-dimensional (3D) dose distributions to more accurately estimate the dose delivered to targets and critical structures during the IMRT process using the anatomical information obtained from the CT scan. Appropriate PTV margins should not only focus on target coverage, but also consider the impact on normal tissue sparing (Ballivy et al., 2006).

Barker et al., (2004) showed that the size of GTVs decreased at a median rate of approximately 2% per treatment day during treatment. In addition, they said that weight loss during the treatment also caused the displacement of the defined organs, and adding an extra margin to the PTV in order to completely eliminate the geometric uncertainty was not fully effective in the mean dose (Dmean) of the OAR tissues (Barker et al., 2004). Dose-Volume Histograms (DVHs) for all anatomical definitions may be affected, as variations in tumour shape or size may cause OARs to enter the treatment field more than desired throughout treatment.

Conclusion

IMRT was first used clinically in the mid-1990s. Since then, the QA in IMRT applications have progressed further, depending on both the development of software programmes and the developments in technology. The most time-consuming aspect of the QA process is still the patient-specific QA procedure based on individual dose measurements. The limitations of the dosimeters used in IMRT and the personnel performing the measurements and controls cause the QA measurements to be insufficient to fully define the IMRT dose distributions. Therefore, significant systematic errors may occur and may not be detected even if existing protocols are used. In order to reduce the error rates in IMRT, the first priority is beam modelling and commissioning tests, which cover the parameters that need to be determined correctly. Especially MLC accuracy, appropriate and precise measurements during modelling, output made with reference to protocols and the accuracy of the given dose have a great effect on reducing the sources of error. Since high doses and complex fields are used in IMRT, besides the correct determination of target and normal tissue contours, the treatment device and equipment, the mechanical parameters of the CTSIM used in patient simulation, the image quality and Hounsfield Unit (HU) values are correctly determined and TPS needs to be defined. In addition, the use of appropriate patient-specific immobilisation systems is also important in reducing error rates. QA of the treatment planning system, treatment plan, and patient-specific evaluation should also be performed and used routinely in clinical practice.

References

Alliasye, A., Wambersie A., Caswell R. S., Adams G.E, Doi K., Feinendegen L., Unokuti M., Isherwood I., Mallard J. R., Paretzke H., Rossi H. H., Whitmore G. F. TaylorL. S. 1999. "The International Commission on Radiation Units and Measurements Report 62 : Prescribing, recording and reporting photon beam therapy (supplement to ICRU report 50)." *ICRU report 62. ICRU Publications* Bethesda, MD, USD.

Astreinidou, E., Bel, A., Raaijmakers, C. P., Terhaard, C. H., & Lagendijk, J. J. (2005). Adequate margins for random setup uncertainties in head-and-neck IMRT. *International Journal of Radiation Oncology* Biology* Physics*, *61*(3), 938-944.

Ballivy, O., Parker, W., Vuong, T., Shenouda, G., & Patrocinio, H. (2006). Impact of geometric uncertainties on dose distribution during intensity modulated radiotherapy of head-and-neck cancer : the need for a planning target volume and a planning organ-at-risk volume. *Current Oncology*, *13*(3), 108-115.

Barker Jr, J. L., Garden, A. S., Ang, K. K., O'Daniel, J. C., Wang, H., Court, L. E., & Dong, L. (2004). Quantification of volumetric and geometric changes occurring during fractionated radiotherapy for head-and-neck cancer using an integrated CT/linear accelerator system. *International Journal of Radiation Oncology* Biology* Physics*, *59*(4), 960-970.

Bayouth, J. E., Wendt D., and Morrill S. M.. 2003. "MLC Quality Assurance Techniques for IMRT Applications." *Medical Physics* 30 (5): 743–50.

Benedict, Stanley H., Yenice Kamil M., Followill David, Galvin James M., Hinson William, Kavanagh Brian, Keall Paul, Lovelock Micheal, Meeks Sanfort, Papiez Lech, Purdie Thomas, Sadagopan Ramaswamy, Schell Michael C., Salter Bill, Schlesinge David J., Shiu Almon S., Solberg Timothy, Song Danny Y., Stieber Volker, Timmerman Robert, Tomé Wolfgang A., Verellen Dirk, Wang Lu, Yin Fang-Fang. Benedict, S. H., Yenice, K. M., Followill, D., Galvin, J. M., Hinson, W., Kavanagh, B., & Yin, F. F. (2010). Stereotactic body radiation therapy : the report of AAPM Task Group 101. *Medical physics*, *37*(8), 4078-4101.

Boyer, A., Biggs P., Galvin J., Klein E., LoSasso T., Low D., Mah K., Yu C. (2001). "Basic Applications of Multileaf Collimators : AAPM Radiation Therapy Committee Task Group No. 50 Report No. 72". *Published for the AAPM by Medical Physics Publishing.* Medison. Printed in the United States of America.

Bortfeld, T. R., Kahler, D. L., Waldron, T. J., & Boyer, A. L. (1994). X-ray field compensation with multileaf collimators. *International Journal of Radiation Oncology* Biology* Physics*, *28*(3), 723-730.

Brahme, A. (1988). Optimization of stationary and moving beam radiation therapy techniques. *Radiotherapy and Oncology*, *12*(2), 129-140.

Burnet, N. G., Thomas, S. J., Burton, K. E., & Jefferies, S. J. (2004). Defining the tumour and target volumes for radiotherapy. *Cancer Imaging*, *4*(2), 153.

Burman, C., Chui, C. S., Kutcher, G., Leibel, S., Zelefsky, M., LoSasso, T., & Ling, C. C. (1997). Planning, delivery, and quality assurance of intensity-modulated radiotherapy using dynamic multileaf collimator : a strategy for large-scale implementation for the treatment of carcinoma of the prostate. *International journal of radiation oncology, biology, physics*, *39*(4), 863-873.

Chang, J., Mageras, G. S., Chui, C. S., Ling, C. C., & Lutz, W. (2000). Relative profile and dose verification of intensity-modulated radiation therapy. *International Journal of Radiation Oncology* Biology* Physics*, *47*(1), 231-240.

Deng, J., Pawlicki, T., Chen, Y., Li, J., Jiang, S. B., & Ma, C. M. (2001). The MLC tongue-and-groove effect on IMRT dose distributions. *Physics in Medicine & Biology*, *46*(4), 1039-1060.

Dieterich, S., Cavedon, C., Chuang, C. F., Cohen, A. B., Garrett, J. A., Lee, C. L., & Yu, C. (2011). Report of AAPM TG 135 : quality assurance for robotic radiosurgery. *Medical physics*, *38*(6Part1), 2914-2936.

Ezzell, G. A., Galvin, J. M., Low, D., Palta, J. R., Rosen, I., Sharpe, M. B., & Yu, C. X. (2003). Guidance document on delivery, treatment planning, and clinical implementation of IMRT : report of the IMRT Subcommittee of the AAPM Radiation Therapy Committee. *Medical physics*, *30*(8), 2089-2115.

Fielding, A. L., Evans, P. M., & Clark, C. H. (2004). Verification of patient position and delivery of IMRT by electronic portal imaging. *Radiotherapy and oncology*, *73*(3), 339-347.

Fraass, B., Doppke, K., Hunt, M., Kutcher, G., Starkschall, G., Stern, R., & Van Dyke, J. (1998). American Association of Physicists in Medicine Radiation Therapy Committee Task Group 53 : quality assurance for clinical radiotherapy treatment planning. *Medical physics*, *25*(10), 1773-1829.

Galvin, J. M., Chen, X. G., & Smith, R. M. (1993). Combining multileaf fields to modulate fluence distributions. *International Journal of Radiation Oncology* Biology* Physics*, *27*(3), 697-705.

Galvin, J. M., Ezzell, G., Eisbrauch, A., Yu, C., Butler, B., Xiao, Y., & Palta, J. (2004). Implementing IMRT in clinical practice : a joint document of the American Society for Therapeutic Radiology and Oncology and the American Association of Physicists in Medicine. *International journal of radiation oncology, biology, physics*, *58*(5), 1616-1634.

Hansen, V. N., Evans, P. M., Budgell, G. J., Mott, J. H., Williams, P. C., Brugmans, M. J., & Brown, K. (1998). Quality assurance of the dose delivered by small radiation segments. *Physics in Medicine & Biology*, *43*(9), 2665-2675.

Hardcastle, N., Metcalfe, P., Ceylan, A., & Williams, M. J. (2007). Multileaf collimator end leaf leakage : implications for wide-field IMRT. *Physics in Medicine & Biology*, *52*(21), N493.

Huq, M. S., Das, I. J., Steinberg, T., & Galvin, J. M. (2002). A dosimetric comparison of various multileaf collimators. *Physics in Medicine & Biology*, *47*(12), N159.

Jaffray, D. A., Yah D., and Wong J. W. (1999). Managing Geometric Uncertainty in Conformal Intensity-Modulated Radiation Therapy. *Seminars in Radiation Oncology* 9 (1): 4–19.

Johnson, T. K. (2007). Commissioning and Quality Assurance of Computerized Planning Systems for Radiation Treatment of Cancer. Technical Reports Series No. 430" *Health Physics* 92 (4): 16-96.

Kamath, S., Sahni, S., Palta, J., Ranka, S., & Li, J. (2004). Optimal leaf sequencing with elimination of tongue-and-groove underdosage. *Physics in Medicine & Biology*, *49*(3), N7.

Kanakavelu, N., & Jebaseelan Samuel, J. (2016). Determination of patient set-up error and optimal treatment margin for intensity modulated radiotherapy using image guidance system. *J BUON*, *21*(2), 505-511.

Khan, F. M., Gibbons, J. P. (2014). *Intensity-Modulated Radiation Therap in The Physics of Radiation Therapy*. 5th ed. by Lippincott Williams & Wilkins, 430-53. ISBN 978-1-4511-8245-3

Klein, E. E., Hanley, J., Bayouth, J., Yin, F. F., Simon, W., Dresser, S., & Holmes, T. (2009). Task Group 142 report: Quality assurance of medical accelerators a. *Medical physics*, *36*(9Part1), 4197-4212.

Kung, J. H., & Chen, G. T. Y. (2000). Intensity modulated radiotherapy dose delivery error from radiation field offset inaccuracy. *Medical Physics*, *27*(7), 1617-1622.

Kutcher, G. J., Coia, L., Gillin, M., Hanson, W. F., Leibel, S., Morton, R. J., & Wingfield, L. (1994). Comprehensive QA for radiation oncology: report of AAPM radiation therapy committee task group 40. *Medical Physics-Lancaster PA-*, *21*, 581-581.

Lanberg, T., Chavaudra J., Dobbs J., Hanks G., Johansson K.-A, Möller T., Purdy J. (2016). The International Commission on Radiation Units and Measurements Report 62: Prescribing, recording and reporting photon beam therapy. *Icru Report 50. ICRU Publications* Bethesda, MD, USD http://jicru.oxfordjournals.org/.

Laub, W. U., & Wong, T. (2003). The volume effect of detectors in the dosimetry of small fields used in IMRT. *Medical physics*, *30*(3), 341-347.

Lee, H. R., Pankuch, M., Chu, J. C., & Spokas, J. J. (2002). Evaluation and characterization of parallel plate microchamber's functionalities in small beam dosimetry. *Medical physics*, *29*(11), 2489-2496.

Ling, C. C., Zhang, P., Archambault, Y., Bocanek, J., Tang, G., & LoSasso, T. (2008). Commissioning and quality assurance of RapidArc radiotherapy delivery system. *International Journal of Radiation Oncology* Biology* Physics*, *72*(2), 575-581.

LoSasso, T., Chui, C. S., & Ling, C. C. (1998). Physical and dosimetric aspects of a multileaf collimation system used in the dynamic mode for implementing intensity modulated radiotherapy. *Medical physics*, *25*(10), 1919-1927.

Low, D. A., Klein E. E. (2005). Technology and Implementation : Capter 14 "Quality Assurance Processes and Future Directions" *Intensity Modulated Radiation Therapy A Clinical Perspective in,* edited by Arno, J. Mundt, John C. Roeske, 198-203. Hamilton • London. ISBN 1–55009–246-4.

Low, D. A., Moran, J. M., Dempsey, J. F., Dong, L., & Oldham, M. (2011). Dosimetry tools and techniques for IMRT. *Medical physics*, *38*(3), 1313-1338.

Low, D. A., Sohn, J. W., Klein, E. E., Markman, J., Mutic, S., & Dempsey, J. F. (2001). Characterization of a commercial multileaf collimator used for intensity modulated radiation therapy. *Medical physics*, *28*(5), 752-756.

Manning, M. A., Wu, Q., Cardinale, R. M., Mohan, R., Lauve, A. D., Kavanagh, B. D., & Schmidt-Ullrich, R. K. (2001). The effect of setup uncertainty on normal tissue sparing with IMRT for head-and-neck cancer. *International Journal of Radiation Oncology* Biology* Physics*, *51*(5), 1400-1409.

Martens, C., De Wagter, C., & De Neve, W. (2000). The value of the PinPoint ion chamber for characterization of small field segments used in intensity-modulated radiotherapy. *Physics in Medicine & Biology*, *45*(9), 2519-2530.

Menzel, H. G. (2014). International commission on radiation units and measurements. Report 83" *Journal of the ICRU* 10 (1): 1–106.

Mileusnić, D. (2005). Verification and correction of geometrical uncertainties in conformal radiotherapy. *Archive of oncology*, *13*(3-4), 140-144.

Mott, J. H., Hounsell, A. R., Budgell, G. J., Wilkinson, J. M., & Williams, P. C. (1999). Customised compensation using intensity modulated beams delivered by dynamic multileaf collimation. *Radiotherapy and Oncology*, *53*(1), 59-65.

Mukherji, A. (2018). Planning a Patient, Deciding on the Volumes and Fields and Plan Verification-A Guide for Students and Practitioners. In *Basics of Planning and Management of Patients during Radiation Therapy* (pp. 79-107). Springer, Singapore.

Mutic, S., Palta, J. R., Butker, E. K., Das, I. J., Huq, M. S., Loo, L. N. D., & Van Dyk, J. (2003). Quality assurance for computed-tomography simulators and the computed-tomography-simulation process: report of the AAPM Radiation Therapy Committee Task Group No. 66. *Medical physics*, *30*(10), 2762-2792.

Neeley, M. L. (2009). TRACE: Tennessee Research and Creative Exchange Patient-Specific Quality Assurance for IMRT. Master Theses https://trace.tennessee.edu/utk_gradthes/5741.

Nill, S., Hinderer R., and Oelfke U. (2006). X-IMRT, in. *New Technologies in Radiation Oncology*, edited by Wolfgang Schlegel, Thomas Bortfeld, Anca-Ligia Grosu, 289–298. Springer-Verlag Heidelberg. ISBN 978-3-540-00321-2.

Palma, D. A., Verbakel, W. F., Otto, K., & Senan, S. (2010). New developments in arc radiation therapy: a review. *Cancer treatment reviews*, *36*(5), 393-399.

Poznanski, A. K., Fischer H. W., Gray, J. E., Hendee, W. R., Kereiakes, J. G., Kundel, H. L., Tuddenham, W. J., and Zagzebski, J. A. (1988). Quality Assurance for Diagnostic Imaging. *National Council on Radiation Protection and Measurement. NCRP Rapor No: 99:*1-250.

Purdy, J. A. (2001). Intensity Modulated Radiation Therapy Collaborative Working Group: Intensity-Modulated Radiotherapy: Current Status and Issues of Interest. *International Journal of Radiation Oncology Biology Physics* 51 (4): 880–914.

Que, W., Kung, J., & Dai, J. (2004). 'Tongue-and-groove'effect in intensity modulated radiotherapy with static multileaf collimator fields. *Physics in Medicine & Biology*, *49*(3), 399-405.

Sharpe, M. B., Miller, B. M., Yan, D., & Wong, J. W. (2000). Monitor unit settings for intensity modulated beams delivered using a step-and-shoot approach. *Medical physics*, *27*(12), 2719-2725.

Spirou, S. V., & Chui, C. S. (1994). Generation of arbitrary intensity profiles by dynamic jaws or multileaf collimators. *Medical Physics*, *21*(7), 1031-1041.

Stroom, J. C., & Heijmen, B. J. (2002). Geometrical uncertainties, radiotherapy planning margins, and the ICRU-62 report. *Radiotherapy and oncology*, *64*(1), 75-83.

Thomas, E., Chapet, O., Kessler, M. L., Lawrence, T. S., & Ten Haken, R. K. (2005). Benefit of using biologic parameters (EUD and NTCP) in IMRT optimization for treatment of intrahepatic tumors. *International Journal of Radiation Oncology Biology Physics*, *62*(2), 571-578.

Ting, J. (2005). Technology and Implementation : Capter 13. Commissioning and Dosimetric Quality Assurance. *Intensity Modulated Radiation Therapy a Clinical Perspective in,* edited by Arno, J. Mundt, John C. Roeske, 186-197. Hamilton London. ISBN 1–55009–246-4.

Van Herk, M. (2004). Errors and Margins in Radiotherapy. *Seminars in Radiation Oncology* 14 (1): 52–64.

Van Herk, M., Bruce, A., Kroes, A. P., Shouman, T., Touw, A., & Lebesque, J. V. (1995). Quantification of organ motion during conformal radiotherapy of the prostate by three-dimensional image registration. *International journal of radiation oncology, biology & physics*, *33*(5), 1311-1320.

Wang, X., Spirou, S., LoSasso, T., Stein, J., Chui, C. S., & Mohan, R. (1996). Dosimetric verification of intensity-modulated fields. *Medical physics*, *23*(3), 317-327.

Xia, P., & Verhey, L. J. (1998). Multileaf collimator leaf sequencing algorithm for intensity modulated beams with multiple static segments. *Medical Physics*, *25*(8), 1424-1434.

Yu, Cedric X. (1998). Design Considerations for the Sides of Multileaf Collimator Leaves. *Physics in Medicine and Biology,* 43 (5): 1335–1342.

Chapter 9

Quality Assurance of Intensity-Modulated Radiotherapy

Aydin Cakir*
Vocational School of Health Service, Istanbul Bilgi University, Istanbul, Turkey

Abstract

In the intensity-modulated radiotherapy (IMRT) technique, high doses and many small complex fields are used. To ensure the accuracy and safety of treatments, a detailed quality control (QA) programme specific to the IMRT technique used should be established and put into clinical practice periodically. The general aim is to increase the patient's quality of life by minimising side effects in normal tissues while providing tumour control. Since IMRT is a rapidly developing treatment technique, it is recommended that Medical Physicists follow the relevant reports published by The American Association of Physicists in Medicine (AAPM) on their QA programmes and participate in national/international training. For QA programmes to be successful, the radiotherapy team must have sufficient technical and clinical practice. In addition, it is necessary to have all dosimetric equipment (water and solid phantoms, ion chambers, diode and diamond detectors, etc.) to be used in the measurements of the treatment device. Appropriate detector selection is important to obtain accurate results. In this chapter, the issue of quality assurance at IMRT will be discussed.

Keywords: intensity-modulated radiotherapy, quality assurance, small field dosimetry

---

*Corresponding Author's Email: aydin.cakir@bilgi.edu.tr.

In: Frontiers in Intensity-Modulated Radiotherapy Research
Editor: Sibel Karaca
ISBN: 979-8-88697-252-8

1. Introduction

IMRT treatment planning plays an important role in the clinical treatment of patients. Today, IMRT is developing rapidly and is used in the planning process with major application changes.

The International Commission on Radiation Units and Measurements (ICRU) recommends that the dose administered to the patient be within ±5% of the prescribed dose. Given the many steps involved in dosing a patient to a target volume, each step must be performed with an accuracy of better than 5% to achieve this recommendation (Kutcher et al., 1994).

The purpose of a QA programme for linear accelerators is to ensure that the machine characteristics do not deviate significantly from the baseline values obtained during acceptance and commissioning. There are several publications describing the procedures and conditions for admission testing and commissioning, and readers refer to the American Association of Physicists in Medicine (AAPM) and the American College of Medical Physicians (ACMP) (IAEA, 2004; Kutcher et al., 1994). Many of these baseline values are entered into treatment planning systems to characterise and/or model the treatment machine and can therefore directly affect the treatment plans calculated for each patient treated on that machine. Deviation from baseline values may therefore result in inadequate treatment of patients. Machine parameters can deviate from their initial values for many reasons. Unexpected changes in machine performance can occur due to machine failure, mechanical failure, physical accidents, or component failure. Changing the main components may also change the machine performance from the original parameters. In addition, gradual changes may occur as a result of the aging of the machine components. These failure patterns must be taken into account when creating a periodic QA programme (Fraas et al., 1998; Klein et al., 2009; Low et al., 2011).

The limitations in treatment planning system (TPS) dose calculation algorithms are important to give the correct dose to the patient. The patient-specific QA programme aims to prevent possible accidents. Every clinic has to create and successfully implement a quality control programme.

2. Commissioning and Beam Data Modelling

Commissioning processes usually start with the collection of basic beam data such as output factors for beam modelling, percent depth dose, and dose profiles for treatment areas. The beam data should be carefully measured with detectors (ion chambers, diodes, diamonds, etc.) suitable for different field sizes and measurement techniques, at all energies from the smallest field to the largest field used. Errors in measurements may result from the dosimeters used and the techniques applied. The detector volume effect is the most important parameter invalidating the IMRT plan. If the ion chamber will be used; In small area ($<4 \times 4$ cm^2) measurements, small volume ion chambers should be preferred, as large volume ion chambers cause lateral electron balance deficiencies (Low et al., 2011; Ting et al., 2005). Laub and Wong determined that the volume effects of the ion chamber increase as the treatment field gets larger (Laub and Wong, 2003). Therefore, while the active volume ~0.1 cm^3 ion chamber is sufficient especially for areas $<4 \times 4$ cm^2, ~0.01 cm^3 ion chambers can be used in small areas of treatments such as SRS and SBRT (Low et al., 2011; Ting et al., 2005). If micro-MLC that can provide a field size of $<5 \times 5$ mm^2 is used, then smaller-volume micro ion chambers (<0.01 cm^3) can be used. It is also recommended to use tissue-equivalent detectors in very small fields. To minimise the effect of position errors on the dose, ion chamber measurements are measured in a region of low dose gradient. Ion chamber measurements should be within ±2%. In addition to ion chambers for profile measurements, a radio-chromic/radiographic (EDR2) film or a high sensitivity small diode, diamond detector, or electronic portal imaging device (EPID; electronic portal imaging device) can also be used for monthly tests.

Output factors that change rapidly depending on the field size should be modelled within 0.5% uncertainty (Dieterich et al., 2011). For 6 MV photon beams, a 2 mm deviation in field size affects the output factor by 2% for a 2 x 2 cm2 area and 15% for a 1×1 cm^2 area. Often in IMRT, an exposure consists of many small areas. In order to add them correctly, the penumbra of the fields must be determined very precisely and measured with special care. To check the off-axis ratios, the profiles of both symmetrical and some asymmetrical areas must be measured. To accurately determine the output factors and beam profiles of small irregular areas, a very detailed treatment device head model and commissioning are required (Sharpe et al., 2000).

The most important factor affecting IMRT treatment planning, are MLC's end-leaf leakage, leaf transmission, inter-leaf leakage, leaf movement length, penumbra modelling, output factor in small fields, percent deep dose values at off-axis points, dose profiles, and dose calculation grid size, etc. should be tested and modelled in the treatment planning system by choosing an appropriate and accurate calculation algorithm. Dose constancy per MU should be controlled throughout the treatment interval for IMRT. Also, for small MU (<2 MU) output, flatness and symmetry stability should be tested in phantom with suitable detectors (diode, diamond, film). It has been reported that some treatment systems have dosimetric differences within the nominal range of use for clinical treatments in small MU due to the communication delay between the MLC control system and the linear axillary console (Ting et al., 2005).

TPS that does not calculate the heterogeneity can result in dose differences that affect some beam fields more than others. The effects of transient electronic instability in air and increased lateral electron scattering may result in a significant reduction in the central axis dose beyond the gap, resulting in a low dose of the tumour. It is especially important when the target is surrounded by low-density tissues such as the lungs. Therefore, dose calculation algorithms that take into account loss of electronic balance and lateral electron scatterings, such as lung tissue interface or tumour margin in a low-density environment, need to be used. The most accurate tissue inhomogeneity corrections are achieved with Monte Carlo dose calculation (Benedict et al., 2010). To calculate heterogeneity corrections in planning systems, an electron-based and/or mass density-based CT density model needs to be introduced to the system. The user should know which density type the system uses for each dose calculation algorithm and should follow the recommendations set out in AAPM TG66 and NCRP Report No: 99 for CT quality control (Mutic et al., 2003; Poznanski et al., 1988). The compatibility of the treatment planning system and data transfer tests should be tested. After creating an acceptable IMRT plan, the intensity profiles for each beam are sent via digital imaging and communications in medicine (DICOM) to the processing accelerator, which is electronically equipped with the appropriate hardware and software to provide the planned intensity-modulated beams. The accuracy of the patient's data must be checked. As a result, the integrity of data transfer over the whole system (CT simulator, treatment planning system, registration and verification system, and IMRT accelerator control system) needs to be verified, as in conventional 3DCRT.

3. Linac Specific Quality Assurances

In order for the optimal plans obtained in TPS to be implemented accurately and completely, the routine quality controls of the treatment devices should be carried out regularly and recorded. General mechanical and dosimetric quality-control tests and limit values for linear accelerators were reported in Task Group 40 published by AAPM (Kutcher et al., 1994). Later, in Task Group 142 published in 2009, detailed mechanical and dosimetric tests including the MLC system, which enables the adjustment of the dose intensities of the treatment areas in IMRT, additional controls specific to Cyberknife and Tomotherapy devices, are given together with the frequency and tolerance values (Klein et al., 2009). Some of the mechanical and dosimetric tests for the treatment device showed in Table 1.

Quality control for the MLC-based IMRT technique plays an important role in IMRT treatment planning and dose delivery, as the treatment field consists of multiple segments as a result of optimisation processes. Specific QA tests are highly dependent on the design of the MLC, and specific tests have been developed for MLC (Lo Sasso et al., 1998). MLC QA tests should be repeated at routine intervals to maintain the tolerance values set during IMRT commissioning testing.

According to the IMRT technique used (static-dynamic), MLC velocity (dynamic), MLC position accuracy and repeatability, MLC leakage, round tip MLC leakage, beam stability at low MUs, some MLC-specific tests should be performed in the IMRT technique. Some important tests are given in Table 2.

Table 1. Some of the mechanical and dosimetric tests for the treatment device

	IMRT	SRS/SBRT
Dosimetric parameters		
X-beam output constancy	%2	
Dose rate/output stability	%2	%2
Photon beam profile	%2	
Mechanical parameters		
Light/beam matching	2 mm or %1	
SSD distance indicator	1 mm	
Jaw position stability	1 mm	
Crosshair	1 mm	
Couch position stability	1 mm	<1 mm/0,5°
Gantry/Coll. indicators	±1°	
Laser indicators	±1 mm	

Dose distribution is provided by MLC movement, the slightest error arising from the MLC position accuracy will affect many points in the PTV and cause an incorrect dose in the patient, since the MLCs are irradiated not only at the edge of the area but also within the treatment area. Losasso et al., reported that an MLC position error of ±1 mm in the sliding window technique could cause a 10% dose error in the 1 cm region (Lo Sasso et al., 1998). Errors in MLC positioning cause output changes and profile irregularities in cold and hot spots, especially in the small area where the beams are adjacent. This may cause underdose in PTV and overdose in OAR. Low et al., For static MLC, when adjacent field segments overlap, for 6 MV and 18 MV photon beams, hot and cold spots may occur at approximately 13% and 17% of the average dose per millimetre in the overlap regions (Low et al., 2001).

To test the MLC position, it can be measured using a film (EDR, GafChromic film), electronic portal imaging device (EPID) dosimetry, or 2D Array dosimeters. For example, the MLC position test is performed with the most commonly used picket fence test method as follows. A radiographic/radio-chromic film is fixed to the block tray. With the gantry at 0°, 90°, 180°, and 270° angles and the collimator 0°, respectively, the distance between the closed MLCs is set to about 0.25 cm and the film is irradiated. Then, irradiations are made by shifting the leaves at 1 cm intervals (Figure 1).

Because of the increased MU numbers (approximately 2-10 times that of conventional treatments) in IMRT, leakage between MLCs is extremely important. The amount of leakage contributed to each IMRT field depends on the intensity of the beam generating the field and the leaf sequencing algorithm used.

Table 2. Some of the MLC tests and tolerance values in step and shoot and dynamic IMRT techniques

MLC	Step and shoot	Dynamic
MLC position accuracy	1 mm	0,5 mm
MLC position repeatability	0,2 mm	0,2 mm
Gap length	0,2 mm	0,2 mm
MLC speed	-	±0,1 mm/s

To minimise inter-leaf leakage, the vertical edges of two adjacent MLCs in MLCs are step-shaped and the MLCs are interconnected by tongue and groove designs (Figure 2). Thus, radiation leakage between adjacent MLC pairs is significantly reduced. However, at the edges of the irregularly shaped segments, either the tongue or groove protrudes into the open portion of the area causing low dose lines between adjacent segments (Que et al., 2004; Yu.,

1998). Depending on the linear accelerator device manufactured by different commercial companies.

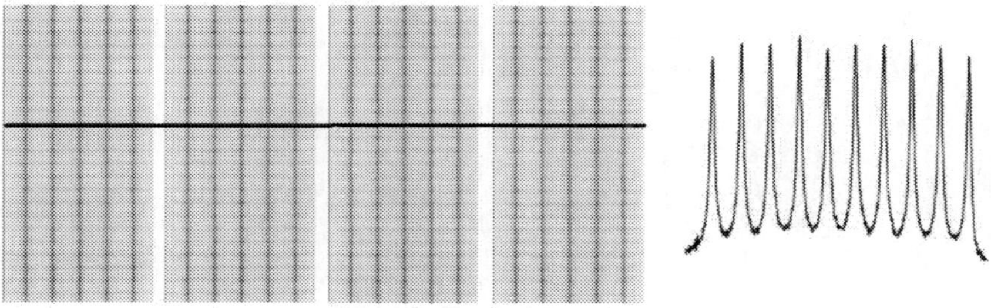

Figure 1. Picket fence test and profiles using the EPID dosimetry method.

In tongue and groove design, if the MLCs are not properly synchronised with the leaf sequencing algorithm, IMRT may cause blocking and dose reduction in small fields of the treatment area (Figure 3). It has been shown that it can be caused in low doses (Kamath et al., 2004). It has been reported that this may be important especially when the number of beams in the treatment plan is low (<5) (Deng et al., 2001). Monte Carlo simulation and an accurate MLC leaf sequencing algorithm with the tongue and groove effect can be significantly reduced (Yu, 1998).

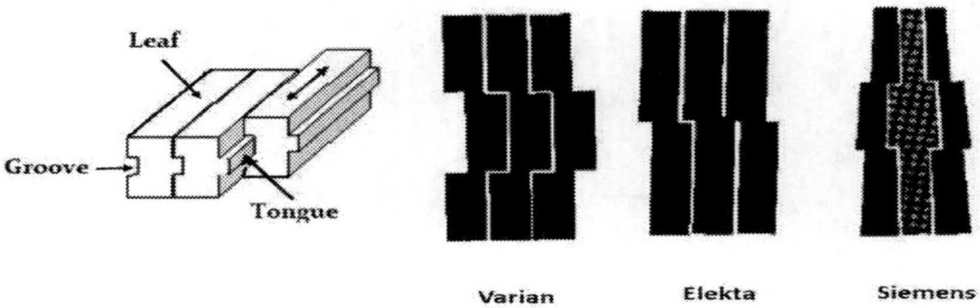

Figure 2. Tongue and groove designs of MLCs for Varian, Elekta, and Siemens linear accelerator therapy devices.

An important point for IMRT is the alignment of the tip of the MLC with the beam receiving edge. When the MLC edges are designed as rounded (single focus), there is an offset with the beam receiving edge. The design of this offset MLC is between 0.4 and 1.1 mm depending on the beam energy and the distance from the central axis (Figure 4). For this reason, hot zones occur in case of overlap due to radiation leakage.

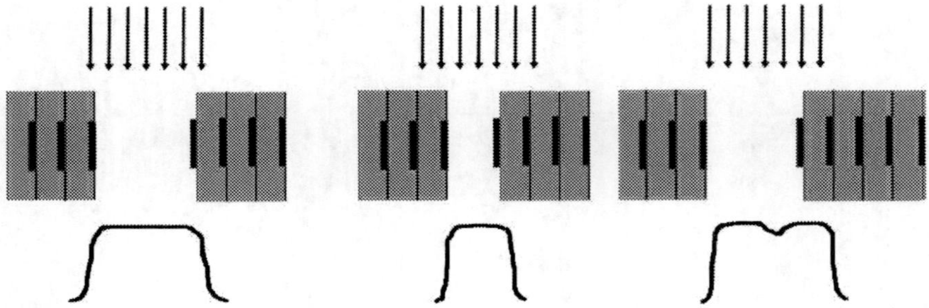

Figure 3. The dose profile resulting from the tongue and groove effect designed to prevent interleaf leakage.

The rounded end of the MLC transmission is more effective, especially in sliding window techniques, and causes small areas to receive higher doses.

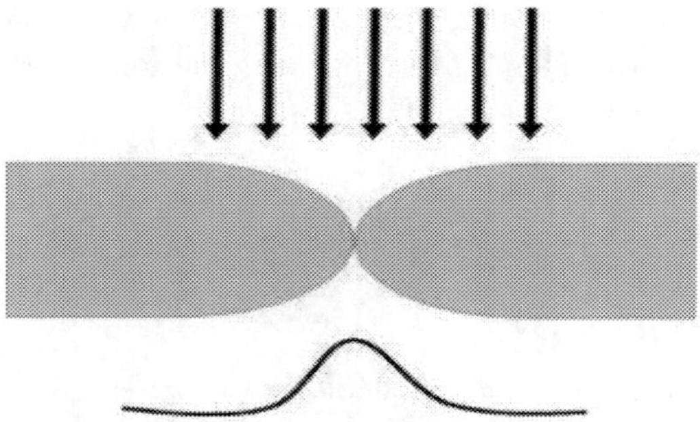

Figure 4. The offset representation and dose leakage between the tips in the rounded MLC design.

For Millennium MLC (Varian, Palo Alto - CA) as a result of inadequate modelling of the penumbra, its leakage may result in an additional absorption dose of 2Gy to 3Gy over a treatment period (Hardcastle et al., 2007; Low et al., 2011). For this reason, the end of the MLC penumbra should be modelled correctly with appropriate algorithms. Small variable gaps between MLCs generate regional output variations. A variation of 0.2 mm in gap width may result in a dose change of ±3% for the dynamic MLC technique.

MLC transmission (intra-leaf) is the amount of radiation that passes under the MLC. MLC permeability is determined by measuring with a film, water phantom, or small volume ion chamber, with the collimators fully open in a certain field size, while the MLCs are closed. It is usually <3%, depending on MLC design and energy. The average permeability value for treatment planning is accepted as 2%.

While the MLC speed must be controlled for dynamic MLC treatments, it is sufficient to investigate the static calibration accuracy when using the static MLC technique. The control system can change the MLC rate, the dose rate, or both to achieve the desired result. MLC speed should be measured by film, portal dosimetry, or array detectors by determining the time taken for leaf movement at a defined distance. MLC sequencing files specially designed to test the stability of MLC speed move MLC pairs at constant speeds varying from low to high. MLCs have a maximum speed set by the manufacturer. Sometimes MLC engines may not be able to maintain this speed during normal operation. Also, the stability of the MLC velocity can be measured by profiling the phantom with a film placed perpendicular to the central axis at a depth greater than the maximum dose. Profiles are homogeneous if the MLC rate is constant. Fluctuations in profiles indicate instability in MLC speed.

Today, depending on the developments in IMRT technologies, the absorbed dose calculations can be simplified; with the removal of the field scattering filter (FFF treatments), scattering from the linac head can be reduced, and the penumbra is sharper and treatment times can also be reduced. It is also recommended to use dose calculation algorithms that accurately account for the effects of collimator scattering, collimator leakage, and charged particle contamination.

QA procedures for volumetric IMRT, in addition to the routine tests for IMRT in conventional linear accelerators, the gravity effect should be checked for all parts including gantry, diaphragm, and MLC position at different gantry angles, especially at 90°/270° angles where gravity has the maximum effect. It must be ensured that the MLC and diaphragms operate with the required precision at all gantry angles and that there are no positional effects when the gantry starts and stops turning. In addition, dose and dose rate linearity, different dose rates during rotation and beam flatness and symmetry at low MUs, and MLC-gantry-dose rate synchronisation tests should also be routinely performed.

4. Patients Specific Quality Assurance

Patient-specific QA is recommended due to the small and complex field of the irradiated treatment areas in IMRT, and the position and velocity change of MLCs depending on time. Unlike 3DCRT, due to the three-dimensional complexity of the dose, the total dose needs to be controlled in more than one place, as it is insufficient to reference the dose measured at a single reference point. For this reason, patient plan-specific dosimetric validation is required for the dose obtained in the treatment planning computer to be given accurately on the treatment device. The differences between the calculated and measured doses depend on the dose calculation algorithm of the planning system, the dosimetric characteristics of the MLC (leakage, penumbra at the end of the leaf, etc.), the choice of dosimetry, and the measurement geometry and technique. To calculate the dose accurately, the parameters affecting the dose distributions such as MLC-related properties, inhomogeneity, and small area dosimetry in treatment planning systems must be modelled correctly using an appropriate algorithm. Before applying the treatment plan to the patient, it is recommended to perform patient-specific QA (Ibbott et al., 2009). To obtain accurate dose distribution and MUs near critical structures, high resolution absolute and relative dosimetry should be used. Although patient-specific quality control procedures are still in development, in the early year's measurements generally relied on point dose measurement with an appropriate small volume ion chamber at one or more points of the patient plan on the IMRT phantom, and isodose distribution measurement with radiographic or radio-chromic film. The film is used to measure the spatial position of the irradiated area, and the ion chambers are used to measure the absorbed dose in the low and high dose regions. More practical 2D/3D array detectors and EPID dosimeters are used for relative dose measurements (Table 3).

The patient-specific QA plan is created with two different techniques using the beam configurations of the patient plan.

4.1. Relative Dose Measurement

The treatment plan calculated for the patient is compared to the intensity maps/profiles by irradiating the QA plan prepared for the patient on the treatment device. Checking the density maps gives information about the spatial alignment of the beamlets. For fixed gantry angle IMRT, it can be measured by placing the film inside a suitable IMRT phantom as mentioned above. However, nowadays, two-dimensional array dosimeters including electronic portal dosimetry (EPID) and ion chamber or diode detectors are used in a more advanced and practical way. With the gantry rotation in VMAT, MLCs also move continuously, and two-dimensional measurement systems are no longer sufficient due to irradiation at varying dose rates and obtaining the dose distribution in three dimensions. Therefore, 3D cylindrical diode detectors should be used. PTW Octavius phantom in VMAT plan measurements is a phantom made for rotational treatment quality control to be used with the PTW Seven 29 2D array ion chamber. These dosimeters also have some advantages and disadvantages according to the technique used (Table 3).

Table 3. Some dosimetric equipment used for IMRT patient QA

	PTW Seven 29/Octavius	**Matrix & Mapcheck**	**Sun Nuclear Arc Check**	**Epid**	**Gaf Chromic (EBT)**	**Radyo Chromik film**	**TLD**
Modality	Ion chamber	Diode detector	Diode detector	Amorf Silikon	Polymer	Silver coated film	LiF
Resolution	Low	Low	Low	Low	High	High	Low
Analysing time	High	High	High	High	Low	Low	Low
Energy dependence	Yes	Yes	Yes	Yes	No	Yes	Yes
Dose rate dependence	Yes	Yes	Yes	Yes	Yes	Yes	Yes
Tissue equivalent	No	No	No	No	Yes	No	Yes

The gamma index (γ) method has been defined to quantitatively evaluate the calculated and measured 2D or 3D dose distribution (Low et al., 1998, 2001, 2003). This method provides a quantitative evaluation of the calculated and measured dose distributions. Gamma analysis expresses the difference between the measured and calculated dose distributions between two doses at the same point and the distance between two isodoses receiving the same dose. In high or low dose areas, these two techniques can give misleading results if used separately. The Gamma analysis method combines these two techniques and gives the most accurate result. The harmony of the distance between isodoses is expressed by Distance to Agreement (DTA) and is the geometric distance from a measurement point to the nearest calculation point with the same dose value. Dose difference (DD) criteria are important in low-dose regions and DTA criteria in high-dose regions (Figure 5).

Geometric criteria, for each point in the measured distribution, there must be a point of the same dose in the determined distribution at a specified tolerance distance. In the AAPM TG-119 report, 3% for dose difference in gamma criteria; 3 mm for DTA; they reported that the gamma index (γ) ≤ 1 was valid (Ezzel et al., 2009). Stereotactic radiosurgery (SRS) was accepted as 2% and 2 mm for stereotactic body radiotherapy (SBRT). (95% for $\gamma \leq 1$) $\gamma > 1$ may be caused by set-up or MLC error. Otherwise, the verification is repeated or the plan is re-optimised.

1. Verification of dose per beam (Area-related method): In this method, planar measurements of all beam areas are made separately or simultaneously for each beam area by using dosimeters such as film, 2D detector array, or EPID. With its simple setup and fast response feature, systematic errors can be detected for specific beams. It is usually done at gantry 0°, so the uncertainties created by exposures at other gantry angles may not be detected. It cannot fully reflect the patient plan.

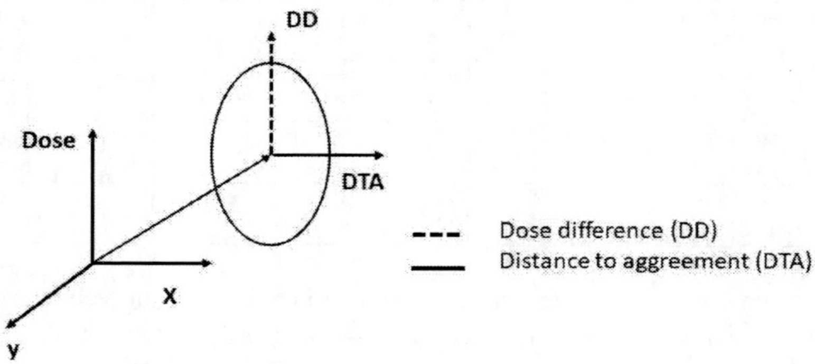

Figure 5. Gamma histogram analysis comparing calculated and measured dose distributions.

2. Cumulative dose verification (Plan related method): It includes cumulative planar measurements, even point dose measurements. Because IMRT beams are generally designed to create a homogeneous dose distribution at the target volume, the dose must be accurately known at every point within the treatment area. For this reason, planar and point dose measurement is recommended for

checking the accuracy of dose flux maps of IMRT fields. For all beams, all effects of the uncertainties present can be determined. In cumulative dose measurement, all the patient plan geometry (gantry, collimator, table angles, etc.) and segment densities for a patient plan are transferred from a phantom treatment planning system. Thus, it is exactly similar to the planned patient treatment, except for the different absolute MU values due to geometric differences between the phantom and the patient. Thus, errors that may occur due to parameters used such as table angle and gantry can also be controlled. Pelvic, thorax, and head-neck phantoms (ellipsoid, cylindrical or spherical shape) used for IMRT are designed to simultaneously measure both the absorbed dose with the ion chamber and the relative dose measurement using the film. Some phantoms may also be used in TLDs. In the treatment plans of inhomogeneous tissues such as lungs or head and neck (especially stereotactic radiosurgery), tissue inhomogeneity should be corrected without error. For this reason, it is recommended to use phantoms containing inhomogeneous structures (e.g., an anthropomorphic lung phantom). Generally, phantom-based patient QA procedures are performed in the order shown in Figure 6.

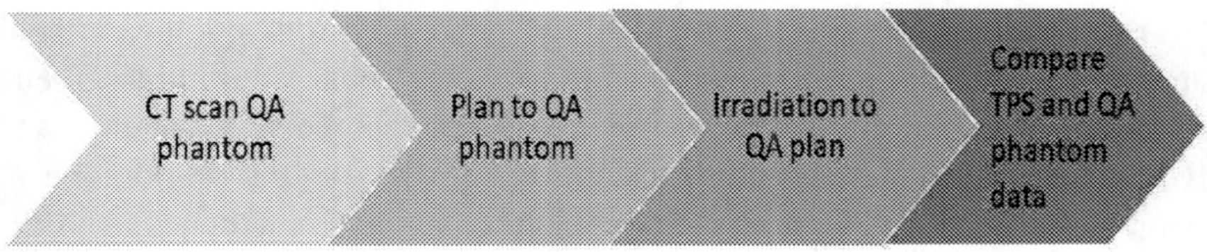

Figure 6. Patient-specific quality control steps.

If both the absorbed dose and the relative measurement are to be made at the same time, this is done in two stages. First, the CT image is taken with the small volume ion chamber to be used for point dose measurement of the phantom and transferred to the QA part of the planning system. In the second stage, the patient is transferred to this phantom with all the features of the treatment plan (gantry, collimator, table angle, segment densities, etc.). In the dose-volume histogram calculated by giving a certain dose to the target created in the phantom, the isocentre and the place where the film will be placed are determined by changing the table positions so that the difference between the maximum and minimum doses received by the ion chamber is less than 5% (Ting et al., 2005). The adjusted hybrid plane phantom, together with the film/Epid and the ion chamber, is irradiated on the treatment device in the same patient geometry and MU in the recording and verification system.

4.2. Absolute Dose Measurement

The reference point dose for IMRT is usually a comparison of the measured point dose (MU comparison) with the calculated point dose at the same point as measured with the ion chamber, and is part of patient-specific quality control. The number of MUs used to provide dose distribution is a strong function of a complex MLC distribution array and therefore cannot be estimated based on patient geometry alone. Direct measurement is small, to avoid volume effects due to the inhomogeneity of dose distributions placed in an anthropomorphic or geometric IMRT phantom as mentioned above. It is based on the planned irradiation of the patient with a voluminous ion chamber.

Since IMRT plans show greater dose inhomogeneity than 3DCRT plans, dose gradients may be higher at modulations up to 1 x 1 cm^2. The ion chamber results obtained for the point dose are considered within ±2-3%. Smaller, tissue-equivalent dosimeters have also become available, requiring less correction for absolute dosimetry. Ion chambers are ideally used in a highly uniform dose region. Thus, the effect of position errors on the dose is minimised. Control of the relationship between beam configuration and patient geometry is achieved by verifying the SSD (source-skin distance) and MU of each beam independently (Kung et al., 2000). It is impossible to perform this verification process by manual calculation method due to the complex and many small areas in the IMRT plan. The treatment devices have a dose calculation algorithm that enables verification without using a phantom by utilising 'log file' based QA system files. The 'log file' based QA system is a system that uses an algorithm to recalculate the dose in the patient's CT using both the planned values and the data found in the log files (Childress et al., 2015).

In SBRT applications with the VMAT technique, it is very important to properly determine the tissue inhomogeneities and dose verification in the created plans (especially in lung SBRT). This is because small areas are often used in combination with high-dose gradients and large tissue heterogeneities near target volumes. If the algorithm of the treatment planning system does not take into account heterogeneities, it may cause inconsistencies between the measured and calculated doses.

Conclusion

IMRT treatment planning plays an important role in the clinical treatment of patients. Today, IMRT is developing rapidly and is used in the planning process with major application changes. For this reason, mechanical and dosimetric controls of the treatment device should be done at certain intervals. The limitations in TPS dose calculation algorithms are important to give the correct dose to the patient. The patient-specific QA programme aims to prevent possible accidents. Each clinic has to implement it successfully by making its own quality control programme. For IMRT applications, AAPM protocols and scientific literature are recommended as educational tools.

References

Benedict, S. H., Yenice, K. M., Followill, D., Galvin, J. M., Hinson, W., Kavanagh, B., Paul Keall, Michael Lovelock, Sanford Meeks, Lech Papiez, Thomas Purdie, Ramaswamy Sadagopan, Michael C Schell, Bill Salter, David J Schlesinger, Almon S Shiu, Timothy Solberg, Danny Y Song, Volker Stieber, Robert Timmerman, Wolfgang A Tomé, Dirk Verellen, Lu Wang & Yin, F. F. (2010). Stereotactic body radiation therapy: the report of AAPM Task Group 101. *Medical physics*, 37(8), 4078-4101.

Childress, N., Chen, Q., & Rong, Y. (2015). Parallel/opposed: IMRT QA using treatment log files is superior to conventional measurement-based method. *Journal of applied clinical medical physics*, 16(1), 4.

Deng, J., Pawlicki, T., Chen, Y., Li, J., Jiang, S. B., & Ma, C. M. (2001). The MLC tongue-and-groove effect on IMRT dose distributions. *Physics in Medicine & Biology*, 46(4), 1039.

Dieterich, S., Cavedon, C., Chuang, C. F., Cohen, A. B., Garrett, J. A., Lee, C. L., Jessica R. Lowenstein, Maximian F. d'Souza, David D. Taylor Jr., Xiaodong Wu & Yu, C. (2011). Report of AAPM TG 135: quality assurance for robotic radiosurgery. *Medical physics*, 38 (6 Part 1), 2914-2936.

Ezzell, G. A., Burmeister, J. W., Dogan, N., LoSasso, T. J., Mechalakos, J. G., Mihailidis, D., Andrea Molineu, Jatinder R. Palta, Chester R. Ramsey, Bill J. Salter, Jie Shi, Ping Xia, Ning J. Yue & Xiao, Y. (2009). IMRT commissioning: multiple institution planning and dosimetry comparisons, a report from AAPM Task Group 119. *Medical physics*, 36(11), 5359-5373.

Fraass, B., Doppke, K., Hunt, M., Kutcher, G., Starkschall, G., Stern, R., & Van Dyke, J. (1998). American Association of Physicists in Medicine Radiation Therapy Committee Task Group 53: quality assurance for clinical radiotherapy treatment planning. *Medical physics*, 25(10), 1773-1829.

Ibbott, G. S. (2009). QA for clinical dosimetry, with emphasis on clinical trials. *Clinical Dosimetry Measurements in Radiotherapy*, 577-604.

International Atomic Energy Agency (2004). *Commissioning and Quality Assurance of Computerize Planning Systems for Radiation Treatment of Cancer*. Technical Reports Series No. 430. Vienna: International Atomic Energy Agency; 16-96.

Kamath, S., Sahni, S., Palta, J., Ranka, S., & Li, J. (2004). Optimal leaf sequencing with elimination of tongue-and-groove underdosage. *Physics in Medicine & Biology*, 49(3), N7.

Klein, E. E., Hanley, J., Bayouth, J., Yin, F. F., Simon, W., Dresser, S., Serago, C., Aguirre, F., Ma, L., Arjomandy, B., Liu, C., Sandin, C. & Holmes, T. (2009). Task Group 142 report: Quality assurance of medical accelerators a. *Medical physics*, 36 (9 Part 1), 4197-4212.

Kung, J. H., Chen, G. T. Y., & Kuchnir, F. K. (2000). A monitor unit verification calculation in intensity modulated radiotherapy as a dosimetry quality assurance. *Medical physics*, 27(10), 2226-2230.

Kutcher, G. J., Coia, L., Gillin, M., Hanson, W. F., Leibel, S., Morton, R. J., Palta, J. R., Purdy, J. A., Reinstein, L. E., Svensson, G. K., Weller, M. & Wingfield, L. (1994). Comprehensive QA for radiation oncology: report of AAPM radiation therapy committee task group 40. *Medical Physics-Lancaster PA-*, 21, 581-581.

Laub, W. U., & Wong, T. (2003). The volume effect of detectors in the dosimetry of small fields used in IMRT. *Medical physics,* 30(3), 341-347.

LoSasso, T., Chui, C. S., & Ling, C. C. (1998). Physical and dosimetric aspects of a multileaf collimation system used in the dynamic mode for implementing intensity modulated radiotherapy. *Medical physics*, 25(10), 1919-1927.

Low, D. A., & Dempsey, J. F. (2003). Evaluation of the gamma dose distribution comparison method. *Medical physics*, 30(9), 2455-2464.

Low, D. A., Harms, W. B., Mutic, S., & Purdy, J. A. (1998). A technique for the quantitative evaluation of dose distributions. *Medical physics*, 25(5), 656-661.

Low, D. A., Moran, J. M., Dempsey, J. F., Dong, L., & Oldham, M. (2011). Dosimetry tools and techniques for IMRT. *Medical physics*, 38(3), 1313-1338.

Low, D. A., Sohn, J. W., Klein, E. E., Markman, J., Mutic, S., & Dempsey, J. F. (2001). Characterization of a commercial multileaf collimator used for intensity modulated radiation therapy. *Medical physics*, 28(5), 752-756.

Mutic, S., Palta, J. R., Butker, E. K., Das, I. J., Huq, M. S., Loo, L. N. D., Salter, B. J., McCollough, C. H., & Van Dyk, J. (2003). Quality assurance for computed-tomography simulators and the computed-tomography-simulation process: report of the AAPM Radiation Therapy Committee Task Group No. 66. *Medical physics*, 30(10), 2762-2792.

Poznanski, A. K., Fischer, H. W., Gray, J. E., Hendee, W. R., Kerciakes, J. G., Kundel, H. L. Tuddenham, W. J., and Zagzebski, J. A. (1988). Quality Assurance for Diagnostic Imaging: National Council on Radiation Protection and Measurement. *NCRP Rapor* No: 99, 1-250.

Que, W., Kung, J., & Dai, J. (2004). 'Tongue-and-groove'effect in intensity modulated radiotherapy with static multileaf collimator fields. *Physics in Medicine & Biology*, 49(3), 399.

Sharpe, M. B., Miller, B. M., Yan, D., & Wong, J. W. (2000). Monitor unit settings for intensity modulated beams delivered using a step-and-shoot approach. *Medical physics*, 27(12), 2719-2725.

Ting, J. Commissioning and dosimetric quality assurance. In: Mundt AJ, Roeske JC, eds. (2005). *Intensity Modulated Radiation Therapy: A Clinical Perspective*. London: BC Decker Inc., 186-97.

Yu, C. X. (1998). Design considerations for the sides of multileaf collimator leaves. *Physics in Medicine & Biology*, 43(5), 1335.

Chapter 10

IG-IMRT

Murat Okutan[1,2,*]

[1]Medical Physics Department, Oncology Institute,
University of Istanbul,Istanbul, Turkey
[2]Radiothetrapy Department, Vocational School of Health Services,
Cerrahpasa University of Istanbul, Istanbul, Turkey

Abstract

Imaging has an important role in both diagnosis and treatment in radiotherapy (RT). The purpose of Image-Guided Radiotherapy (IGRT) can be expressed in two steps. The first step is to increase the accuracy of the determination of target and normal tissues during RT planning. The second step is to ensure that the location of the target is fully verified during treatment. With the development of technology, techniques such as Intensity Modulated RT (IMRT) and Intensity Modulated Arc Therapy (IMAT) are used in RT. With these techniques, the radiation dose given to the target covers the shape of the target in three dimensions, depending on the location, shape and movement of the target. Therefore, the accuracy of tumour location is very important. Reducing the margin of Planned Target Volume (PTV), called target, is possible with IGRT. Thus, more normal tissue volume can be preserved during RT and accordingly, the dose to be given to the target can be increased. IGRT also informs us about the uncertainties associated with systematic and random errors during treatment. In addition, it also guides us about the weight change that will occur during the treatment, the growth or shrinkage of the tumour. Thanks to this information, continuous evaluation of PTV can be made and adaptive treatment techniques can be applied to ensure that PTV receives the required dose. The reliable

[*]Corresponding Author's Email: mokutan@istanbul.edu.tr.

In: Frontiers in Intensity-Modulated Radiotherapy Research
Editor: Sibel Karaca
ISBN: 979-8-88697-252-8

applicability of advanced RT techniques such as Stereotactic Radiosurgery (SRS), Stereotactic Body RT (SBRT), in which we give high doses per fraction, is only possible with IGRT. In conclusion, in this chapter, it will be discussed that RT improves the quality of treatment with imaging performed for tumour follow-up before and during treatment.

Keywords: IGRT and set-up, IGRT techniques, IMRT

1. Introduction

In this chapter, the importance of Image Guided Radiotherapy (IGRT) in radiotherapy (RT), image and set-up correction approaches and IGRT techniques will be discussed. Imaging plays an important role in both diagnosis and treatment in RT. IGRT is referred to as the use of images to provide precise and accurate treatment throughout the RT process. For this precise and accurate treatment, images taken during treatment are compared with images taken during simulation. This process is known as set-up. With this process, it is possible to determine the location of the target, control the tumour location and follow the tumour movement, and deliver the radiation dose to the target exactly (Li et al., 2012). In conformal RT, portal films have been replaced by Electronic Portal Images Device (EPID) with the development of technology. Portal films and EPID images have poor image quality and are two-dimensional (2D). In these images, localisation is made according to the bone structure. Tumours are usually found in soft tissue in the body and are physiologically mobile. For this reason, it is making the patient's set-up according to the anatomical structure (e.g., bone structure) causes errors. Considering all possible positions of the tumour and set-up errors, large margins are used when creating the planned target volume (PTV) in order not to be off-target the tumour. This situation causes the normal tissues to receive unnecessarily more radiation doses during the treatment. However, the use of the PTV margin has been the most common method used to account for geometric uncertainties until recent years. However, due to the increased likelihood of normal tissue side effects, the use of large margins has limited the safe increase of radiation doses delivered to the tumour. Especially today, with the increase in computer and software technology, imaging systems such as Computed Tomography (CT), Magnetic Resonance Imaging (MRI) and Positron Emission Tomography (PET-CT) are used in treatment planning systems. In this way, tumour volume and microscopic spread can be accurately determined in three-dimensional (3D). Accordingly, with the help of this technology used during treatment, it is possible to increase the dose of radiation delivered to the monitored target. Therefore, tumour margins can be reduced. Accordingly, with the help of this technology used during treatment, it is possible to increase the dose of radiation delivered to the monitored target. By increasing the dose given to the tumour, the possibility of local control with superior treatment success can be achieved and side effects can be reduced (Jaffray et al., 1999). With the development of treatment techniques such as Intensity Modulated RT (IMRT), Intensity Modulated Arc Therapy (IMAT), Stereotactic Radiosurgery (SRS), and Stereotactic Body RT (SBRT), these treatment options are frequently applied and the targeted PTV margins are gradually getting smaller. So, every pre-treatment check of the accuracy of the PTV and the location of critical organs in or near the treatment area has become mandatory. This is possible with IGRT. This requirement is tried to be met with imaging instruments mounted in the treatment room or on the LINAC device (Korreman et al., 2010). In order to deliver the planned treatment dose to the target more accurately, there are both (inter-fractional) set-up differences between treatments and tumour position changes due to (intra-fractional) organ movements during treatment.

The main source of uncertainty during treatment is respiratory movements. Especially in radiotherapy of the thorax and abdomen regions, the displacement of the organs during respiration varies up to 1-3 cm, but the change according to the bone structure can be seen as 3-5 mm (Santos et al., 2013). Different IGRT solutions are used to reduce the dosimetric uncertainties that arise due to the displacement of the target volume with respiration. During therapy, there are systems that allow the beam to follow the target throughout the entire respiratory cycle or to irradiate during a certain respiratory stage. In addition, it is aimed to minimise respiratory uncertainties with systems that suppress respiratory movement. With IGRT, it is possible to monitor the changes in the patient and therefore the target throughout the treatment process. It can be detected that the tumour shrinks or grows, the shape of the tumour changes, or the normal tissue anatomy around it changes. During the treatment period, the treatment can be adapted to this new condition of the patient. Thus, clinical advantage can be provided in terms of patient treatment.

2. Setup Errors in IGRT

The sources of errors in radiotherapy are examined in two groups: systematic and random. Errors that exist in any of the treatment planning stages in radiotherapy and affect all patients are called systematic errors. Systematic errors are repeatable and permanent errors. These errors occur in the same way and at the same rate throughout the treatment. For instance; incorrect target volume definition, errors in room lasers, mechanical and dosimetric errors of the device, and information transfer errors are called systematic errors. Unnoticed systematic errors affect all patients undergoing treatment. Random errors, on the other hand, are one-time errors that occur at any stage of treatment, regardless of systematic error. For instance; errors related to the patient's position or organ movement are random errors. Set-up uncertainty includes the fixation and positioning systems used for the treated area. To determine the margins of PTV, the average values of systematic and random errors in the patient group are used. By using set-up errors, systematic and random errors of the clinic should be followed, and target volume margin and IGRT usage protocols should be determined for the treatment techniques used (Van Herk et al., 2000). Apart from systematic and random errors, it should not be forgotten that the physiological movements of the organs in the irradiated volume also cause uncertainties. Dosimetric uncertainty arises when periodic movements such as breathing or irregular movements such as swallowing are not taken into account. Uncertainties are tried to be eliminated by using systems that restrict or follow respiration during the application. The correct implementation of the planned treatment is carried out with the help of IGRT systems located in the treatment room.

There are 3 different set-up correction approaches in IGRT applications; on-line method, off-line method and online real-time method.

2.1. On-line Method

Just before the treatment, the image is taken and the set-up correction is made. The patient is taken into treatment from the corrected set-up position. It eliminates both random and systematic errors on a daily basis. It is difficult for the patient to keep the time spent on the treatment table to a minimum during the acquisition, analysis, and implementation of the correction decision (Korreman et al., 2010). It is recommended to perform a set-up correction with IGRT before each treatment, especially when the fraction number is low.

2.2. Off-line Method

Pre-treatment imaging is performed, but no correction is made in the set-up position. The images are then examined, and the position that needs to be corrected is determined after the patient's treatment is finished. The purpose of the off-line method is to eliminate the systematic errors of the patient. With this method, systematic errors belonging to the patient group are detected, and protocols are created in which the imaging frequency and correction limits of the clinic specific to the treatment area are determined (Korreman et al., 2010).

2.3. Online, Real-Time Method

It is the imaging performed simultaneously during the treatment that monitors the anatomical mobility of the target. In tumour follow-up, different methods are used that monitor respiratory movements, the patient's body surface or markers placed on the patient. During treatment, kilovoltage (kV) Fluoroscopic imaging or Megavoltage (MV) Cine imaging methods allow simultaneous monitoring of target and normal tissues displaced by respiration. In addition, the set-up correction made before the treatment and the systems that monitor the change during the treatment (markers placed on the prostate and the tracking systems in the Cyberknife device, etc.) increase the accuracy of the treatment (Korreman et al., 2010).

3. IGRT Techniques

Depending on the imaging methods used, IGRT systems can generally be divided into two with and without radiation (Balter et al., 2007, Santos et al., 2013).

3.1. Non-Radiation Systems

These systems include ultrasound, camera-based systems, electromagnetic systems, and MRI systems integrated into the treatment room.

3.1.1. Ultrasound-Based Systems

These systems (e.g., BAT, SonArray, Clarity) are used to correct inter-fractional errors. It can be preferred especially for localising soft tissue structures and targets in the abdomen, pelvis and breast. It is a non-invasive real-time 3D imaging technique. Geometric accuracy is 3-5 mm. Its biggest advantage is that it does not contain ionising radiation. The difference in user usage is quite large. It has low image quality. During application with the probe, anatomical changes occur depending on the probe pressure. In addition, correct use will vary from person to person, with the user's training and experience. Transabdominal ultrasound systems are widely used for the localisation of the prostate (Fung et al., 2006; Lattanzi et al., 2000).

BAT system Best-NOMOS (Pittsburgh, PA); it is a quick method of localising the prostate before each treatment. It makes corrections for inter-fraction variation of prostate position. The main problem of ultrasound imaging methods is poor image quality which makes images difficult to interpret. Therefore, wider planning margins have been suggested in the literature (Chandra et al., 2003; Langen et al., 2003).

SonArray system Varian Medical System (Ashland, MA); it is an optically directed three-dimensional ultrasound target localisation system. The user applies the ultrasound probe to the anatomical region to obtain two-dimensional images that will be automatically transferred to the computer via a video link. The position and angle of the ultrasound probe are monitored by four infrared light-emitting diodes (IRLEDs). The ultrasound probe position determined by the IRLEDs is combined with the acquired images. A new 3D ultrasound image volume is created (Tome et al., 2002).

Clarity system Electa (Montreal, QC); during the treatment of the prostate patient, the perineal US probe continuously monitors the position of the prostate. If the amount of shift in the prostate position exceeds the threshold value determined by the doctor, the treatment is discontinued. The table is repositioned according to the new position of the prostate. Afterwards, the treatment is continued from where it left off (Robinson et al., 2012).

3.1.2. Camera-Based (Infrared) or Optical Surface Tracking Systems

These systems provide real-time monitoring of non-motile tumors such as intracranial tumours and superficial tumours such as breast. One of these systems, Align RT-Vision RT, works with 2-3 stereo-camera pods placed on the ceiling. Each pod contains 2 cameras and a "speckle pattern" projector. The triangle between them and the skin point is used to calculate the position of this skin point in space. The patient's skin surface is reconstructed from visible surface points. The accuracy of surface imaging is within 1-2 mm. Since Optical Surface Tracking systems cannot visualise the tumour, it needs to be confirmed with a second radiographic imaging method. This method; It is used in breast, lung, brain and head and neck patients. The surface images taken during the patient set-up are overlapped with the reference surface image of the relevant region contoured from the patient's planning CT. With real-time feedback, the patient's position is constantly corrected throughout the treatment (Bert et al., 2006).

3.1.3. Electromagnetic Tracking Systems

In this system (e.g., Calypso), continuous tracking of the target is possible without using ionising radiation. It is a system that detects signals from wireless implant transmitters (beacons) induced by alternating current (AC) electromagnetic fields.

Calypso system (Seattle, WA); consists of a console, an optical tracking system and a tracking station. The main feature of the Calypso System is the Beacon® electromagnetic transmitters. Three Beacon® transponders, each the size of a small grain of rice, are implanted into the patient's prostate before starting radiation therapy in a biopsy-like procedure. They work with the Calypso System and 4D Tracking Station™. It can continuously detect the slightest movement of the prostate during each radiation treatment. Calypso sends an alert when it detects transponder movement. Radiation therapy stops until the target is back in range. The presence of transponders may cause artifacts in MRI. Calypso's area of use is prostate radiotherapy and it works with an accuracy of < 2 mm (Liebenberg et al., 2007).

3.1.4. MRI Systems

These systems (e.g., ViewRay, ViewRay MRIdian Linac, Unity MR-Linac) are gamma and X-ray IMRT systems integrated into MRI guidance. ViewRay system (Oakwood Village, OH); consists of a low magnetic field (0.35 Tesla) open MRI and three sources of Cobalt-60 device. The Cobalt-60 device was chosen because of its compatibility with the MRI system. The computerised MLC system provides gamma-ray IMRT, similar to the Linac-based IMRT system. The system works with an accuracy of 1-2 mm. MRI has some disadvantages, such as the formation of motion-induced artifacts. If the patient has a pacemaker or a metal implant, its use is not preferred. It is widely used in brain, lung and prostate radiotherapy (Saenz et al., 2014). MR-Linac systems are in use today, with the introduction of a linear accelerator system instead of Cobalt-60 sources in 2017. These MR-Linac systems are systems consisting of 6 MV linear accelerators integrated with MRI with different magnetic field sizes. Better soft tissue separation is possible with MR imaging, and adaptive radiotherapy is possible with online, real-time imaging (Hunt et al., 2018).

ViewRay MRIdian Linac (Oakwood Village, OH); the system has a 0.35 Tesla split superconducting magnet (double ring) and a 6 MV flattening filter free (FFF) linear accelerator. The MRI part of the system enables pre-and post-treatment MRI of the patient. Thus, it provides good target localisation thanks to its superior soft tissue contrast (Kashani et al., 2018). In addition, MRI images can be taken in one or three planes (sagittal, coronal, transverse) for automatic beam control (gating) during treatment (Green et al., 2018).

Unity MR-Linac Elekta (Stockholm, Sweden); the system has a 1.5 Tesla Philips large diameter MRI (Philips Healthcare, Amsterdam Netherlands) with a single energy 7 MV FFF linear accelerator. MRI can be used to capture both between fractions and intra-fractional movement (Kleijnen et al., 2016). It is very convenient to use for adaptive radiotherapy. Thus, MR images taken in treatment can be used for location verification or daily real-time replanning (Kontaxis et al., 2017; Stemkens et al., 2017).

3.2. Radiation-Based Systems

These systems can be broadly classified as Gantry-mounted systems, Free-standing systems in the Treatment room, and Fluoroscopy-based monitoring systems.

3.2.1. Gantry Mounted System

3.2.1.1. Electronic Portal Imaging Device

EPID was developed to replace the port film for treatment area verification. Although it was used in clinical practice in the early 1980s, widespread use of this system began in the 1990s. Flat panel amorphous silicon (aSi) detectors are mostly used in EPIDs. These detectors first convert the X-rays into visible light by scintillation, and then this light into electrons that will activate the pixels in the photodiode plane aSi layers. Pixels read in consecutive lines are processed and displayed on the computer screen. This resulting image is called MV portal imaging. It is made with the lowest photon energy found in Linac. It is a useful method as it provides radiographic localisation according to the patient's anatomy. The treatment centre Digitally Reconstructed Radiography

(DRR) image created on the patient's treatment planning computer is superimposed on the MV portal image taken from the patient. This procedure is performed by taking both anteroposterior and lateral images, respectively. Thus, the treatment accuracy is determined in two dimensions. Since the contrast difference between tissues decreases in imaging using MV energies, localisation is generally made according to bone structures such as vertebrae and pelvis. However, bone structure is not a good reference for many treatment sites. Therefore, there may be possible setup errors in the target localisation according to the bone structure. To avoid these errors, Fiducial Markers can be used due to their appearance in MV energies. They can be used as a reference by placing them in the soft tissues of the target structure (e.g., prostate and lung). Therefore, this can reduce image registration errors. If the EPID device has the appropriate software programme, it may be possible to take an image of the patient and evaluate this image while the treatment is ongoing. By keeping the detector on during the treatment, images can be taken at certain intervals from the rays passing through the patient for treatment (Cine mode). For example, for a prostate patient with Fiducial Markers, treatment may be stopped when the patient's rectum suddenly fills with gas during treatment. In addition, the follow-up of left breast patients treated by holding their breath in deep inspiration can be done with the Cine mode (Göksel et al., 2013). Because EPID uses produced X-rays for treatment, the disadvantage is that the patient is given high doses of radiation (1-5 cGy). Also, poor image quality occurs due to Compton scattering, as high-energy X-rays are used. Image control is performed with a geometric accuracy of 2 mm (Walter et al., 2007). The report of the American Association of Physicists in Medicine Task Group 58 (AAPM TG-58) provides a review of commissioning procedures for EPID. This report includes routine quality assurance (QA) of MV EPIDs, especially mechanical, electrical safety checks and image quality tests on a routine basis (Herman et al., 2001).

3.2.1.2. Megavoltage Cone Beam CT (MV CBCT)

MV CBCT uses X-rays and EPID systems in the treatment energy of the linear accelerator. Especially with the development of aSi plane panel detectors, it has become possible to quickly take a large number of 2D image projections with the treatment device. The amount of scattered radiation reaching the detector; depends on photon energy, field size, and thickness of the imaged object (Li et al., 2012). In MV CBCT, 3D volumetric images are created by software using a filtered back-projection algorithm. MV CBCT filming area information is transferred from the imaging computer to the treatment control console. Then system parts such as the gantry, jaw and detector come to starting conditions. During this process, patient reference information such as CT, anatomical contours and treatment isocentre are automatically loaded into the 3D registration application in the treatment control console. Later the gantry makes a 200° arc from 270° to 110° and takes a low dose portal view for each "1" angle. While the gantry rotates continuously, the device irradiates as beam-on, beam-off one after the other. A total of 200 projection images are recorded and the merging process begins. The time from the start of shooting to the completion of the image is approximately 2 minutes. The resulting MV CBCT image is overlaid with the planning CT image. A patient is exposed to a dose of approximately 1.2-0.6 cGy in MV CBCT (anterior arc) acquisition. Compton Effect is more dominant in the interaction of MV energy X-rays with matter. Therefore, soft tissue contrast is low in MV CBCT. However, bone structures around the target, high atomic number materials such as metal implants, and fiducials implanted in the patient appear better without artifacts.

3.2.1.3. Kilovoltage (kV) Systems

These systems consist of aSi detectors with a retractable X-ray tube mounted opposite the Gantry (Elekta Synergy, Varian OBI). The dose delivered in kV imaging is typically in the low dose range of 0.01-0.1 cGy. For this reason, it is more preferred to be used in daily patient setup. Since the kV X-ray plane is not the same as the MV beam plane, the difference between isocentres should be checked in the QA programme (Walter et al., 2007).

3.2.1.4. Kilovoltage Cone Beam BT (kV CBCT)

Gantry-mounted kV imaging systems offer nearly all the necessary solutions for IGRT, such as fluoroscopy and CBCT. In kV CBCT, the gantry is created from projections of images taken as it arcs around the patient. 3D volumetric images are obtained by reconstructing these images by a computer using a filtered back-projection algorithm (Feldkamp et. al., 1984). The quality of the images is affected by problems such as the flexing of the supporting arm holding the X-ray tube and the detector due to gravity, small movements of the gantry during its rotation, X-ray scattering effect. This means low contrast, false registration and artifact formation (Jaffray et al, 2002). CBCT image quality is affected by respiratory motion due to limitations in gantry rotation speed. IGRT set-up prolongs the treatment time by 5 minutes (1-2 minutes scanning time and 1-3 minutes image registration and validation time) (IGRT set-up prolongs the treatment time by 5 minutes (1-2 minutes scanning time and 1-3 minutes image registration and validation time). kV CBCT images provide acceptable soft tissue contrast for localisation of target and at-risk organs (Li et al., 2012). The plane panel detector size of the Elekta Synergy system is 41x41 cm^2, and in the Varian True Beam device, the active image area of the aSi detector is 39.7 x 29.8 cm2. This panel detector size limits the scan length to 15 cm in "full-fan" scan mode. When scanning in the "half-fan" technique, the scanning area (Field of view-FOV) can be expanded up to at least 40 cm. In the OBI system, mean doses of 1.1-8.3 cGy and the highest dose were measured in the head phantom when the "full-fan" protocol was used (Song et al., 2008).

3.2.2. Free Standing Systems in the Treatment Room

3.2.2.1. Fan Beam kV CT (CT-on-Rails)

This system consists of a single treatment table that can be rotated towards the CT or gantry, respectively, for imaging and treatment. The treatment room includes a CT and a Linac. While the patient is on the table, both the CT image is taken and the treatment is performed. For accuracy and applications, it is similar to CBCT with an average dose of 1–5 cGy per image (Crevoisier et al., 2006). Examples of in-room CT system devices are Siemens Primatom AG (Erlangen, Germany) and GE-Varian Medical Systems (Waukesha, WI).

Siemens Primatome In-Room System; the primatome system is a multifunctional, hybrid configuration system. This system consists of a "Siemens Primus" linac and a "Somatome" diagnostic CT scanner moving on two parallel rails in the treatment room. The CT gantry is placed on a motorised carrier. This CT gantry runs on rails above ground. Linac and CT gantry are placed at opposite ends of the treatment couch. The upper part of the treatment couch is made of carbon fiber to prevent scattering artifacts on CT. CT gantry diameter is 70 cm and FOV is 50 cm. Somatom is a CT scanner capable of 16 slices and 4D acquisition (Mundt et al., 2011).

GE-Varian In-Room CT System; this system consists of a combination of "ExaCT Couch," a "Varian 21EX" linac with a slightly modified couch and "GE Smart Gantry" CT systems. In the GE in-room CT system, the CT gantry moves on three rails. The gantry opening of the CT device is 70 cm and the rotation speed is 1 rotation per second. The CT unit is a single section helical CT scanner and the scanning time takes less than 2 minutes (Mundt et al., 2011).

3.2.2.2. Fan Beam MVCT (TomoTherapy)

This system includes a built-in imaging system for acquiring MVCT images of the patient in the treatment position. It is a treatment device in which the features of LINAC and helical CT scanner are used together. A Linac producing 6 MV FFF X-rays is mounted on a CT-like gantry. Like the CT, the gantry 3600 can rotate. With the rotation of the gantry, the treatment couch slowly enters into the bore. Thus, a helical movement is created according to the patient. The same LINAC is used to generate both the treatment (6MV) and the imaging beam (3MV). Helical tomotherapy is the only device that allows IMRT and IGRT to be applied in the same treatment geometry. Despite the poor image quality, MVCT images provide sufficient contrast to confirm the patient's position at the time of treatment using a low dose (typical scanning dose 1 to 2 cGy). In addition, image artifacts caused by high atomic number of objects such as surgical clips, hip implants or dental fillings occur less (Meeks et al., 2005).

3.2.3. Fluoroscopy-based Monitoring Systems

3.2.3.1. Hybrid Systems for Real-Time 4D Monitoring

Most monitoring systems use fluoroscopy to detect metal fiducial points implanted in the tumour. Fiducials are continuously displayed during irradiation. Radiation is given or interrupted depending on whether it is within the predefined gating window. Some of these systems are gantry mounted while others are room mounted. A few of these systems are given below as examples.

Optical Imaging and 2D KV Orthogonal Imaging (Novalis Exactrac); Exactrac (Brain Lab, Feldkirchen, Germany) is a 6D automated patient positioning and verification system using infared (IR) reflectors and stereoscopic X-ray imaging. The system can provide image guidance with sub-millimetre precision in cranial and extra-cranial SRS treatments. Brain Lab image guidance system consists of two main components. These are; a positioning system with infrared patient tracking and a radiographic kV X-ray imaging system. In the infrared system; a ceiling mounted IR video camera sends low-intensity signals to spherical IR reflectors placed above the patient. In general, 4-6 reflectors are placed on the patient so that they are not in the same plane. External reflectors must be placed in a stable location for correct set-up. The IR camera retracts the reflected signal from the reflector. Therefore, position information is obtained. The IR system samples the position of the reflectors with a frequency of 20 Hz with an accuracy of better than 0.3 mm. Thus, the position of the patient is constantly monitored in real time during the treatment. The system can also automatically move the treatment couch to the desired position by using a table-mounted robotic system by matching the IR reflectors. In addition to the IR tracking system, the video camera image can be used as a stand-alone patient position verification tool. In the first set-up of the patient, the video image is recorded and compared with the images taken in other fractions (Gevaert et al., 2012). The Exactrac X-ray system consists of two floor-mounted X-ray tubes and two ceiling-mounted aSi plane panel detectors. Varian (Palo Alto, CA) has integrated the Exactrac Aurora IGRT system with the Varian on board imager (OBI). This system facilitates localisation of both fixed and moving targets that can be volumetrically visualised with CBCT. In addition, respiratory-controlled treatment can be performed under image guidance with the Exactrac system. The goal of respiratory-controlled therapy (RCT) is to irradiate the tumour during a defined phase of respiration. Thus, the amount of irradiated normal tissue can be reduced. The end-expiratory phase, which is generally considered to be the most stable and reproducible phase, is chosen for treatment. For the irradiation time, 20-30% of the whole respiration can be selected as the irradiation window. In order to perform RCT, external IR reflectors should be placed on the patient and fiducials near the isocentre within the tumour. With the time dependent movement of the reflectors, Exactrac displays the patient's respiratory movement curve. The reference level and irradiation range for the RCT can be adjusted individually on this curve. While IR reflectors provide the respiratory monitoring signal required for RCT; The X-ray system periodically verifies the patient's position relative to the irradiation range throughout RCT. Typically, the kV X-ray image is taken for target locaation as soon as the curve enters the irradiation range. Fiducials are determined in each X-ray image and compared to the DRR image obtained from the selected phase of 4DCT for planning. For adaptive RCT, a high degree of correlation between Fiducials and external reflectors is assumed (Willoughby et al., 2006).

3.2.3.2. 2D kV Stereoscopic Imaging (Cyberknife)

The CyberKnife (Accuray Inc., Sunnyvale, CA) intelligent IMRT system is a 6 MV X-ray generating linear accelerator mounted on a 6D robotic arm. There is a 6D robotic couch for patient positioning. The imaging system in CyberKnife consists of two diagnostic x-ray tubes mounted perpendicular to the ceiling and two opposing a-Si flat panel detectors. Stereoscopic X-ray imaging system; It provides real-time tumour tracking in both image-guided patient positioning and image-guided radiosurgery applications. In order to follow the target, the slice thickness should be <1.25 mm while the planning CT is scanned. A maximum of 512 images should be scanned with no gaps between sections (Antypas et al., 2008). Synchrony respiratory monitoring system is used especially in the treatment of lung tumours that are mobile due to respiration. The robotic arm can follow the tumour's movement due to breathing, thanks to its ability to move at a speed of several centimetres per second. The system uses a combination of infrared (IR) light emitting fiber optics placed on a vest worn on the patient and surgically placed fiducials markers. When the vest is worn by the patient, the external IR emitters are positioned to coincide with the abdominal region so that they can reflect the movement of the diaphragm and lungs. Since the tumour is in constant motion, an online radiograph is taken to follow the tumour. Cyberknife periodically takes snapshots of internal markers at regular intervals and at other times predicts the future location of the tumour position by tracking the movements of the external IR emitters. The IR emitted from the external IR emitters is continuously monitored by the charge-coupled device (CCD) camera. A computer algorithm models the motion correlation between external IR emitters and fiducials. Based on the movement of external IR emitters, the "Synchrony" system tracks the location of the internal markers and thus the location of the tumour. If breathing patterns change during treatment, the correlation model can be renewed (Ozhasoglu et al., 2008).

Conclusion

With the development of treatment techniques, IGRT has become a more effective treatment method today. IGRT is very important in terms of determining the accuracy of the treatment, especially in clinics where IMRT, VMAT, SRS and SBRT treatment techniques are frequently used. However, it should not be forgotten that in practice, the patient is given an extra dose, albeit a small one. Therefore, the IGRT technique and frequency should be adjusted based on clinical gain. It should also be considered that the QA of these IGRT systems is important to avoid treatment errors. In order to maintain the quality reliability of IGRT systems, daily, weekly, monthly and annual quality control tests should be carried out regularly. Each clinic should perform these tests for appropriate periods with forms specific to its own device and keep these tests after the approval of the responsible person.

References

Antypas, C., & Pantelis, E. (2008). Performance evaluation of a CyberKnife® G4 image-guided robotic stereotactic radiosurgery system. *Physics in Medicine & Biology*, *53*(17), 4697.

Balter, J. M., & Cao, Y. (2007, October). Advanced technologies in image-guided radiation therapy. In *Seminars in Radiation Oncology* (Vol. 17, No. 4, pp. 293-297). WB Saunders.

Bert, C., Metheany, K. G., Doppke, K. P., Taghian, A. G., Powell, S. N., & Chen, G. T. (2006). Clinical experience with a 3D surface patient setup system for alignment of partial-breast irradiation patients. *International Journal of Radiation Oncology* Biology* Physics*, *64*(4), 1265-1274.

Chandra, A., Dong, L., Huang, E., Kuban, D. A., O'Neill, L., Rosen, I., & Pollack, A. (2003). Experience of ultrasound-based daily prostate localization. *International Journal of Radiation Oncology* Biology* Physics*, *56*(2), 436-447.

de Crevoisier, R., Kuban, D., & Lefkopoulos, D. (2006). Image-guided radiotherapy by in-room CT-linear accelerator combination. *Cancer Radiotherapie: Journal de la Societe Francaise de Radiotherapie Oncologique*, *10*(5), 245-251.

Feldkamp, L. A., Davis, L. C., & Kress, J. W. (1984). Practical cone-beam algorithm. *Josa a*, *1*(6), 612-619.

Fung, A. Y., Ayyangar, K. M., Djajaputra, D., Nehru, R. M., & Enke, C. A. (2006). Ultrasound-based guidance of intensity-modulated radiation therapy. *Medical Dosimetry*, *31*(1), 20-29.

Gevaert, T., Verellen, D., Tournel, K., Linthout, N., Bral, S., Engels, B., & De Ridder, M. (2012). Setup accuracy of the Novalis ExacTrac 6DOF system for frameless radiosurgery. *International Journal of Radiation Oncology* Biology* Physics*, *82*(5), 1627-1635.

Göksel, E. O., Şenkesen, Ö., Tezcanlı, E., Garipağaoğlu, M., Küçücük, H., Şengoz, M., & Aslay, I. (2013). Monitoring the maintainability of deep inspiration phase with cine acquisition in patients with left-sided breast carcinoma receiving radiotherapy. *Nucl Med Radiat Ther*, *4*(1).

Green, O. L., Rankine, L. J., Cai, B., Curcuru, A., Kashani, R., Rodriguez, V., & Santanam, L. (2018). First clinical implementation of real-time, real anatomy tracking and radiation beam control. *Medical physics*, *45*(8), 3728-3740.

Herman, M. G., Balter, J. M., Jaffray, D. A., McGee, K. P., Munro, P., Shalev, S., & Wong, J. W. (2001). Clinical use of electronic portal imaging: report of AAPM Radiation Therapy Committee Task Group 58. *Medical Physics*, *28*(5), 712-737.

Hunt, A., Hansen, V. N., Oelfke, U., Nill, S., & Hafeez, S. (2018). Adaptive radiotherapy enabled by MRI guidance. *Clinical Oncology*, *30*(11), 711-719.

Jaffray, D. A., Drake, D. G., Moreau, M., Martinez, A. A., & Wong, J. W. (1999). A radiographic and tomographic imaging system integrated into a medical linear accelerator for localization of bone and soft-tissue targets. *International Journal of Radiation Oncology* Biology* Physics*, *45*(3), 773-789.

Jaffray, D. A., Siewerdsen, J. H., Wong, J. W., & Martinez, A. A. (2002). Flat-panel cone-beam computed tomography for image-guided radiation therapy. *International Journal of Radiation Oncology* Biology* Physics*, *53*(5), 1337-1349.

Kashani, R., & Olsen, J. R. (2018, July). Magnetic resonance imaging for target delineation and daily treatment modification. In *Seminars in radiation oncology* (Vol. 28, No. 3, pp. 178-184). WB Saunders.

Kleijnen, J. P. J., Van Asselen, B., Burbach, J. P., Intven, M., Philippens, M. E., Reerink, O., & Raaymakers, B. W. (2015). Evolution of motion uncertainty in rectal cancer: implications for adaptive radiotherapy. *Physics in Medicine & Biology*, *61*(1), 1.

Kontaxis, C., Bol, G. H., Kerkmeijer, L. G., Lagendijk, J. J., & Raaymakers, B. W. (2017). Fast online replanning for interfraction rotation correction in prostate radiotherapy. *Medical physics*, *44*(10), 5034-5042.

Korreman, S., Rasch, C., McNair, H., Verellen, D., Oelfke, U., Maingon, P., & Khoo, V. (2010). The European Society of Therapeutic Radiology and Oncology–European Institute of Radiotherapy (ESTRO–EIR) report on 3D CT-based in-room image guidance systems: a practical and technical review and guide. *Radiotherapy and Oncology*, *94*(2), 129-144.

Langen, K. M., Pouliot, J., Anezinos, C., Aubin, M., Gottschalk, A. R., Hsu, I. C., & Roach Iii, M. (2003). Evaluation of ultrasound-based prostate localization for image-guided radiotherapy. *International Journal of Radiation Oncology* Biology* Physics*, *57*(3), 635-644.

Lattanzi, J., McNeeley, S., Donnelly, S., Palacio, E., Hanlon, A., Schultheiss, T. E., & Hanks, G. E. (2000). Ultrasound-based stereotactic guidance in prostate cancer—quantification of organ motion and set-up errors in external beam radiation therapy. *Computer Aided Surgery*, *5*(4), 289-295.

Li, G., Mageras G. S., Dong L., Mohan R. (2012). Image guided radiation therapy. In: Khan M. F., Gerbi B. J. *Treatment Planning in Radiation Oncology*. 3rd Philadelphia, PA: Lippincott Williams & Wilkins, 229-258.

Litzenberg, D. W., Willoughby, T. R., Balter, J. M., Sandler, H. M., Wei, J., Kupelian, P. A., & Pouliot, J. (2007). Positional stability of electromagnetic transponders used for prostate localization and continuous, real-time tracking. *International Journal of Radiation Oncology* Biology* Physics*, *68*(4), 1199-1206.

Meeks, S. L., Harmon Jr, J. F., Langen, K. M., Willoughby, T. R., Wagner, T. H., & Kupelian, P. A. (2005). Performance characterization of megavoltage computed tomography imaging on a helical tomotherapy unit. *Medical physics*, *32*(8), 2673-2681.

Mundt, A. J., & Roeske, J. C. (Eds.). (2010). *Image-guided radiation therapy: A clinical perspective*. PMPH-USA.

Ozhasoglu, C., Saw, C. B., Chen, H., Burton, S., Komanduri, K., Yue, N. J., & Heron, D. E. (2008). Synchrony–cyberknife respiratory compensation technology. *Medical Dosimetry*, *33*(2), 117-123.

Robinson, D., Liu, D., Steciw, S., Field, C., Daly, H., Saibishkumar, E. P., & Amanie, J. (2012). An evaluation of the Clarity 3D ultrasound system for prostate localization. *Journal of applied clinical medical physics*, *13*(4), 100-112.

Saenz, D. L., Paliwal, B. R., & Bayouth, J. E. (2014). A dose homogeneity and conformity evaluation between ViewRay and pinnacle-based linear accelerator IMRT treatment plans. *Journal of medical physics/Association of Medical Physicists of India*, *39*(2), 64.

Santos, J., Popple, R., Agazaryan, N., Bayouth, J. E., Bissonnette, J. P., Bucci, M. K., & Chetty, I. J. (2013). Image guided radiation therapy (IGRT) technologies for radiation therapy localization and delivery. *International journal of radiation oncology, biology, physics*, *87*(1), 33-45.

Song, W. Y., Kamath, S., Ozawa, S., Al Ani, S., Chvetsov, A., Bhandare, N., & Li, J. G. (2008). A dose comparison study between XVI® and OBI® CBCT systems. *Medical physics*, *35*(2), 480-486.

Stemkens, B., Glitzner, M., Kontaxis, C., De Senneville, B. D., Prins, F. M., Crijns, S. P., & Tijssen, R. H. (2017). Effect of intra-fraction motion on the accumulated dose for free-breathing MR-guided stereotactic body radiation therapy of renal-cell carcinoma. *Physics in Medicine & Biology*, *62*(18), 7407.

Tomé, W. A., Meeks, S. L., Orton, N. P., Bouchet, L. G., & Bova, F. J. (2002). Commissioning and quality assurance of an optically guided three-dimensional ultrasound target localization system for radiotherapy. *Medical physics*, *29*(8), 1781-1788.

Van Herk, M., Remeijer, P., Rasch, C., & Lebesque, J. V. (2000). The probability of correct target dosage: dose-population histograms for deriving treatment margins in radiotherapy. *International Journal of Radiation Oncology* Biology* Physics*, *47*(4), 1121-1135.

Walter, C., Boda-Heggemann, J., Wertz, H., Loeb, I., Rahn, A., Lohr, F., & Wenz, F. (2007). Phantom and *in-vivo* measurements of dose exposure by image-guided radiotherapy (IGRT): MV portal images vs. kV portal images vs. cone-beam CT. *Radiotherapy and Oncology*, *85*(3), 418-423.

Willoughby, T. R., Forbes, A. R., Buchholz, D., Langen, K. M., Wagner, T. H., Zeidan, O. A., & Meeks, S. L. (2006). Evaluation of an infrared camera and X-ray system using implanted fiducials in patients with lung tumors for gated radiation therapy. *International Journal of Radiation Oncology* Biology* Physics*, *66*(2), 568-575.

Chapter 11

Respiratory Motion Management in Intensity Modulated Radiotherapy

Murat Koylu*

Department of Radiation Oncology, Ege University School of Medicine, Izmir, Turkey

Abstract

Intensity modulated radiotherapy (IMRT), which provides an increase in the treatment dose and a decrease in morbidity, improves the results of the treatment. Especially in the irradiation of mobile region tumours such as thorax and abdomen, the application of IMRT with high accuracy poses a problem. In these tumours, it is important to monitor and manage the movement of the patient's breathing. There are many respiratory monitoring methods and devices developed for this purpose. We can classify the methods developed for monitoring respiratory movement in radiotherapy in four major categories as respiratory gating techniques, breath-hold techniques, forced shallow breathing techniques, and respiration synchronised techniques. Using these techniques, respiration-related tumour displacement is detected and extra margins that will be given to the tumour due to movement are eliminated. In this way, better protection of normal healthy tissues, which is among the goals of IMRT, can be achieved. In this chapter, the management of respiratory movements in IMRT will be examined.

Keywords: breath, intensity modulated radiotherapy, motion management, respiratory

---

*Corresponding Author's Email: murat.koylu@ege.edu.tr.

In: Frontiers in Intensity-Modulated Radiotherapy Research
Editor: Sibel Karaca
ISBN: 979-8-88697-252-8

1. Introduction

Intensity-modulated radiation therapy (IMRT) is a widely used radiotherapy method to deliver high doses to tumours in many regions (Smith et al., 2009). Treatment outcomes improve with IMRT, which increases the treatment dose and reduces morbidity (Yorke et al., 2000). IMRT achieves this by allowing dose increase to the target volume and dose decrease in close normal tissues. The most important and unique characteristic feature about IMRT is that each area consists of lots of subfields or segments that will be applied sequentially (Chen et al., 2009). The main principle in advanced treatment techniques like IMRT is that complex dose distributions can be applied with high accuracy (Zhang et al., 2008). To protect an organ at risk (OAR) close to the tumour, a characteristic steep dose gradient must be established and applied exactly as planned. A more accurate patient setup and target position information is an important requirement for more precise radiotherapy techniques. It is therefore important to properly account for the interfractional and intrafractional movement of the target (Tacke et al., 2010). In image-guided radiotherapy (IGRT), the determination of intrafractional motion of the tumour has become an increasingly important issue (Keall and Mageras, 2004). Respiratory motion or gastrointestinal fluctuations induce intrafractional movement of the target. The intrafractional movement of the tumour causes significant dosimetric and geometric uncertainties in the dose delivery and treatment planning stages of radiotherapy (Sawant et al., 2008).

In thoracic and abdominal IMRT respiratory motion is the major problem. Induction of target motion by breathing in the abdominal and thoracic region increases the uncertainty of the target position (Hugo et al., 2002). Such motion and uncertainties cause significant limitations during the entire radiotherapy process (Ahunbay and Li, 2007). The fact that patient breathing increases target motion in imaging and treatment is one of the main challenges in dose escalation in thoracic tumours (Zhang et al., 2008). Intrafractional tumour motion can adversely affect the benefits of IMRT treatments with a high dose gradient. As a result, healthy tissues are irradiated more than desired and the increase in tumor dose may be limited. Many publications have shown that respiratory induced motions can be as large as 3-5 cm (Brandner et al., 2017; Chen et al., 2009; Keall et al., 2006b). But, the motion of lung tumours is generally less than 5 mm. It is known that liver, spleen and kidneys in the upper abdomen move more than 10 mm as a result of respiration (Brandner et al., 2017). Increasing the margin given to the target to enclose the maximum range of movement is a common solution. However, these widening margins, which cause neighbouring healthy tissues or critical structures to enter the treatment field, cause an increase in radiation-related complications. Continuous online adaptation of dose delivery is required to eliminate intra-fractional motion (Tacke et al., 2010).

There is no general model of breathing behaviour that can be used prior to observation for a given patient, as respiratory movement patterns can vary between and even within fractions. Respiratory movement is patient specific, and characteristics of respiratory may differ in amplitude, regularity and period (Brandner et al., 2017). Respiration-induced motion of tumours and healthy critical structures in the lung and upper abdominal region should be monitored and taken into account. To effectively manage intrafractional motion, radiation delivery techniques such as breath hold techniques, respiratory gating, manual beam gating, and four-dimensional (4D) planning/tracking have been developed (Smith et al., 2009). Different technologies have been developed to monitor respiration and target movements. These are, target motion surrogates, respiratory air flow monitoring, surface tension variations record devices, and camera-based passive and active motion monitor markers positioned on a patient's skin (Solberg et al., 2006). These techniques, which require patient cooperation in practice, have the potential to use a smaller internal margins and thus irradiate less healthy tissue (Abbas et al., 2014). The techniques used to predict the target's location are based on, internal anatomic structures, implanted internal markers, or imaging external markers (Sawant et al., 2008).

One of the ways used to manage breathing movement during radiotherapy is the respiratory gating method. Respiratory gating is a commercially used respiratory motion management system. Respiratory gating, commonly referred to as a "gate," involves administration of radiation during both treatment application and imaging during a specific portion of the patient's respiratory cycle (Keall et al., 2006b). Gating system only reduces the motion during radiotherapy, it cannot eliminate the interaction between the multi leaf collimator and residual organ movement. More residual movement during IMRT delivery, the greater the motion artifacts in the resulting doses. Using the gating method, the patient's breathing is monitored and target motion is reduced by activating the radiation of the linear accelerator at a chosen part of the breathing cycle (Yorke et al., 2000). The limitation of gating that if the tumour has moved outside of the gating volume for an extended period of time, the gating system cannot take this into account, and treatment is paused until the patient can be readjusted manually (Smith et al., 2009).

Respiratory movement characterised by two variables which are recorded as respiratory signal or internal anatomy movement (Keall et al., 2006b). Gating method is implemented in two ways as phase gating and displacement gating. In displacement of respiratory signal, the relative displacement gating position between the extreme respiratory motions, called exhalation and inhalation, is measured. Displacement gating, the radiation beam activated when the respiratory signal within a preset relative position screen.

2. Respiratory Motion Management Techniques

Breathing motion in radiotherapy divided into four main categories: breath-hold techniques, respiratory gating techniques, respiration synchronised methods, and forced shallow respire techniques.

2.1. Shallow Breathing with Abdominal Compression

The magnitude of intrafractional movement is decreased using forced shallow breathing techniques. This method is frequently used approach in the control of tumour or organ movement. There are several commercially available abdominal compression devices in clinical use. The compression device has of a compression belt that can be attached to the treatment table top and a compression plate that presses against the abdomen (Abbas et al., 2014). With the pressure applied to the abdomen, the motion of the diaphragm is minimised and thus, the circulating gas volume during normal breathing decreases, allowing limited normal breathing (Keall and Mageras, 2004). The used arch position can be adjusted both longitudinally and vertically accommodate patient anatomy. The pressure apparatus used is typically positioned 2-3 cm below the triangular rib cage boundary. The magnitude of the pressure on the abdominal region can be regulated with the help of a screw that can be adjusted up and down. Thanks to this applied pressure, the motion of the diaphragm decreases and the target localisation in the abdomen is improved.

Another way to apply pressure to the abdominal region is to use a compression belt instead of a hard compression arch. This belt includes an air bag that fits over the abdomen. In order to create a desired pressure on the abdomen, this air bag is inflated and creates a compression on the patient's abdominal region. The amount of pressure applied and the reproducibility of the pressure plate position between simulation and daily therapy determine the effectiveness of the use of abdominal compression (Abbas et al., 2014).

2.2. Breathing Control

2.2.1. Breath Hold

Breath-holding techniques can restrict respiratory movement. Motion during CT imaging and treatment is effectively reduced by breath-hold techniques. CT simulation or radiotherapy is delivered within the breath-hold interval, with the patient voluntarily holding his/her breath. In this method, treatment machines with a controlled beam turn-off interlock are used that can automatically stop the treatment delivery when the patient's breath goes out of the specified tolerance range (Abbas et al., 2014). Although the technical requirements are similar to free-breathing gating, this method is more efficient where radiation is delivered continuously during breath-hold (Abbas et al., 2014).

In this method, where patient selection is very important, the patient must be able to hold his/her breath for at least 10 seconds reproducibly. It should be verified that the anatomy of the patient has minimum movement while breath-hold. Uncertainty in the reproducibility of breath-hold, residual anatomical motion, and setup uncertainties must be taken into account when constructing the PTV. Maximum benefit is obtained from the breath-hold technique during the inhalation and exhalation phases of the respiratory cycle, where mobility of the internal organ is minimised. The exhalation phase of breath-hold is more reproducible than the inhale phase (Solberg et al., 2006). The repeatability and stability of breath-hold should be verified by tracking the breathing of the patient (Abbas et al., 2014).

Various respiration monitoring tools have been developed to preserve the reproducibility of breath-hold techniques. Among these monitors spirometers, thermal sensors near nostrils, cameras tracking reflective markers, strain gages affixed to the torso, fluoroscopic images of implanted fiducials, and implanted transponders (Brandner et al., 2017). Breath-hold can be limited to a certain volume by attaching valves to spirometers, which are used to measure breath volume.

2.2.1.1. Active Breathing Control

One of the methods that facilitate reproducible breath-hold is the active-breathing control (ABC) method (Keall et al., 2006b). This method does not require the patient to reach the highest inspiration capacity to be used, thus facilitating reproducible breath-hold (Keall and Mageras, 2004). Simulation, treatment planning and delivery are performed using the same active breath-hold conditions and minimum margin for breathing motion. The active breathing control method was commercialised by ELEKTA company with an active breathing coordinator device (Keall and Mageras, 2004; Keall et al., 2006b). The active breath coordinator can be used to prop up temporarily take a breath during inspiration (Ahunbay and Li, 2007). It is generally used in deep inhales or moderate breathing. The device bonded to a balloon valve and measures the respiratory trace via a spirometer (Frazier et al., 2004) (Figure1).

In the ABC procedure, the patient breathes normally while connected to the device. In this phase, the valve inflates for a pre-defined duration time and the patient's breath is held. The patient's breath hold duration is typically chosen between 15-30 seconds to provide repeatable breath hold without causing unnecessary patient distress.

The processing and control of the data obtained by the system is carried out on the laptop computer outside the treatment room. The patient watches through the prism glass provided in the room and follows the respiratory trace and breath-hold duration on the flat panel screen (Remouchamps et al., 2003). The same screen and command functions are also seen by the team outside the treatment room.

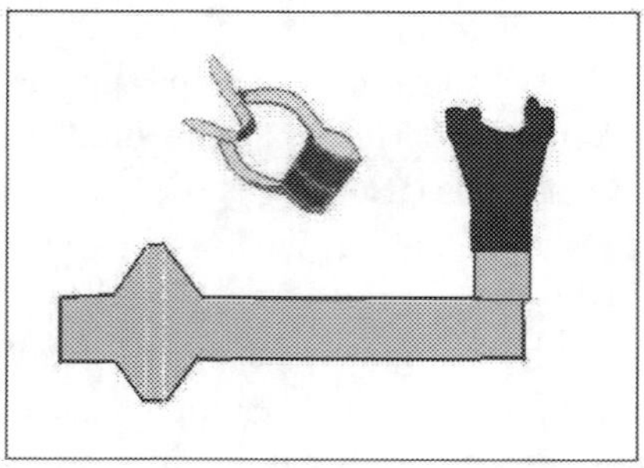

Figure 1. Active breathing coordinator device mouthpiece and filter kid.

2.2.1.2. Deep Inspiration

Deep inspiration breath-hold (DIBH), a type of self-held breath-hold technique, is used in the treatment of left breast and lung cancer (Abbas et al., 2014). The reproducible deep breath-hold technique is advantageous in the treatment of breast tumours. Since it reduces tumour movement and changes the anatomy in a way that protects organs at risk (Keall and Mageras, 2004).

Although the DIBH technique is mostly used in lung, breast and abdominal cancers.

The patient should be verbally coached to ensure reproducible deep inhale breath-hold during simulation and treatment in the DIBH technique (Keall et al., 2006b). Many methods have been developed for the implementation of the DIBH technique. All methods developed require patient compliance, active participation and the use of extra therapists (Keall and Mageras, 2004). In this method, the patient breathes using a mouthpiece connected by soft pipes to a spirometer. The nose is closed with a nose clip so that breathing is done only through the mouth. The airflow rate from the spirometer is converted into a respiratory signal as a function of time with the help of a computer programme (Keall et al., 2006b). When the target is at the breath-hold level, the therapist turns on the beam and instructs to stop the therapy if it goes out of this level.

2.2.1.3. Breath-Hold without Respiratory Monitoring

In self-held breath-hold techniques, the patient holds their breath at one point in the respiratory cycle (Keall and Mageras, 2004). The irradiation is done during the breath-hold and the required dose is administered to the tumour. According to the amount of time the patient can hold their breath, one or more breath-holds may be required for irradiation from that field. An effective control system for the linear accelerator is required to effectively deliver the radiation to the patient during breath-hold.

For Varian C series linear accelerators, a control system using the "customer minor (CMNR)" interlock was developed and used in the implementation of the self-breath-hold technique (Keall and Mageras, 2004). In this system, the patient is given a hand-held switch connected to the CMNR interlock circuit. The therapist's ability to activate the beam depends on the patient unlocking the CMNR interlock on the console by pressing the switch. If the switch is released, the CMNR interlock will be activated and irradiation will be disabled up to the switch is pressed again.

2.2.1.4. Breath-Hold with Respiratory Monitoring

This technique, which requires patients to hold their breath for a specific part of the respiratory cycle, makes use of a device (Varina RPM) to track the breath of the patient. The ideal of self-breath-hold treatment delivery is the monitoring of active respiratory (Abbas et al., 2014). An advantage of this technique is that it possibly be applied more effective than respiratory-gated techniques since the radiation is not stopped applied during breath-hold. Another advantage is that the irradiation is automatically held in case the breath-holding level deviates from what is intended as a result of continuous monitoring of the patient's respiration constantly.

2.3. Respiratory Gating

In the respiratory gating method, the aim is to irradiate the tumour while it reaches a predefined position in the respiratory cycle. In this way, the margins required to create CTV-PTV can be greatly reduced (Abbas et al., 2014). The respiratory signal or the movement of the internal anatomy can be used to characterise respiratory motion. The respiratory gating technique, often called a "gate," involves delivering radiation during a specific part of the patient's breathing cycle (Keall and Mageras, 2004; Keall et al., 2006b). The location and amplitude of the gate to be used in the breathing cycle is determined by monitoring the patient's breathing movement. The task cycle, which is a measure of the effectiveness of the method used, is the ratio of the time spent by the signal in the "gate" to the total treatment time (Keall and Mageras, 2004). In this method, unlike the self-breath-hold technique, radiation is triggered when the respiratory signal enters the defined range in the predefined breathing cycle and the patient continues to breathe normally. Since there is no obligation to hold the breath, respiratory gating methods are much easier for patients. In this technique, gating takes longer to deliver the same prescribed dose as the radiation is given only during certain segment (30-50%) of the breathing cycle (Abbas et al., 2014; Keall et al., 2006b).

Respiratory gating treatments using external surrogates are more common. The respiratory signal is usually obtained by respiratory movement of the chest wall. Examples of these external surrogates are the chest wall surface, lung air volume exchange measured by spirometry and infrared markers placed on surface of abdomen. Reproducible respiratory patterns and accurate representation of target/organ location time-depend by surrogates monitored by the gating system are required in external gating (Abbas et al., 2014). Natural respiration always involves some disorder. Visual or auditory coaching increases the reproducibility of the respiratory cycle.

Real-time display of target or reference marker placed in target volume creates internal surrogates. Internal surrogates enable us to obtain the most correct information about the target/organ location to be used in beam gating.

When it comes to the use of gate radiotherapy, several issues need to be considered. The gating method is generally referred a phase gating or displacement gating (amplitude) (Brandner et al., 2017; Keall et al., 2006b).

Computed tomography (CT) obtainment and treatment are delivered within the same respiratory window depending on the patient's amplitude or respiratory phase (Abbas et al., 2014). The relative position between two extreme respiratory movements (inhalation and exhalation) is measured by the displacement of the respiratory signal. Activation of radiation in displacement-based gating occurs when the respiratory signal is within the pre-set relative position window. The second variable, the phase, is calculated with the help of the algorithm, which is the periodicity criteria that must be met by using the respiratory signal. Radiation beam in the phase-based gate is activated while the phase of the breathing signal is within the preset phase window (Keall et al., 2006b). While there is less residual motion in amplitude-based gating, gating is easier to coach in phase-based gating. Amplitude-based binning is more accurate and consistent than the phase-based binning.

Treatments can be gated by synchronising the respiratory motion with a breathing monitor to be used. Thresholds can be set on the breathing monitor so that the beam can be turned on and off at certain respiratory phases and amplitudes (Brandner et al., 2017). With the help of the acquired 4D CT, it is determined which phases or amplitudes will be included in the gating window. While determining the window to be chosen, attention is paid to keeping the target or critical structure movement within acceptable limits. Cantering of the gating window is done on the end-exhalation, where it is most stable.

2.3.1. Residual Tumour Motion within the Gating Window

Breath-hold respiratory gating reduces movement but some residual movement will remain (Solberg et al., 2006). If some tumour motion still remains in the gate, it is called "residual motion." The gate amplitude is selected by looking at the balance between the residual amount of movement and the duty cycle. Reducing the size of the window, which negatively affects the gated treatments by causing longer treatment times, reduces the size of the residual motion. With the use of audio-visual breathing coaching, residual movement is reduced, increasing the effectiveness and efficiency of respiratory-gated treatments (Solberg et al., 2006).

2.3.2. Gating Using an External Respiration Signal

Active gating is one of the external radiotherapy methods operated on areas affected by intra-fractional movement (Solberg et al., 2006). Respiratory gating includes the application of radiation inside a specific window in the patient's breathing cycle. In order to apply this method, the respiratory motion of the patient should be monitored using external or internal fiducial markers.

One of the sources of error is that the tumour motion monitored doesn't match target location timed by gating system. The difficulties in real-time detection of the moving tumour position along the treatment constitute the biggest barrier to active gating. Respiratory motion management is also performed using three-dimensional video cameras.

Some of the respiratory gating systems used commercially are the Varian RPM system and the BrainLab Exactrac gating system. The RPM system uses an infrared reflective plastic box. This box is positioned in the midline between the xyphoid process and the umbilicus. The optimal position of the reflector box is chosen to maximise respiration-induced motion. The position of the marked box is adjusted horizontally so that the in-room camera can detect reflective markers correctly (Keall et al., 2006b)

The RPM gating system, which detects tumour motion using an external IR marker, may not always be associated with internal movement (Solberg et al., 2006). The ExacTrac gating system is combined with external markers and a radiography system. This device which has x-ray imaging system to check the reproducibility of internal anatomy during treatment uses external markers in radiation beam gating (Keall et al., 2006a; Keall et al., 2006b). This system determines the respiratory model using an IR camera and reflective markers. When this system detects a respiratory model, it can use each of the diagnostic x-ray units at a user-specified point in the respiratory cycle. The three-dimensional (3D) position of the internal radio-opaque fiducial can be determined from these two images. At this point the patient is moved to the true treatment position using internal markers. Because these markers are so close to tumour, they are more advantageous than positioning with external fiducial points (Solberg et al., 2006). Besides, the system can trigger the accelerator at the point of respiratory cycle point where localisation x-rays are acquired. In the latest versions of Exactrac, there is no need for fiducial markers placed on the surface. In this new version, the skin surface is followed by both a digital camera and a thermal camera (Figure 2).

2.3.3. Gating Using Internal Fiducial Markers

Real-time tumour monitoring radiotherapy system that uses radiography of implanted fudicial markers to gate the deliver beam. The fiducial location is monitored in three times per second using a dual x-ray imaging system. Linear accelerator delivers radiation when each fiducial is in limits for both x-ray cameras.

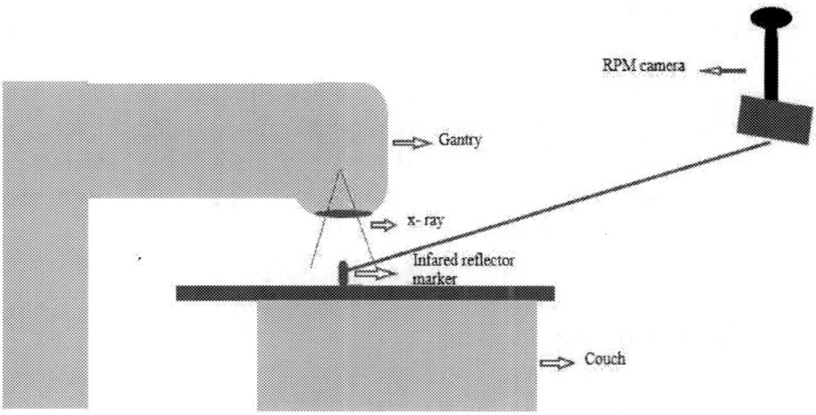

Figure 2. Reel time position manager system.

At the start of each treatment, the patient's breathing cycle is monitored with the aid of the reference marker. At the beginning of each treatment, the fiducial marker pathway is monitored several times in the patient's breathing cycle and the patient is repositioned if necessary. In this way, the fiducial marker passes near the predicted position in the breathing cycle. The beam is enabled when a total of two gates from each imaging system overlap. In this method whole treatment takes more than 30 minutes, but this time varies depending on the patient-dependent duty cycle and the choosing breathing cycle part to be used in the treatment (Keall et al., 2006b).

2.3.4. Gated IMRT

The duration of treatment is prolonged when respiratory gating is applied. This results in a 4 to 15-fold increase in treatment time over a conventional therapy for gated IMRT. The dose rate can be increased to reduce this increase in treatment time. By increasing the dose rate from 300 MU/min to 600 MU/min, the clock time can be reduced by approximately 40% (Keall et al., 2006b). Depending on patient compliance, gated treatment session times increase between 2 to 10 minutes. The increase in delivery time results in patient comfort, the possibility of increased patient motion. It is suggested that the increase in the duration of treatment sessions will lead to a reduce in tumour control due to the increase in intrafraction repair of sublethal damaged tumour cells (Keall et al., 2006b).

The dosimetry of the movable gated IMRT is the same as the immobile. Deformation of the target isn't taken into account. Gated treatment can be applied in both arc therapy and tomotherapy. In this scenario, the accelerator is gating by repeating an arc or continuous rotation until the radiation that needs to be delivered from each beam is applied (Keall et al., 2006b). The couch remains stationary until all pulses of the beam have been delivered and then indexed to its next position. The same method applies to helical delivery. In this case, the treatment helix is repeated until all pulses have been delivered for each angle.

2.4. Real Time Tumour Tracking

The best way to adapt to the motion caused by breathing is to follow the change in tumour location along with the free aspiration. Nevertheless, clinical experience with this is limited (Keall and Mageras, 2004). This technique is also called the respiratory-synchronised or real-time tracking method. The most advanced breath monitoring methods are tumour monitoring or respiratory synchronisation (Solberg et al., 2006). In the condition that organ/tumour movement can be monitored continuously, the system that will deliver radiation should also be designed to follow the moving target (Abbas et al., 2014; Keall and Mageras, 2004). In this method, a "dose distribution" in three dimension is shifted to follow the tumour's location in space. In this way, the margin to be given for tumour motion is eliminated and the amount of irradiated normal tissue is reduced. It provides the most efficient dose delivery (100% duty cycle) by eliminating the need for gating and breath- hold methods. In this method it is necessary to define the target location accurately in real time. In this technique, target volume or internal surrogates must be monitored directly. The correlation between the external surrogate's location and the tumour should be maintained and confirmed throughout the respiratory cycle.

Tracking tumour location using real-time tracking is a difficult task. Tumour tracking is technologically difficult for many reasons. There are four possible ways of tumour position along with the treatment,

1. Real-time imaging of the target
2. Real-time imaging of artificial fiducial markers
3. Extraction of the tumour location from surrogate respiratory movement signals
4. Non-radiographic monitoring of a signalling device implanted in the tumour.

Although all of them are used clinically, the improvement phases are still ongoing (Solberg et al., 2006; Keall et al., 2006b). Accurate target motion prediction is a necessity due to the time delay between determining the tumour's location and the system's answer to this modification (Solberg et al., 2006).

In addition, it should be checked whether the normal tissue protection is as planned by confirming the relationship of the adjacent structures with the target (Abbas et al., 2014). Dynamically adjusting the beam according to the detected target motion is another major requirement of this approach. This method should have the following properties,

1. Determine the target location in real time
2. Making up time delays in the response of the beam by predicting target motion
3. Reposition the beam
4. Customise the dosimetry to allow for changing lung volume and critical structure positions during the respiratory cycle.

Another technique of adapting to breathing movement is real-time tumour tracking. In this method, the changing location of the tumour is followed by dynamically repositioning the radiation beam. Real-time tumour tracking can be performed with the robotic arm linear accelerator (Keall et al., 2006b). Another real-time tumour tracking method is collimate the target to the beam by moving the couch. A good example is the Synchrony respiratory monitoring system, which creates a model of target motion by associating both the reference marker implanted in tumour and the external markers (Brandner et al., 2017).

Understanding respiratory target motion by following its anatomy has become a widely used method because it is practical and non-invasive. Organ motion is determined by following the reflective markers placed on the chest surface with a camera-based system. This method, which uses infrared illumination of reflective markers, used by the real-time position management RPM system (Solberg et al., 2006). A major drawback of the RPM system with a single camera is that it cannot determine the position of a single marker in absolute spatial coordinates. So, it doesn't offer much additional gain from a strain gauge or spirometer. In addition, the 1D signal cannot adequately characterie patient respiratory motion. Three-dimensional location of an object can be determined more than two-dimensional image with the stereophotogrammetry method used to overcome this deficiency.

The ExacTrac gating system uses passive infrared (IR) reflecting spheres instead of active LEDs (Hugo et al., 2002; Solberg et al., 2006). Consisting of two IR cameras that reflect and detect a low infrared signal, this system is quick and simple to calibrate. An amplitude-based gating window is selected with the help of respiratory trace and amplitude calculated from marker positions (Hugo et al., 2002). The system has subsequently been adopted for use in respiratory correlated imaging and gated radiotherapy (Solberg et al., 2006). The latest version of the Exactrac system does not require a fiducial marker. While monitoring the surface with thermal and video cameras, can provide internal anatomical control with x-rays (Figure 3).

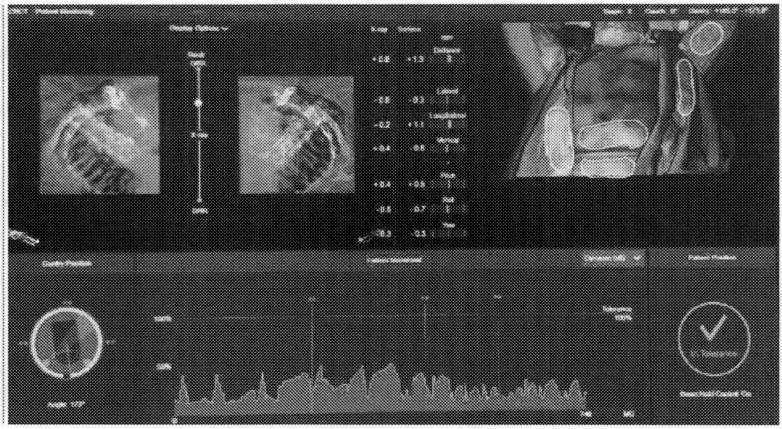

Figure 3. Exactrac internal and surface tracking system working.

Target motion is tracked in real time thanks to the dynamic multi-leaf collimator used to constantly align and reshape the treatment machine apertures (Brandner et al., 2017). This allows the dose distribution to be adapted to the tumour motion by applying tighter margins.

Conclusion

IMRT in which increasing the treatment dose and reducing morbidity is the main goal, improves treatment results (Yorke et al., 2000). With the help of its characteristic steep dose gradient, it is necessary to give the planned dose exactly in order to maintain the organ at risk adjacent to the tumour (Tacke et al., 2010). Since it is a more precise radiotherapy technique than conformal techniques, it requires a more accurate patient setup and target position information (Hugo et al., 2002). Geometric and dosimetric uncertainties occur in radiotherapy as a result of the intrafraction motion (Sawant et al., 2008). Respiratory movement is a big problem in IMRT of abdominal and thoracic tumours. Continuous momentary modification of dose delivery is required to compensate for intrafractional movement. External markers used to predict target position are internal anatomic structures, imaging external markers and implanted internal markers. Breathing movement can be represented by two factor registered as breathing signal or internal anatomy movement (Keall et al., 2006a). The gating methods are called displacement gating or phase gating. Motion from breathing can be restricted using breath-hold techniques. Different respiratory monitoring tools have been developed for the reproducible application of breath-hold methods. These monitors consist of spirometers, cameras tracking reflective markers, laser systems, mechanical devices tracking the torso, strain gages, thermal sensors, implanted fiducials and implanted transponders (Brandner et al., 2017). Active Breath Control facilitates repeatable breath-hold without the need for maximum inspiration (Keall and Mageras, 2004). One form of self-held-breath hold technique is the deep inspiratory breath-hold technique used for left breast and lung cancers. With the respiratory gating methods, irradiation is performed only when the target volume reaches the predefined location in the respiratory cycle (Abbas et al., 2014). Motion management in IMRT gains importance especially in regions with respiratory motion. Selecting and using the most suitable respiratory monitoring device within the available means is necessary for the success of the treatment.

References

Abbas, H., Chang, B., & Chen, Z. J. (2014). Motion management in gastrointestinal cancers. *Journal of gastrointestinal oncology*, *5*(3), 223.

Ahunbay, E., & Li, X. A. (2007). Investigation of the reliability, accuracy, and efficiency of gated IMRT delivery with a commercial linear accelerator. *Medical physics*, *34*(7), 2928-2938.

Brandner, E. D., Chetty, I. J., Giaddui, T. G., Xiao, Y., & Huq, M. S. (2017). Motion management strategies and technical issues associated with stereotactic body radiotherapy of thoracic and upper abdominal tumors: a review from NRG oncology. *Medical physics*, *44*(6), 2595-2612.

Chen, H., Wu, A., Brandner, E. D., Heron, D. E., Huq, M. S., Yue, N. J., & Chen, W. C. (2009). Dosimetric evaluations of the interplay effect in respiratory-gated intensity-modulated radiation therapy. *Medical physics*, *36*(3), 893-903.

Frazier, R. C., Vicini, F. A., Sharpe, M. B., Yan, D., Fayad, J., Baglan, K. L., & Wong, J. W. (2004). Impact of breathing motion on whole breast radiotherapy: a dosimetric analysis using active breathing control. *International Journal of Radiation Oncology* Biology* Physics*, *58*(4), 1041-1047.

Hugo, G. D., Agazaryan, N., & Solberg, T. D. (2002). An evaluation of gating window size, delivery method, and composite field dosimetry of respiratory-gated IMRT. *Medical physics*, *29*(11), 2517-2525.

Keall, P., & Mageras, G. (2004). Managing respiratory motion in radiation therapy. *American Association of Physicists in Medicine*.

Keall, P. J., Mageras, G. S., Balter, J. M., Emery, R. S., Forster, K. M., Jiang, S. B., & Yorke, E. (2006a). The management of respiratory motion in radiation oncology report of AAPM Task Group 76 a. *Medical physics*, *33*(10), 3874-3900.

Keall, P., Vedam, S., George, R., Bartee, C., Siebers, J., Lerma, F., & Chung, T. (2006b). The clinical implementation of respiratory-gated intensity-modulated radiotherapy. *Medical Dosimetry*, *31*(2), 152-162.

Remouchamps, V. M., Letts, N., Vicini, F. A., Sharpe, M. B., Kestin, L. L., Chen, P. Y., & Wong, J. W. (2003). Initial clinical experience with moderate deep-inspiration breath hold using an active breathing control device in the treatment of patients with left-sided breast cancer using external beam radiation therapy. *International Journal of Radiation Oncology* Biology* Physics*, *56*(3), 704-715.

Sawant, A., Venkat, R., Srivastava, V., Carlson, D., Povzner, S., Cattell, H., & Keall, P. (2008). Management of three-dimensional intrafraction motion through real-time DMLC tracking. *Medical physics*, *35*(5), 2050-2061.

Sawant, A., Smith, R. L., Venkat, R. B., Santanam, L., Cho, B., Poulsen, P., & Keall, P. J. (2009). Toward submillimeter accuracy in the management of intrafraction motion: the integration of real-time internal position monitoring and multileaf collimator target tracking. *International Journal of Radiation Oncology* Biology* Physics*, *74*(2), 575-582.

Solberg, T. D., Wink, N. M., Tenn, S. E., Kriminski, S., Hugo, G. D., & Agazaryan, N. (2006). Control of breathing motion: Techniques and models (gated radiotherapy). In *New Technologies in Radiation Oncology* (pp. 299-319). Springer, Berlin, Heidelberg.

Tacke, M. B., Nill, S., Krauss, A., & Oelfke, U. (2010). Real-time tumor tracking: automatic compensation of target motion using the Siemens 160 MLC. *Medical physics*, *37*(2), 753-761.

Yorke, E., Mageras, G., LoSasso, T., Mostafavi, H., & Ling, C. (2000, July). Respiratory gating of sliding window IMRT. In *Proceedings of the 22nd Annual International Conference of the IEEE Engineering in Medicine and Biology Society (Cat. No. 00CH37143)* (Vol. 3, pp. 2118-2121). IEEE.

Zhang, Peng, Geoffrey D. Hugo, and Di Yan. (2008). Planning Study Comparison of Real-Time Target Tracking and Four-Dimensional Inverse Planning for Managing Patient Respiratory Motion. *International Journal of Radiation Oncology Biology Physics* 72 (4): 1221–27.

Chapter 12

IMRT Treatment Planning

Ayse Gulbin Kavak*

Radiation Oncology Department, Gaziantep University, Gaziantep, Turkey

Abstract

Radiotherapy is one of the treatments that can be applied before or after surgery, together with chemotherapy or alone for most types of cancer. The aim of radiotherapy is to preserve healthy structures as much as possible while treating cancerous cells. Although radiotherapy treatment techniques are increasing day by day, Intensity Modulated Radiation Therapy (IMRT) and Intensity Modulated Arc Therapy (IMAT) are the most used techniques. These techniques try to find the best result for planning by using the optimisation method. Many factors can affect the quality of the desired plan. The first of these is the experience of the planner. Accurate identification of dose constraints significantly improves plan quality. Even if the planner has sufficient planning experience, it is not possible to try all alternative possibilities for the plan due to clinical intensity. Therefore, the multi-criteria optimisation (MCO) method was developed to solve this problem. MCO is a software feature that generates different Pareto plans in a single optimisation calculation. In this method, plans with different dose distributions can be viewed at the same time. Thanks to this feature, the decision-making process of the radiation oncologist is accelerated, and as a result, the clinical workload of the planner is reduced. The MCO method is an applicable feature that provides a time advantage in terms of clinical use. This book chapter, it is aimed to explain the multi-criteria optimisation method developed as an alternative to the standard optimisation method in radiotherapy treatment planning.

---

*Corresponding Author's Email: gkavak@gantep.edu.tr.

In: Frontiers in Intensity-Modulated Radiotherapy Research
Editor: Sibel Karaca
ISBN: 979-8-88697-252-8

Keywords: IMAT, IMRT, multicriteria optimisation, radiotherapy

1. Introduction

Intensity Modulated Radiation Therapy (IMRT) is a planning technique that produces irregular beams and intensities using different commercial optimisation methods. IMRT is still the most exciting form of treatment in radiation oncology since the use of computed tomography imaging (Bentzen, 2005; Nutting, 2003). In the IMRT method, the aim is to shape the irregular target volume by varying the photon intensity along the beam field to obtain the desired dose distribution. In this treatment method, although a wide variety of different plan optimisations are used, there is the same goal to achieve the plan (Alber, 2000).

Intensity Modulated Arc Therapy (IMAT) is another technique with a similar working principle to IMRT. It allows selectively giving the radiation dose on the move from different optimal beam angles (Duthoy et al., 2004). It can be said that the first IMAT technique started with the invention of Tomotherapy, which used a rotational beam of radiation. Tomotherapy can be characterised as a new concept for the application of dynamic conformal radiotherapy. (Mackie et al., 1993). As an alternative to tomotherapy, IMAT with dynamic multi-leaf collimation was developed using a cone radiation beam. This technique is called the rotational IMRT or IMAT technique.

Varian Eclipse treatment planning system (Varian Medical Systems, Palo Alto, CA) implements the IMAT planning module using a technique called Direct Aperture Optimisation. The name of this module is called RapidArc in Varian systems. The RapidArc module in Varian Systems is used both as planning software and as a solution to transmit the plan to the linear accelerator device (Korreman et al., 2009; Shepard et al., 2011)

The SmartArc module in the Pinnacle treatment planning system (Philips Medical, Bothell, Wash., USA) can be utilised as another alternative to building the IMAT module in Varian and Elekta linear accelerator devices. The IMAT module integrated with the Pinnacle system is very similar to the IMRT module in terms of planning workflow.

Elekta systems (Elekta Oncology Systems, Crawley, UK) have two different systems for IMAT planning solutions. The first of these is the IMAT module integrated into the Ergo++ system, with aperture shapes defined based on the patient's anatomy. This system uses anatomy-based semi-reverse planning. With this feature, it is closer to dynamic conformal arc conduction.

The main difference is that weights can change from one beam angle to another within a spring. This allows a higher percentage of radiation to be transmitted at more preferred beam angles. (Haga et al., 2009; Shepard et al., 2012).

Elekta systems created the Monaco treatment planning system as a second commercial solution for the IMAT planning algorithm. The working principle of the Monaco system is based on biology-based IMRT optimisation and Monte Carlo dose calculation. Monaco generates plans using a 'sweeping leaf sequencer' in which leaves move unidirectionally across the field. Leaf movement tends to vary between arc sectors. (Cameron et al., 2005).

RayPlan (RaySearch Laboratories, Stockholm, Sweden) is a planning software programme that can work with linear accelerator devices of different commercial companies. RayPlan; can perform IMRT, Volumetric Modulated Arc Therapy (VMAT), TomoTherapy, and electron beam radiation therapy for different devices. It supports all treatment planning activities. Using the Direct optimisation of the step-by-step segments feature, it can make high-quality IMRT plans with a minimum number of segments. This feature speeds up both the planning and implementation processes.

Many publications have been published by many researchers comparing the pros and cons of IMAT techniques in Tomotherapy, Elekta, and Varian therapy devices. (Cao et al., 2007; Fogliata et al., 2008; Palma et al., 2008; Rao et al., 2010; Yu. 1995,).

IMAT techniques implement greater capability to dynamically change gantry speed, dose rate, and multi-leaf collimator (MLC) leaf positions during rotational beam delivery. There are restrictions on changes to be made from one beam angle to another in an arc to create beam shapes. These are mainly due to the MLC leaf rate limitation. Reducing these constraints is crucial to the quality of the plan. Thanks to the new features developed by commercial systems, both IMRT and IMAT techniques can meet the treatment requirements to a large extent. Regardless of which commercial therapy devices and software programmes that work with them are preferred, it is crucial to determine the correct dose constraints in the treatment planning system to obtain effective plans (Ling et al., 2008).

2. Dose Constraints

Treatment planning systems are software programmes that can work integrated with treatment devices to plan patient treatment. Although the working principles of software programmes are based on different algorithms, their basic functions are similar. The purpose of creating a treatment plan is to obtain dose distribution appropriate for the desired dose targets for the target volume and the tolerance doses of the surrounding healthy tissues. The setting of certain mathematical expressions by the planner on the treatment planning system is called dose constraints. First of all, the beam weights should be arranged in a way to ensure the proper distribution of the dose for the desired treatment plan. The software system used for this job takes time to find the best beam weight solution. The best solution is dose constraints with a lower described mathematical objective function. The most advanced planning system is the one that realises what is desired to be planned and what the planner wants in a short time. The dose-volume histogram (DVH) is used to analyse the suitability of the resulting plan. DVHs are shown as a graphical representation of the radiation dose delivered to the target volume and critical structures.

The resulting dose homogeneity in the planning target volume (PTV) and the dose distribution in organs at risk (OAR) may depend on the specific combination of planning delivery systems. In addition, site-specific strategy can also affect the final result (Claus et al., 2002). Therefore, evaluation of the performance, characteristics, and limitations of these different combinations of equipment installed at different centres, with their inherent variability, is only possible by evaluating the resulting treatment plans. Unlike most treatment planning studies in which some aspect of treatment planning is evaluated, such as dose calculation, delivery technique, or optimisation procedure, the concept proposed in this chapter aimed to reveal whether a combination of software and hardware yields acceptable results at any given centre (Fogliata et al., 2003; Mattia et al., 2004).

Dose homogeneity is a specific parameter that depends on the size of the PTV and the dose distribution of critical organs. (Claus et al., 2002). Dose homogeneity indicates the quality of the planning and differs depending on the system used in the clinic (Fogliata et al., 2003; Mattia et al. 2004).

The most important criterion for making a good IMRT or IMAT plan is to define the correct dose criteria for the target volume and critical organs. OARs adjacent to the target volume should be identified and subtracted from the target volume. Thanks to the dose definitions given, it should be ensured that the target volume receives the desired dose while trying to protect critical structures as much as possible. In most cases, one will have to choose between the target dose range and the doses received by normal constructs. In this case, the most optimal plan should be preferred. When choosing the appropriate treatment plan, not only the dose-volume histograms should be reviewed, but also the slice-by-slice dose distribution should be carefully reviewed. The traditional way in IMRT or IMAT plans is a trial-and-error approach, where the planner manually adjusts a set of plan parameters to reach the target volume. As a result, a good treatment plan largely depends on the experience and effort of the planner.

Although treatment planning systems (TPS) have different working principles, they basically achieve the same purpose. The plan created in TPS is directly dependent on the selected beam, beam weight, and defined dose constraints. The IMRT technique aims to increase the control over the three-dimensional dose distribution by physically superimposing a large number of fields that are distributed over one or more arcs and are divided independently of a set of fixed directions. IMRT planning requires dose specifications for both the target volume and surrounding healthy structures. The TPS software creates a series of modulation patterns at each beam angle to achieve the desired dose definition goals. This created process is called "inverse planning". Inverse planning can describe a technique using a software program to automatically achieve a treatment plan which has optimal merit. Inverse planning is less dependent on the geometric parameters but more on the specification of volumes of target and critical structures, as well as their dose constraints. As a different alternative to external beam radiotherapy, two different inverse planning methods with advanced features were developed that allow planning in a shorter time. This method is an optimisation method that can make both IMRT and IMAT plans and is compatible with different treatment devices. It is called multi-criteria optimization in terms of offering different plan options. It can be defined as an alternative workflow for optimisation.

3. Multi Criteria Optimisation

IMRT plan optimisation is a multi-criteria problem that aims to provide dose coverage, homogeneity, and conformity to PTV while sparing OARs. (Craft, 2013). Goals and weights are firstly defined for each structure in traditional commercial systems (Bortfeld, 1999; Webb, 2015). Then a plan is optimised by treatment planning software until plan goals provide dose constraints as well as possible. Finally, the plan is computed by software. This process is completed when the ideal plan is acquired. This is a step-by-step manual method to obtain a desired treatment plan. Because of poor modeling of optimisation problems, improving one aspect can lead to deteriorating other aspects.

It is not always straightforward to solve multi-objective problems mathematically directly. It is more reliable to use weighted and summed single-objective optimisation instead. (Craft et al., 2005). Current commercial systems require users to enter some optimisation parameters, including ideal dosimetric targets and organ-based weighting factors. These factors illustrate the importance of certain organs that are difficult to assign prior to optimisation. Therefore, dosimetrists must manually adjust these parameters by trial and error, which makes the quality of the plan depends on the experience of the dosimetrist (Potrebko et al., 2017).

Multicriteria optimisation (MCO) is a sophisticated feature of the optimisation method. It is based upon the approximation of the Pareto surface-based technique that refers to a state where one parameter cannot be improved without negatively affecting another (Craft et al., 2005). MCO has the capability to see all plans in one optimisation-derived Pareto plan (Figure 1). MCO plans eliminate the time-consuming trial-and-error process of selecting appropriate weighting factors in conventional IMRT planning and calculate these dosimetric trade-offs (Breedveld et al., 2009; Monz et al., 2008).

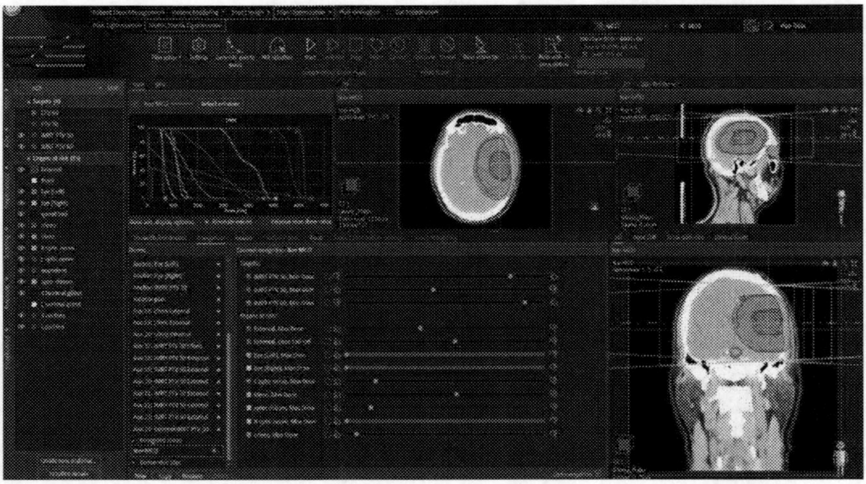

Figure 1. An example of creating Pareto plans was obtained using the MCO method.

The MCO creates so-called anchor plans for each critical organ and target volume. These anchor plans consist of different templates that will deliver the lowest possible dose to critical structures while maintaining target coverage.

A single optimisation calculation, it creates Pareto optimal plans that show the different balances between the criteria at once. In this way, you can see the scenario in which the target volume dose best covers and the scenario in which critical organs are best protected at the same time. Once these are created, the dosimetrist or planner can adjust the weight tradeoff between the different Pareto plans and monitor the dose distributions in real-time. This event gives an idea of how the dose is distributed without completely rescheduling the case (Bodensteiner, 2018).

Traditional IMRT planning, it tries to predict which system optimisation parameters might provide the best balance between multiple conflicting objectives. This process can be quite time-consuming. It is not possible for planner to try all plan possibilities in their clinical routine in terms of time constraints. The multi-criteria optimisation method greatly simplifies the work in clinical use. This method allows the planner to navigate the swap area with one click and decide on the right plan faster. Compared to the normal optimisation planning method, in the MCO method, the radiation oncologist and the dosimetrist can see more plan options and choose the best-desired plan (Craft and Bortfeld, 2008).

4. Multi Criteria Optimisation Workflow

In the MCO clinical workflow, beam angles are first determined as in normal optimisation. Then, objectives and targets for critical structures are loaded into protocols. For the MCO to plan correctly, it is necessary to define at least one constraint for the target volume or volumes. The next step is to create Pareto plans based on the number of targets. In the Pareto plan generation method, the system asks the user to specify how many plans will be created. The number of these created plans can be increased or decreased by the user. Plans navigation can be performed when Pareto plans are created.

Clinical goals show with red and green light what has been achieved and what has not been achieved in the current plan. From the clinical target indicators, the planner identifies sites and structures where further dose reduction is required. Dose values can be changed by means of a slider on the obtained Pareto plans. By moving the corresponding slider to decrease the dose, the planner can update the isodose lines, DVH, and clinical target values in real-time. Once the planner is satisfied with the dose delivered to the critical structure, they can lock the slider and prevent the negative impact of crawling on that structure (Bodensteiner, 2018). By locking the slider, we can create a resolution space on the chart that will produce the most reasonable results. When we get the plan we want, we calculate it to get the final dose values. If changes are requested in the decision-making process, changes are made between plans without re-optimisation calculation.

A four-step remediation procedure was developed for multi-criteria planning and used to evaluate head and neck cases. In this process, it was primarily aimed to obtain homogeneous dose distributions for PTV. Secondly, doses for critical structures (spinal cord, brain stem, parotid, oral cavity, etc.) were reduced. In the third, the doses of the remaining normal tissues were reduced. Fourthly, the correction of fluency maps was performed (Wilkens et al., 2007). This procedure is prostate, etc. applied in other cases as well. (Jee et al., 2007). Unlike these studies, it has adopted a restraint strategy based on a predefined priority list to create a plan where all restraints can be made as far as possible. (Breedveld et al., 2007). This strategy includes four stages. The first one is an initial solution that is tried to find by software. When the constraints of the first solution in the first stage are not met, it loosens the constraints in the second stage. In the final stages, it tries to tighten all restrictions as much as possible without higher priority restrictions. As a result, an advanced automatic multi-criteria plan optimisation model based on more lexical sorting was developed. This method is closer or better plan quality than the original plans of the dosimetrists. (Breedveld et al., 2012).

However, the voxel-based optimisation method has been developed as an alternative to an organ-based optimisation model, which has an incomplete area of the mathematical solution. (Holdsworth et al., 2012). Subsequent studies have shown that a refined voxel-based optimisation model is more helpful in navigating the solution from partial space to the entire Pareto surface, compared to the organ-based optimisation model. (Zarapisheh et al., 2014). In this condition, it is more practical to create an optimal treatment plan with a voxel-based optimisation model. It has been shown that the DVH can be greatly improved when the voxel-based optimisation model is preferred. (Cotrutz et al., 2002; Wu et al., 2003).

To create an efficient and high-quality plan at voxel-based optimisation, the optimisation engine needs to define appropriate constraints based on clinical planning experience. Given very tight constraints, it becomes difficult for the optimisation engine to find satisfactory solutions. However, if the constraints given are too loose, the resulting plans may be insufficient. Therefore, it is important to try to set automatic dose restrictions. Before these adjustments, a constraint priority list with some initial values should be given. The constraint priority list is an important shift from clinical bias to a scientific trade-off. The restriction priority list is classified by critical organ severity. Constraints are divided into two classes, hard and soft. Hard constraints cannot be violated and relaxed during optimisation. Conversely, flexible constraints can be loosened more during optimisation or raised to strict constraints during optimisation. As a result, when these steps are done in voxel-based optimisation, it is highly possible to achieve the desired results. Based on the plan strategy of the voxel-based optimisation method based on auto-tuning and constraint, the multi-criteria optimisation framework was successfully developed. The multi-criteria optimisation method is very important for radiation therapy, in terms of appropriate dosimetric target determination and adjustment methods. Both optimisation methods have been shown to significantly reduce the existing trial-and-error planning workload and provide an efficient method to ensure high plan quality consistency.

5. Multi Criteria Optimisation Dose Constraints for Cases

Although the choice of a good treatment plan depends on the guidelines, the decision-making process is controversial. Different hospitals may apply different protocols. While there are guidelines and protocols for many critical structures at a treatment site, it is not always easy to find an appropriate starting point. This section will provide some guidelines that allow the reader to focus on the multi-criteria problem. In this section, it will be tried to define the optimising methods that help to overcome the difficulties in the clinic. Although the guidelines given in this section provide tools for clinical plan solutions, it should be stated that they do not represent a gold standard in any way.

A general guideline for prescribing PTV is that at least 99% of the volume should receive a dose that is between 95% and 107% of the prescribed dose. And also structures and doses for PTVs and OARs are determined according to International Commission on Radiation Units and Measurements (ICRU) 50, 62, and 83 reports and clinical observation (Chavaudra et al., 2001; Gregoire et al. 2011; Purdy, 2004). While it is not always possible to obtain desired dose criteria for each treatment plan, defining these dose criteria can be considered a good starting point.

Radiation therapy aims to destroy malignant cells while preserving critical structures in the surrounding. The radiation dose to be defined varies according to the tumour pathology, stage, and location. For example, in cancer types such as brain tumours, taking the upper limit value is more beneficial in terms of eliminating the malignancy. In cancer types such as liver, pancreas, and adrenal tumours, when using the optimisation method, the dose to be given to the target volume should be increased and the surrounding healthy structures should be better protected. (Petit et al., 2012). In terms of multi criteria optimisation, a prostate treatment plan may be simpler than a head and neck plan. As the dose to be delivered to the tumour increases, it will be difficult to achieve dose tolerance for OARs. Below are sample dose definitions and critical organ doses for specific cases from some studies. The prescription dose to be given to the patient will always be determined by the radiation oncologist in clinical applications, and it is given here only to represent the clinical procedure as an example.

6. Prostate Cases

IMRT is considered a standard treatment technique for prostate cancer. In this technique, it is desired to give highly compatible dose distributions. Therefore, it is desirable to keep critical organ doses to a minimum in order to reduce the undesirable side effects of IMRT. When determining the target volume in prostate cancer, the PTV can be either the prostate itself or a volume containing seminal vesicles. A lower dose of 72.2 Gy is defined for the seminal vesicles, while a prescription dose of 76 Gy is generally defined for the prostate. The most critical structure during prostate treatment is the rectum. The rectum dose provides that D50% (dose 50%) should not receive more than 50 Gy, D35% should not receive more than 65 Gy and D20% should not receive more than 70 Gy. The bladder dose provides that D35% should not receive more than 65 Gy. D5% of femoral heads should be less than 50 Gy. The maximum dose of the penile bulb should be less than 50 Gy (Müller et al., 2017; Voet et al., 2014). The image of the prostate plan obtained by using MCO method is given in Figure 2.

7. Lung Cases

In the treatment of IMRT for the lungs, a standard daily dose of 2 Gy fractions is given. While the dose defined for the target volume is generally defined as between 60 Gy and 66 Gy. The lung dose that receives 20 Gy should remain below 35% of volume. The maximum dose value of the spinal cord should not exceed 45 Gy. For the esophagus, V30Gy < 30% and V60Gy < 13%, and the mean dose value should be below 34 Gy. The cardiac maximum dose should not exceed 40 Gy and V30Gy < 10%. Keeping the average dose value below 26 Gy for the heart will be beneficial in terms of preventing future complications (Liu et al., 2004).

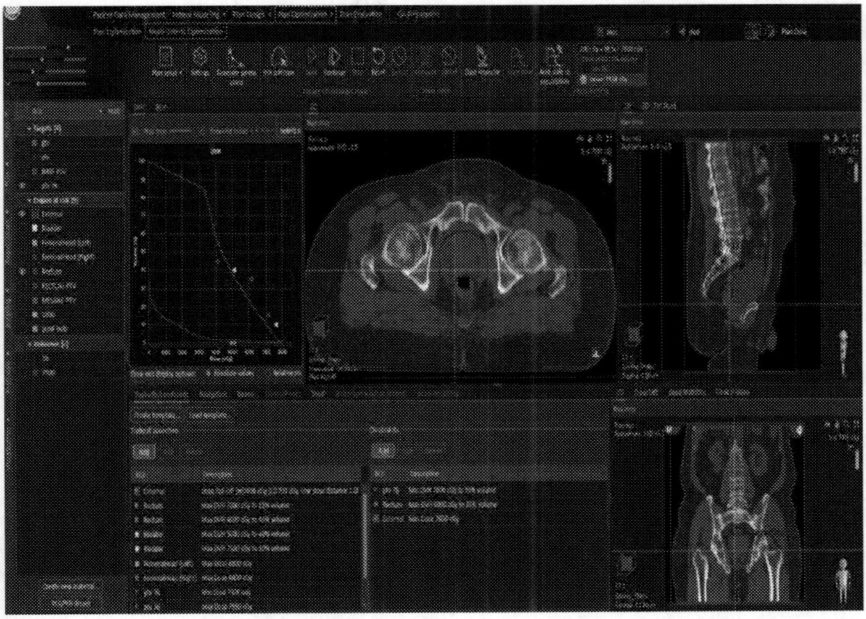

Figure 2. An example of the prostate case plan was obtained by using the MCO method.

8. Liver Cases

The liver therapeutic dose is generally defined as from 10 Gy per fraction to at least 50 Gy in 5 fractions. The maximum dose to the liver should not exceed 75 Gy. Using this dose definition, maximum doses should not exceed 22 Gy for the spinal cord dose, 20 Gy for the heart, and 42 Gy for the chest wall. V15Gy for each kidney should be <33%. Maximum doses for stomach, duodenum, esophagus, and intestine should be below 30 Gy. For the healthy tissue of the liver, there is a dose-volume restriction not to exceed V15Gy < 700 cc. (Sharfo et al. 2017).

9. Head and Neck Cases

It is very difficult to plan the head and neck treatment area due to the proximity of the target volume to many organs. (Voet et al., 2013). Tumour size and location may differ from patient to patient. sometimes different dose definitions may be prescribed to different parts of the tumour. In some cases, a higher dose (such as 66 Gy-70Gy, etc.) can be given to the primary PTV, while a lower dose (46 Gy) may be given to the elective lymph nodes (Van Haveren et al. 2017).

The salivary gland, oral cavity, larynx, spinal cord, brain stem, and optic nerves are among the OARs that need protection. Larger PTVs may also reach near the lungs and the lungs should be added to the OAR list. Critical organ dose restrictions used in the dose optimisation process, dose values for brain D(33%) ≤60 Gy, D(66%)≤50 Gy, D(100%)≤45 Gy, maximum dose value for brainstem and optic nerves 54 Gy, for the Spinal Cord, the maximum dose value should be defined as 48 Gy. Average dose values should be determined as 26 Gy for salivary glands, 40 Gy for the oral cavity, and 45 Gy for the larynx, respectively (Van Haveren et al., 2017).

10. Glioma Cases

Brain tumours can occur at various locations within intracranial anatomical regions. Gross tumour volume (GTV) is defined based on integrated CT and magnetic resonance imaging from preoperative and postoperative studies. After this identification, clinical target volumes (CTV) to cover additional regions of potential microscopic involvement and PTV are created by giving it a 3mm margin in all directions. The defined dose is defined as a total of 60 Gy, in 2 Gy fractions per day. The brainstem, optic nerves, chiasma, eyes, lenses, cochlea, and lacrimal glands are designated as OARs as standard for all cases. Tolerance doses are defined as 2 Gy per day, with a maximum of 54 Gy for the brainstem, optic nerves, and chiasm. It is requested that the maximum dose taken by the lenses should not exceed 6 Gy. It is desired that the maximum dose for the eyes should not exceed 45 Gy, and the maximum dose for the lacrimal gland should not exceed 40 Gy (Müller et al., 2017). Depending on the location of the brain tumour, some values can be stretched a little. The image of the brain tumour plan obtained by using the MCO method is given in Figure 3.

Whether standard optimisation or MCO is used in IMRT plans, it is necessary to define the dose objective for each PTV and critical organ. The dose objective for PTV is defined to receive 100% of the prescribed dose, at least 95% of the target volume. After that, the minimum and maximum dose objectives for PTV are defined in the order. Based on the dose tolerance values given for the different cases mentioned above, similar dose objectives values are defined for critical organs. For each defined dose objective, its priority value must be given. Creating a priority value between 10 and 100 is important for a balanced plan. In general, priority value 100 is given for the target volume, while decreasing values are generated sequentially for other organs. The critical structure given high priority means that more emphasis will be placed on reaching the desired value for the dose restriction. For example, in the prostate case, the rectum is the priority critical structure. The priority value can be defined as 60 for the rectum, 50 for the bladder, and 40 for the femoral heads. Likewise, the most important structure to be protected in head-neck cases is the spinal cord. Therefore, a high priority value such as 70 can be defined for the spinal cord, while decreasing priority values of 60 for the brainstem, 50 for the parotids, and decreasing for other structures, respectively. If the PTV is in the neighbourhood of another critical structure, the high priority value can be determined for this critical structure. Entering the maximum dose to be given to the PTV for the external body structure as a dose objective will prevent the formation of undesired maximum doses in the body. A value of 100 can be created as a priority value in the external body structure.

Conclusion

This book chapter, it is aimed to explain the multi-criteria optimisation method developed as an alternative to the standard optimisation method in radiotherapy treatment planning. The IMRT method uses multiple beam angles, each of which is split into multiple beams of varying intensity, allowing for an infinite number of treatment plans. Although IMRT offers endless plan options in treatment planning, there may not be time to try too many plans as a result of the process inefficiency created by the clinical workload. Therefore, physician participation in the IMRT planning process cannot be encouraged. The physician has to evaluate the plans made by the planner or request another plan. This means that the whole process is done again and takes time. MCO is a good method to avoid the disadvantages that

IMRT offers. In multi-criteria optimisation, unlike standard optimisation, you can see all treatment plan alternatives at the same time. This provides great convenience for the planner and the radiation oncologist. The fact that all plans that can be given to the patient can be seen in a single optimisation calculation provides a serious advantage in terms of timing. It has been shown that the Pareto surface-based MCO approach provides effective, faster, and better plans. In many studies, it has been reported that the time spent for optimisation can be reduced and the performance of the treatment plan can be improved by using MCO (Craft et al., 2012; Craft et al., 2007). In conclusion, it can be stated that the MCO planning method is effective method in terms of both planning efficiency and dosimetric quality.

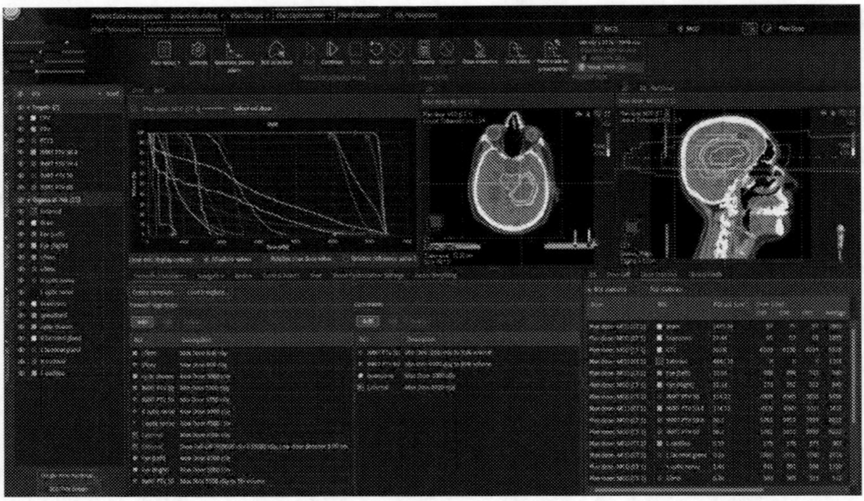

Figure 3. An example of the brain tumour plans was obtained by using MCO method.

References

Alber, M. (2000). Hyperion—an integrated IMRT planning tool The Use of Computers in Radiation Therapy ed W Schlegel and T Bortfeld.

Bentzen, S. M. (2005). Radiation therapy: intensity modulated, image guided, biologically optimized and evidence based. *Radiotherapy and Oncology*, *77*(3), 227-230.

Bodensteiner, D. (2018). RayStation: External beam treatment planning system. *Medical Dosimetry*, *43*(2), 168-176.

Bortfeld, T. (1999, January). Optimized planning using physical objectives and constraints. In *Seminars in radiation oncology* (Vol. 9, No. 1, pp. 20-34). WB Saunders.

Breedveld, S., Storchi, P. R., & Heijmen, B. J. (2009). The equivalence of multi-criteria methods for radiotherapy plan optimization. *Physics in Medicine & Biology*, 54(23), 7199.

Breedveld, S., Storchi, P. R., Keijzer, M., Heemink, A. W., & Heijmen, B. J. (2007). A novel approach to multi-criteria inverse planning for IMRT. *Physics in Medicine & Biology*, 52(20), 6339.

Breedveld, S., Storchi, P. R., Voet, P. W., & Heijmen, B. J. (2012). iCycle: Integrated, multicriterial beam angle, and profile optimization for generation of coplanar and noncoplanar IMRT plans. *Medical physics*, 39(2), 951-963.

Cameron, C. (2005). Sweeping-window arc therapy: an implementation of rotational IMRT with automatic beam-weight calculation. *Physics in Medicine & Biology*, 50(18), 4317.

Cao, D., Holmes, T. W., Afghan, M. K., & Shepard, D. M. (2007). Comparison of plan quality provided by intensity-modulated arc therapy and helical tomotherapy. *International Journal of Radiation Oncology Biology Physics*, 69(1), 240-250.

Chavaudra, J., & Bridier, A. (2001). Definition of volumes in external radiotherapy: ICRU reports 50 and 62. *Cancer radiotherapie: journal de la Societe francaise de radiotherapie oncologique*, *5*(5), 472-478.

Claus, F., Mijnheer, B., Rasch, C., Bortfeld, T., Fraass, B., De Gersem, W., ... & De Neve, W. (2002). Report of a study on IMRT planning strategies for ethmoid sinus cancer. *Strahlentherapie und Onkologie*, 178(10), 572-576.

Cotrutz, C., & Xing, L. (2002). Using voxel-dependent importance factors for interactive DVH-based dose optimization. *Physics in Medicine & Biology*, 47(10), 1659.

Craft, D. (2013). *Multi-criteria optimization methods in radiation therapy planning: a review of technologies and directions*. arXiv preprint arXiv:1305.1546.

Craft, D. L., Hong, T. S., Shih, H. A., & Bortfeld, T. R. (2012). Improved planning time and plan quality through multicriteria optimization for intensity-modulated radiotherapy. *International Journal of Radiation Oncology* Biology* Physics*, 82(1), e83-e90.

Craft, D., & Bortfeld, T. (2008). How many plans are needed in an IMRT multi-objective plan database? *Physics in Medicine & Biology*, 53(11), 2785.

Craft, D., Halabi, T., & Bortfeld, T. (2005). Exploration of tradeoffs in intensity-modulated radiotherapy. *Physics in Medicine & Biology*, 50(24), 5857.

Craft, D., Süss, P., & Bortfeld, T. (2007). The tradeoff between treatment plan quality and required number of monitor units in intensity-modulated radiotherapy. *International Journal of Radiation Oncology* Biology* Physics*, 67(5), 1596-1605.

Duthoy, W., De Gersem, W., Vergote, K., Boterberg, T., Derie, C., Smeets, P., ... & De Neve, W. (2004). Clinical implementation of intensity-modulated arc therapy (IMAT) for rectal cancer. *International Journal of Radiation Oncology Biology Physics*, 60(3), 794-806.

Fogliata, A., Bolsi, A., & Cozzi, L. (2003). Comparative analysis of intensity modulation inverse planning modules of three commercial treatment planning systems applied to head and neck tumour model. *Radiotherapy and oncology*, 66(1), 29-40.

Fogliata, A., Clivio, A., Nicolini, G., Vanetti, E., & Cozzi, L. (2008). Intensity modulation with photons for benign intracranial tumours: a planning comparison of volumetric single arc, helical arc and fixed gantry techniques. *Radiotherapy and Oncology*, 89(3), 254-262.

Grégoire, V., & Mackie, T. R. (2011). State of the art on dose prescription, reporting and recording in Intensity-Modulated Radiation Therapy (ICRU report No. 83). *Cancer/Radiothérapie*, 15(6-7), 555-559.

Haga, A., Nakagawa, K., Shiraishi, K., Itoh, S., Terahara, A., Yamashita, H., ... & Pellegrini, R. (2009). Quality assurance of volumetric modulated arc therapy using Elekta Synergy. *Acta Oncologica*, 48(8), 1193-1197.

Hatano, K., Araki, H., Sakai, M., Kodama, T., Tohyama, N., Kawachi, T., ... & Ishigaki, H. (2007). Current status of intensity-modulated radiation therapy (IMRT). *International journal of clinical oncology*, *12*(6), 408-415.

Holdsworth, C., Stewart, R. D., Kim, M., Liao, J., & Phillips, M. H. (2011). Investigation of effective decision criteria for multiobjective optimization in IMRT. *Medical Physics*, 38(6Part1), 2964-2974.

Jee, K. W., McShan, D. L., & Fraass, B. A. (2007). Lexicographic ordering: intuitive multicriteria optimization for IMRT. *Physics in Medicine & Biology*, 52(7), 1845.

Korreman, S., Medin, J., & Kjaer-Kristoffersen, F. (2009). Dosimetric verification of RapidArc treatment delivery. *Acta oncologica*, 48(2), 185-191.

Ling, C. C., Zhang, P., Archambault, Y., Bocanek, J., Tang, G., & LoSasso, T. (2008). Commissioning and quality assurance of RapidArc radiotherapy delivery system. *International Journal of Radiation Oncology* Biology* Physics*, 72(2), 575-581.

Liu, H. H., Wang, X., Dong, L., Wu, Q., Liao, Z., Stevens, C. W., ... & Mohan, R. (2004). Feasibility of sparing lung and other thoracic structures with intensity-modulated radiotherapy for non–small-cell lung cancer. *International Journal of Radiation Oncology* Biology* Physics*, 58(4), 1268-1279.

Mackie, T. R., Holmes, T., Swerdloff, S., Reckwerdt, P., Deasy, J. O., Yang, J., ... & Kinsella, T. (1993). Tomotherapy: a new concept for the delivery of dynamic conformal radiotherapy. *Medical physics*, 20(6), 1709-1719.

Mattia, M., Del Giudice, P., & Caccia, B. (2004). IMRT optimization: Variability of solutions and its radiobiological impact. *Medical Physics*, 31(5), 1052-1060.

Monz, M., Küfer, K. H., Bortfeld, T. R., & Thieke, C. (2008). Pareto navigation—algorithmic foundation of interactive multi-criteria IMRT planning. *Physics in Medicine & Biology*, 53(4), 985.

Müller, B. S., Shih, H. A., Efstathiou, J. A., Bortfeld, T., & Craft, D. (2017). Multicriteria plan optimization in the hands of physicians: a pilot study in prostate cancer and brain tumors. *Radiation Oncology*, 12(1), 1-11.

Nutting, C. (2003). Intensity-modulated radiotherapy (IMRT): the most important advance in radiotherapy since the linear accelerator? *The British journal of radiology*, 76(910), 673-673.

Palma, D., Vollans, E., James, K., Nakano, S., Moiseenko, V., Shaffer, R., ... & Otto, K. (2008). Volumetric modulated arc therapy (VMAT) for delivery of prostate radiotherapy: Reduction in treatment time and monitor unit requirements compared to intensity modulated radiotherapy. *International journal of radiation oncology, biology, physics*, 72(1), S312.

Petit, S. F., Wu, B., Kazhdan, M., Dekker, A., Simari, P., Kumar, R., ... & McNutt, T. (2012). Increased organ sparing using shape-based treatment plan optimization for intensity modulated radiation therapy of pancreatic adenocarcinoma. *Radiotherapy and Oncology*, 102(1), 38-44.

Potrebko, P. S., Fiege, J., Biagioli, M., & Poleszczuk, J. (2017). Investigating multi-objective fluence and beam orientation IMRT optimization. *Physics in Medicine & Biology*, 62(13), 5228.

Purdy, J. A. (2004, January). Current ICRU definitions of volumes: limitations and future directions. *In Seminars in radiation oncology* (Vol. 14, No. 1, pp. 27-40). WB Saunders.

Rao, M., Yang, W., Chen, F., Sheng, K., Ye, J., Mehta, V., ... & Cao, D. (2010). Comparison of Elekta VMAT with helical tomotherapy and fixed field IMRT: plan quality, delivery efficiency and accuracy. *Medical physics*, 37(3), 1350-1359.

Sharfo, A. W. M., Dirkx, M. L., Breedveld, S., Romero, A. M., & Heijmen, B. J. (2017). VMAT plus a few computer-optimized non-coplanar IMRT beams (VMAT+) tested for liver SBRT. *Radiotherapy and Oncology*, 123(1), 49-56.

Shepard, D. M., & Cao, D. (2011). Clinical implementation of intensity-modulated arc therapy. *Front Radiat Ther Oncol*, 43, 80-98.

Shepard, D., & Popple, R. (2012). MO-A-211-01: Volumetric Modulated Arc Therapy. *Medical Physics*, 39(6Part20), 3858-3858.

Van Haveren, R., Ogryczak, W., Verduijn, G. M., Keijzer, M., Heijmen, B. J., & Breedveld, S. (2017). Fast and fuzzy multi-objective radiotherapy treatment plan generation for head and neck cancer patients with the lexicographic reference point method (LRPM). *Physics in Medicine & Biology*, 62(11), 4318.

Voet, P. W., Dirkx, M. L., Breedveld, S., Al-Mamgani, A., Incrocci, L., & Heijmen, B. J. (2014). Fully automated volumetric modulated arc therapy plan generation for prostate cancer patients. *International Journal of Radiation Oncology* Biology* Physics*, 88(5), 1175-1179.

Voet, P. W., Dirkx, M. L., Breedveld, S., Fransen, D., Levendag, P. C., & Heijmen, B. J. (2013). Toward fully automated multicriterial plan generation: a prospective clinical study. *International Journal of Radiation Oncology* Biology* Physics*, 85(3), 866-872.

Webb, S. (2015). Intensity-modulated radiation therapy. CRC Press.

Wilkens, J. J., Alaly, J. R., Zakarian, K., Thorstad, W. L., & Deasy, J. O. (2007). IMRT treatment planning based on prioritizing prescription goals. *Physics in Medicine & Biology*, 52(6), 1675.

Wu, C., Olivera, G. H., Jeraj, R., Keller, H., & Mackie, T. R. (2003). Treatment plan modification using voxel-based weighting factors/dose prescription. *Physics in Medicine & Biology*, 48(15), 2479.

Yu, C. X. (1995). Intensity-modulated arc therapy with dynamic multileaf collimation: an alternative to tomotherapy. *Physics in Medicine & Biology*, 40(9), 1435.

Zarepisheh, M., Uribe-Sanchez, A. F., Li, N., Jia, X., & Jiang, S. B. (2014). A multicriteria framework with voxel-dependent parameters for radiotherapy treatment plan optimization. *Medical physics*, 41(4), 041705.

Chapter 13

Adaptive Radiation Therapy for IMRT

Serap Çatlı Dinç*

Gazi University Faculty of Medicine, Radiation Oncology Department, Ankara, Turkey

Abstract

Assuming that the anatomy of the treatment site remains unchanged throughout treatment, the treatment plan is usually calculated once initially, and the same plan is used throughout the entire treatment. However, there may be daily changes in the shape and location of the tumour. For example, there may be shrinkage or growth in the tumour, differences in the filling of organs with anatomical spaces or cavities, movements of organs, changes in the patient's weight during treatment, or differences due to hypoxic changes that may occur in the tumour. These differences may cause changes in doses planned to be delivered to the tumour and the organ at risk. Adaptive radiation therapy (ART) is the modification of the treatment plan using image guidance according to the needs during the treatment process, taking into account these changes in the radiotherapy (RT) field. ART is an approach that provides highly personalized radiation therapy for cancer patients, taking into account patient-specific anatomical and biological differences. Furthermore, ART measures the changes in the treatment process and makes the dose distribution equal to the planned optimal dose distribution with the readjustment of the plan. ART application is carried out in three steps: (1) detection of anatomic and biological changes, (2) treatment plan optimization to account for the patient-specific biological changes, and (3) technologies to precisely deliver the optimized plan to the patient. ART can be applied both online and offline. The clinical data have

*Corresponding Author's Email: serapcatli@hotmail.com.

In: Frontiers in Intensity-Modulated Radiotherapy Research
Editor: Sibel Karaca
ISBN: 979-8-88697-252-8

demonstrated the need for ART in clinical settings, assisted by using intensity-modulated RT (IMRT) and image-guided RT (IGRT). ART technology and methodology have advanced significantly over the past few years and are beginning to be used frequently in clinics. This chapter focuses on the ART for IMRT.

Keywords: adaptive radiotherapy, cancer, IMRT

1. Introduction

The word adaptation comes from the Latin word adaptatre, which means fit. Adaptive Radiation Therapy (ART) was first described in 1997 (Yan et al., 1997). In conventional radiotherapy (RT), a safety margin was routinely defined around the target volume to account for anatomical changes (ICRU 50, 1993). Consequently, with increasing margins, the volume of normal tissue exposed to radiation increased, and thus, side effects increased. Furthermore, while the volume of irradiated normal tissue increased due to the treatment volume increased, it was limited to the tumour dose to a higher radiation dose (Witte et al., 2017). As a result, the high irradiated normal tissue caused toxicity (Figure 1).

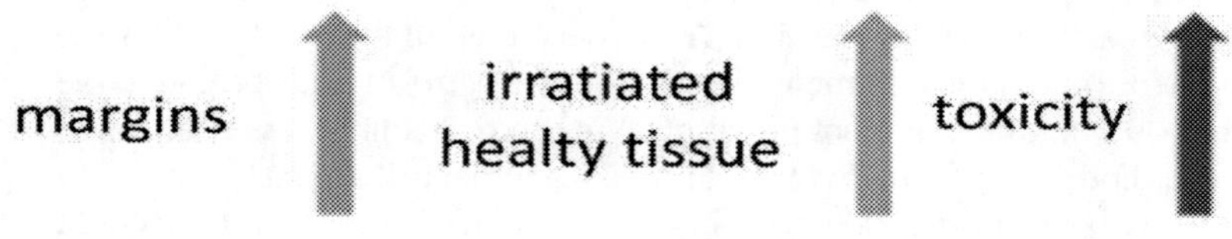

Figure 1. The schematic representation of normal tissue toxicity.

This problem has been solved with intensity-modulated RT (IMRT) by protecting normal tissues with rapid dose reduction around the target (Figure 2).

IMRT is a development of three-dimensional conformal RT (3DCRT), in which the optimization process is used to determine inhomogeneous flow distributions. The IMRT technique is currently the most advanced of conformal RT. IMRT increases the probability of tumour control and decreases the likelihood of the normal tissue complication probability (NTCP). However, the success of IMRT depends on the correct application of the RT dose. Changes in the daily anatomy and shape and position of the target volume during IMRT treatment can cause a sharp drop in radiation dose, resulting in differences between the delivered dose and the planned dose, resulting in an underdose of the target volume and an overdose of normal tissue. That is why "image-guided radiation therapy" (IGRT) methods have been developed during the treatment (Yoo et al., 2010).

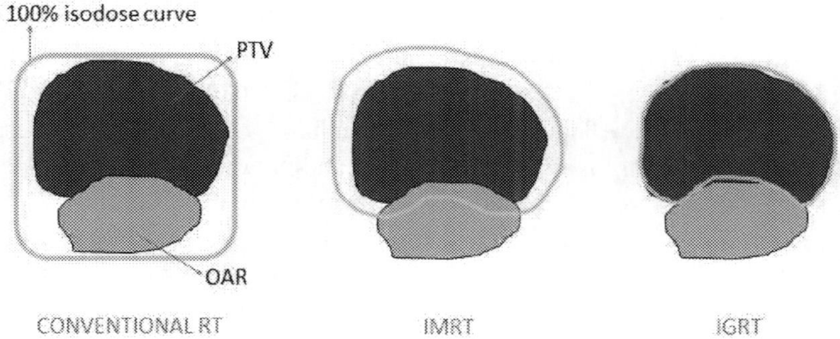

Figure 2. The schematic representation of dose reduction around the target.

IGRT uses imaging during treatment to improve treatment accuracy. Treatment machines are equipped with imaging instruments to allow the doctor to image the tumour and normal tissue during treatment. The patient's position and treatment plan are adjusted to precisely deliver the radiation dose to the tumour by comparing these images with the reference images acquired during the simulation. ART is a more advanced IGRT (Wu et al., 2011). However, anatomical changes frequently occur between radiation treatment planning and during RT. As a result, the dose delivered differs from the planned radiation dose. In ART, the goal is to account for these differences and accurately deliver the radiation dose to the tumour. ART has replaced the traditional notion of stable anatomy in external RT (EBRT) with the concept of changing anatomy. The basic principle in ART is to detect the anatomical change and modify the treatment plan accordingly, ensuring optimal target coverage and protection of critical organs (OAR) in both planning and daily therapy. However, external contour changes, tumour shrinkage, displacement, and shape changes in normal tissues can be observed depending on the patient's weight change during radiation therapy. There are many studies on the anatomical changes that occur during RT. For example, a shift of up to 5 mm has been reported in brain metastases (Hessen et al., 2017).

Posture changes of 3-4 mm (systematic and random) have been reported in head and neck RT (Kranen et al., 2009). Measurable anatomic changes occurred throughout treatment for head and neck cancers. The decrease in tumour volume was reported as 1.8%, and the change in parotid volume was 0.19 cm3 per day (Barker et al., 2004). An average of 16% increase in tumour volume was reported between simulation and initial treatment (Kishan et al., 2014). For bladder cancer, while inter-fraction bladder wall movement was 1 mm in the caudal direction, it increased to 12 mm in the anterior cranial direction, despite water drinking protocols (Dees et al., 2014). Changes in bladder fullness cause displacement of the tip of the uterus up to 50 mm and shape changes in cervical cancer (Bondar et al., 2012). These anatomical changes indicate residual geometric errors that have not been corrected despite the use of IGRT. Margins from 5 mm (head and neck) to 40-50 mm (bladder and stomach) are given to account for such geometric uncertainties (Witte et al., 2017). Figure 3. shows the reduction in tumour volume, the change in tumour volume due to adjacent organs, and the position change in the tumour and adjacent organs.

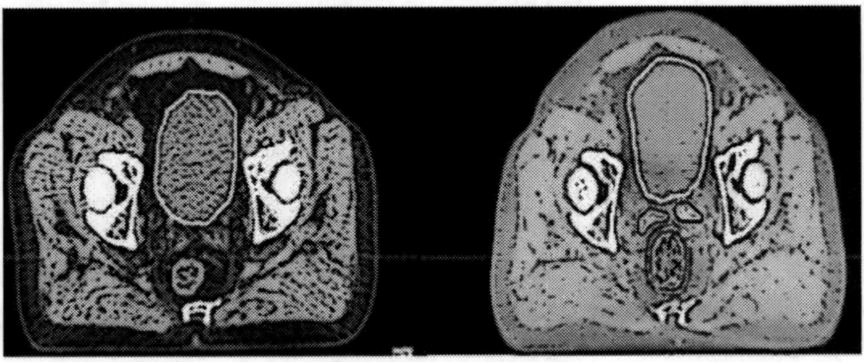

Figure 3. Anatomical changes during radiation therapy.

These changes are patient-specific events, and most of them are dose-dependent. These differences can lead to clinically critical dosimetric changes. Therefore, this problem cannot be solved by pre-treatment imaging. Also, IGRT cannot correct potential variations in the dose delivered to the patient and dosimetric errors. ART is necessary to solve these problems. ART has the potential to reduce OAR doses and toxicity and improve tumour control by increasing the target dose. Obtaining volumetric images is the most critical step. Devices capable of performing 3D volumetric computed tomography (3D CBCT and 3D MVCT) have been put into service in many RT clinics. These devices generate three-dimensional images while the patient is lying in the treatment room and can compare to the images acquired for pre-treatment planning purposes. However, although it is a new technology, it has not been satisfactory for medical physicists and radiation oncologists due to the significant differences between the images. ART is performed in three steps: image guidance, treatment adaptation, and dose verification (Wu et al., 2011). The components of adaptive RT are given in Figure 4.

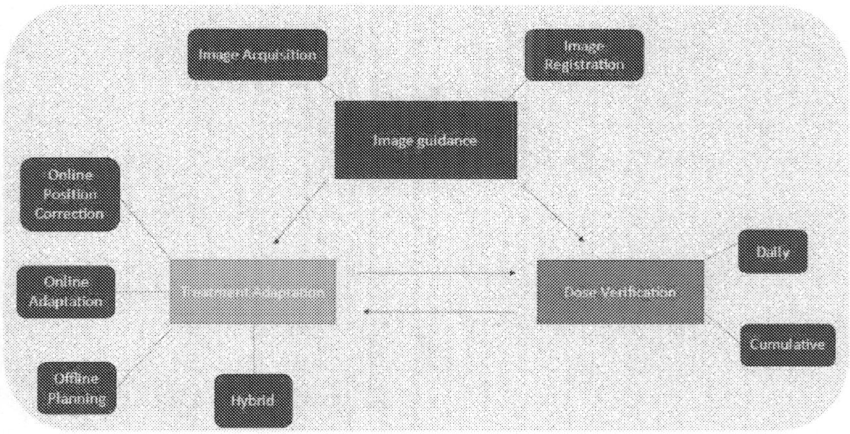

Figure 4. The components of adaptive radiotherapy.

2. Image Guidance

Imaging has become used in almost every aspect of radiation therapy, from staging and contouring to treatment evaluation. The image guidance not only provides information on the daily patient position and allows verifying the consistency of planned and treatment geometry. Image guidance is usually performed in 2 steps; image acquisition and image matching (Wu et al., 2011).

2.1. Image Acquisition

The acquisition and processing of image data are now fundamental parts of patient management in radiation therapy. Image data is acquired and analyzed to aid patient monitoring during and after treatment. In most RT centers, there is a 4D-CT scan. Many centers also have MR and PET/CT scanners. In addition, there are more in-room imaging methods. The hybrid MR scanner/treatment units have just come into use. With kilovoltage (KV) imaging or megavoltage (MV) cone-beam computed tomography (CBCT) imaging, the patient is imaged in the treatment position. It gives information about daily anatomy (Court et al., 2003; Kuriyama et al., 2003).

2.2. Image Matching

Image matching determines the difference between planning CT images and daily anatomy images. It is applied in two ways: rigid Matching and deformable Matching (Non-Rigid).

2.2.1. Rigid Matching

Rigid matching is the matching of daily acquired images with reference images (planning CT) in a 3D planar or 3D planar and rotational way. This matching is used to reposition the patient to confirm the target's location. Furthermore, the matching is done manually. Daily target fix provides speed and performance. Therefore, today IGRT has been widely adapted to clinical practice. However, in the presence of target/organ deformation, the rigid matching may not be sufficient to provide information about anatomical changes. Therefore, it is insufficient to adapt to the anatomical shape and volume changes (Wu et al., 2008).

2.2.2. Deformable Matching (Non-Rigid)

The deformable matching technique carries the organ position in the simulation CT data to the cone Beam CT data acquired during treatment by voxel-to-voxel matching between planning and log image sets. Finding the geometric equivalent of a point in two images is applied with different approaches. First, atlas-based matching is performed with a particular operating system. Then, deformable matching is performed automatically by geometric mapping between daily and planning images (Wang et al., 2005).

3. Treatment Adaptation

Treatment adaptation is another essential component of ART. Several methods have been developed for aiming for optimal target coverage and OAR sparing. These methods are divided into four groups:

3.1. Online Position Correction

It is a technique widely used in clinics with IGRT technology. First, the patient's position is corrected using daily images for possible target position differences from the planned anatomy (Figure 5). For this purpose, portal imaging (bone), CBCT (bone and soft tissue), and fiducial markers (soft tissue) are used (Barney et al., 2011; Chung et al., 2004).

Although it is effective and widely used, online position correction alone is not sufficient for position correction caused by daily target/organ deformation. In such changes, the plan needs to be modified.

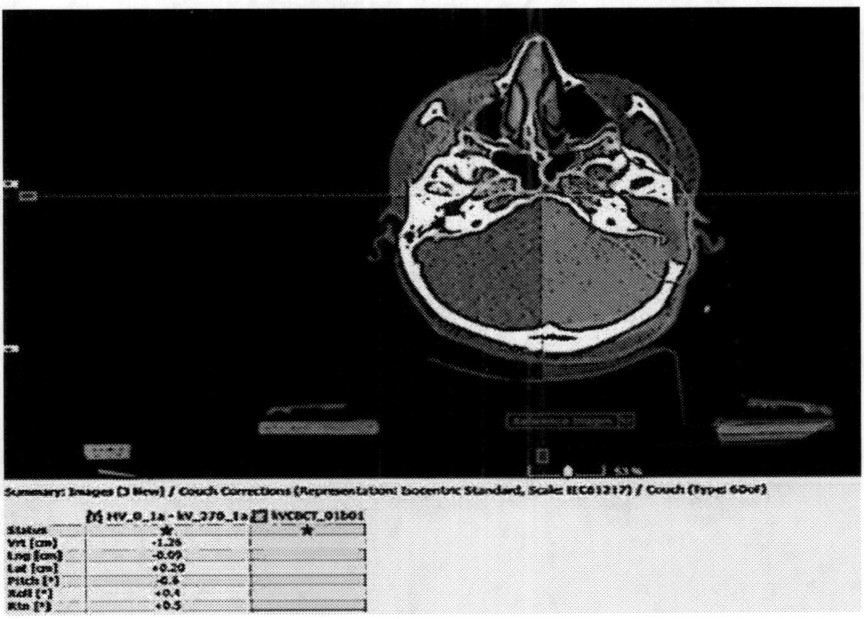

Figure 5. The corrected with online re-positioning.

3.2. Online Adaptation

Online adaptation is typically performed by imaging before each treatment and then adapting treatment to changing anatomy daily. Daily online replanning accounts for complex anatomical changes, both systematic and random. With such an approach, the treatment plan is re-optimized for each faction. Imaging is acquired while the patient is on the treatment table (Tisher et al., 2003). The online adaptive recontouring and replanning processes are repeated for each fraction without moving the patient. Today, RT technology is trying to progress toward online adaptive applications (Li et al., 2010). The most promising technology in online adaptive applications is MR Linac devices. Online replanning technology on CBCT will take place in clinical applications soon. However, its clinical use is limited due to the time-consuming quality control and plan approval.

The steps of Online ART:

- Creation of the original plan
- Imaging in the treatment room just before the treatment
- Matching newly acquired images with simulation images to ensure the patient is in the correct position
- Creating a new treatment plan by automatically creating and re-optimizing contours
- Evaluation of the treatment plan and its application to the patient (Figure 6).

This technique, which requires special utilities for its implementation, seems to be the correct technique for ART.

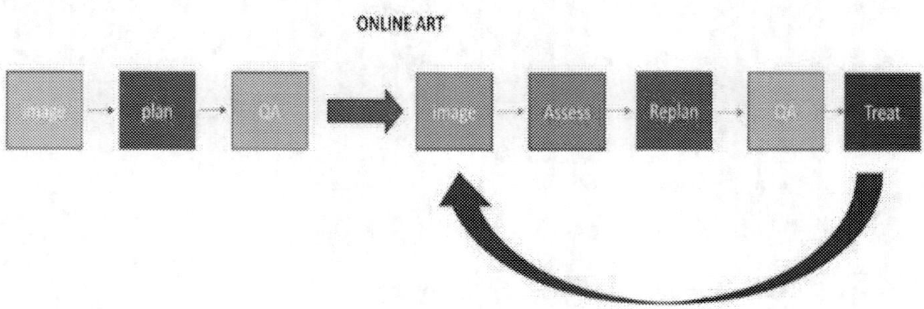

Figure 6. The steps of Online ART.

3.3. Offline Planning

The most frequently used one of these techniques is the Offline ART technique. The plan is reoptimized for the remaining fractions according to the new contours on the image (Nuver et al., 2007; Wu et al., 2002). The critical point of the offline optimization technique is that it is used in the following fractions, not for the fraction in which the daily image is acquired (Figure 7). Thus, it is possible to prevent set-up errors and systematic errors caused by organ movement. The imaging system used: is a conventional CT scanner or an in-room CT scanner.

Adaptive planning application conditions:

- As protocol (for example, after 20 fractions)
- Clinical observations of masks not fitting, weight loss, other surface chances, or changes observed on an in-room imaging system.

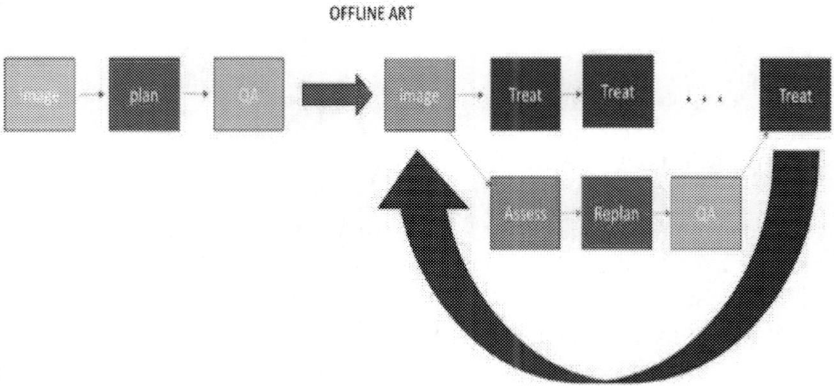

Figure 7. The steps of Offline ART.

3.4. Hybrid Method

Online position correction is still the most straightforward and frequently applied technique for daily anatomic changes. However, in cases with significant target deformation, it is optimal to replan using the new anatomy to ensure tumour volume coverage and protection of OAR. Therefore, combining online repositioning and offline optimizing will likely maximize the benefit of both techniques. Several studies showed that the hybrid methods could offer better target coverage and improved sparing of OAR compared to the current repositioning of IGRT (Li et al., 2011). In addition, the reuse of previously delivered plans increased the efficiency of online ART by reducing unnecessary optimizations during treatment by an average of 43%.

4. Dose Verification

Dose verification is of paramount importance in providing information about the dosimetric accuracy of the treatment process. Dose verification in ART is divided into two groups daily dose verification and cumulative dose analysis.

4.1. Daily Dose Verification

The dose distribution is calculated based on daily anatomy, and the daily dose-volume histogram (DVH) is compared to the planned DVH. The primary goal is to ensure that the target is covered.

4.2. Cumulative Dose Analysis

It analyses the total dose distribution up to that fraction. However, the increasing workload and uncertainty in validation make it challenging to apply in clinical practice. An adaptive process in radiation therapy plays an important role in customizing the treatment plan for the individual patient. Clinical assessment, formation of a gap between immobilization device and skin, reviewing image registration, and the patient complaints about pain or reaction show the need for adaptive.

Improvements in imaging and re-optimization algorithms have made it possible to monitor dynamically changing anatomy throughout treatment and customize RT. However, there are problems in the full integration of ART into clinical practice (image quality and number, time and cost, system integration). Although the dosimetric results reported in the studies are promising, they are not yet sufficient.

Optimizing the new anatomy to refresh the plan is a radical solution to correct any deviations. Therefore, ART needs to be able to optimize IMRT quickly. The most time-consuming factor in optimization is adjusting the plan objectives by trial and error by the operator during IMRT planning rather than the optimization itself. Recently, several methods have been introduced to automate IMRT planning. ART optimization may not be affected much by this problem since it can also use created to optimize the previous original plan. However, it can be advantageous for the most critical step in adaptive RT to check the compatibility of the image acquired in the treatment room with the CT data for simulation purposes.

5. Clinical Application of ART

After the first studies on ART, the different ART techniques started to be applied in clinics. Some institutions have clinically performed the ART technique for prostate cancer treatment. When treating prostate and seminal vesicles, bladder, rectum and even target volume can show significant position/volume change inter-fractionally (Liang et al., 2009). This change makes it challenging to achieve a homogeneous dose distribution in the target volume. Nevertheless, long-term results reported with adaptive therapy in prostate cancer promise clinical responses and toxicity reduction.

Head and neck cancer is another site that will benefit significantly from ART due to dose response-related organ deformation and volume reduction, tumoural/nodal volume reduction, weight loss, change in normal tissue/gland, regression of post-operative changes, and edema.

Although most research on ART focuses on prostate and head-and-neck cancer, researchers have also reported using ART in other disease sites. For example, physiological and radiation dose-dependent morphological changes in tumours and normal tissues during cervical cancer RT are essential. Therefore, ART application is of great importance (Pötter et al., 2007).

In the treatment process of lung cancer, internal organ movement, reduction in tumour volume, change in respiratory pattern, and weight loss are observed. These changes cause a shift in dosimetry. As a result, it can be said that ART can reduce the side effects in critical structures and increase tumour control (Vlachaki et al., 2009).

Liver tumours are also a group that may benefit from ART due to respiratory-related organ movement and the low radiation tolerance of the liver (Velec et al., 2011).

The bladder is a mobile and hollow organ. Up to 0.5-1 cm of movement can be observed in an average of 10 minutes of treatment (Foroudi et al.,

2011). This movement causes a change in dosimetry. Therefore, ART application has excellent benefits.

Most patients with oesophageal cancer choose to come to the clinic for treatment at an advanced stage. Large target volume, presence of critical structures such as lung, heart, and liver, and respiratory-related organ movement increase the importance of ART in oesophageal cancer (Hawkins et al., 2010).

6. Quality Control in the ART Process

ART consists of simulation, contouring, planning evaluation, and patient QA phases. Implementation of complex treatment plans increases the uncertainty in the process and makes it difficult to detect errors. AAPM TG 100 recommends identifying and eliminating the causes of high-priority errors in the clinic (Huq et al., 2016). The TG 132 report is recommended (Brock et al., 2017). End to End test by each clinic using their systems is the right step to verify the whole system. It ensures that every chain link is controlled from the simulation stage to the treatment application. It allows testing the connections between systems and the control of individual devices or systems. After each upgrade, this test should be recommended.

Conclusion

ART is one of the most researched application techniques in RT today. Its contribution to the quality of treatment cannot be underestimated. It is expected that especially online and real-time ART applications will enter daily practice with the technological developments in imaging systems, image registration, auto segmentation, rapid plan optimization programs, and target tracking systems in the treatment room.

References

Barker Jr, J. L., Garden, A. S., Ang, K. K., O'Daniel, J. C., Wang, H., Court, L. E., ... & Dong, L. (2004). Quantification of volumetric and geometric changes occurring during fractionated radiotherapy for head-and-neck cancer using an integrated CT/linear accelerator system. *International Journal of Radiation Oncology* Biology* Physics*, *59*(4), 960-970.

Barney, B. M., Lee, R. J., Handrahan, D., Welsh, K. T., Cook, J. T., & Sause, W. T. (2011). Image-guided radiotherapy (IGRT) for prostate cancer comparing kV imaging of fiducial markers with cone beam computed tomography (CBCT). *International Journal of Radiation Oncology* Biology* Physics*, *80*(1), 301-305.

Bondar, M. L., Hoogeman, M. S., Mens, J. W., Quint, S., Ahmad, R., Dhawtal, G., & Heijmen, B. J. (2012). Individualized nonadaptive and online-adaptive intensity-modulated radiotherapy treatment strategies for cervical cancer patients based on pretreatment acquired variable bladder filling computed tomography scans. *International Journal of Radiation Oncology* Biology* Physics*, *83*(5), 1617-1623.

Brock, K. K., Mutic, S., McNutt, T. R., Li, H., & Kessler, M. L. (2017). Use of image registration and fusion algorithms and techniques in radiotherapy: Report of the AAPM Radiation Therapy Committee Task Group No. 132. *Medical Physics*, *44*(7), e43-e76.

Chung, P. W., Haycocks, T., Brown, T., Cambridge, Z., Kelly, V., Alasti, H., ... & Catton, C. N. (2004). On-line aSi portal imaging of implanted fiducial markers for the reduction of interfraction error during conformal radiotherapy of prostate carcinoma. *International Journal of Radiation Oncology* Biology* Physics*, *60*(1), 329-334.

Court, L. E., & Dong, L. (2003). Automatic registration of the prostate for computed-tomography-guided radiotherapy. *Medical Physics*, *30*(10), 2750-2757.

Court, L., Rosen, I., Mohan, R., & Dong, L. (2003). Evaluation of mechanical precision and alignment uncertainties for an integrated CT/LINAC system. *Medical Physics*, *30*(6), 1198-1210.

Dees-Ribbers, H. M., Betgen, A., Pos, F. J., Witteveen, T., Remeijer, P., & van Herk, M. (2014). Inter-and intra-fractional bladder motion during radiotherapy for bladder cancer: a comparison of full and empty bladders. *Radiotherapy and Oncology*, *113*(2), 254-259.

Foroudi, F., Wong, J., Kron, T., Rolfo, A., Haworth, A., Roxby, P., ... & Duchesne, G. (2011). Online adaptive radiotherapy for muscle-invasive bladder cancer: results of a pilot study. *International Journal of Radiation Oncology* Biology* Physics*, *81*(3), 765-771.

Hawkins, M. A., Brooks, C., Hansen, V. N., Aitken, A., & Tait, D. M. (2010). Cone beam computed tomography–derived adaptive radiotherapy for radical treatment of esophageal cancer. *International Journal of Radiation Oncology* Biology* Physics*, *77*(2), 378-383.

Hessen, E. D., van Buuren, L. D., Nijkamp, J. A., de Vries, K. C., Mok, W. K., Dewit, L., ... & Borst, G. R. (2017). Significant tumor shift in patients treated with stereotactic radiosurgery for brain metastasis. *Clinical and translational radiation oncology*, *2*, 23-28.

Huq, M. S., Fraass, B. A., Dunscombe, P. B., Gibbons, J. P., Ibbott, G. S., & Medin, P. M. (2016). Application of risk analysis methods to radiation therapy quality management: report of AAPM Task Group 100. *Med Phys*, *43*(7), 4209-4262.

ICRU. (1993). *Prescribing, Recording, and Reporting Photon Beam Therapy. Bethesda, MD:* (No. 50). ICRU Report.

Kishan, A. U., Cui, J., Wang, P. C., Daly, M. E., Purdy, J. A., & Chen, A. M. (2014). Quantification of gross tumour volume changes between simulation and the first day of radiotherapy for patients with locally advanced malignancies of the lung and head/neck. *Journal of Medical Imaging and Radiation Oncology*, *58*(5), 618-624.

Kranen, S., Beek, S., Rasch, C., van Herk, M., & Sonke, J. J. (2009). Setup uncertainties of anatomical sub-regions in head-and-neck cancer patients after offline CBCT guidance. *International Journal of Radiation Oncology* Biology* Physics*, *73*(5), 1566-1573.

Kuriyama, K., Onishi, H., Sano, N., Komiyama, T., Aikawa, Y., Tateda, Y., ... & Uematsu, M. (2003). A new irradiation unit was constructed of self-moving gantry-CT and linac. *International Journal of Radiation Oncology* Biology* Physics*, *55*(2), 428-435.

Li, T., Thongphiew, D., Zhu, X., Lee, W. R., Vujaskovic, Z., Yin, F. F., & Wu, Q. J. (2011). Adaptive prostate IGRT combining online re-optimization and re-positioning: a feasibility study. *Physics in Medicine & Biology*, *56*(5), 1243.

Li, T., Zhu, X., Thongphiew, D., Lee, W. R., Vujaskovic, Z., Wu, Q., ... & Wu, Q. J. (2010). On-line adaptive radiation therapy: feasibility and clinical study. *Journal of oncology*, *2010*.

Liang, J., Wu, Q., & Yan, D. (2009). The role of seminal vesicle motion in target margin assessment for online image-guided radiotherapy for prostate cancer. *International Journal of Radiation Oncology* Biology* Physics*, *73*(3), 935-943.

Nuver, T. T., Hoogeman, M. S., Remeijer, P., van Herk, M., & Lebesque, J. V. (2007). An adaptive off-line procedure for radiotherapy of prostate cancer. *International Journal of Radiation Oncology* Biology* Physics*, *67*(5), 1559-1567.

Pötter, R., Dimopoulos, J., Georg, P., Lang, S., Waldhäusl, C., Wachter-Gerstner, N., ... & Kirisits, C. (2007). Clinical impact of MRI-assisted dose volume adaptation and dose escalation in brachytherapy of locally advanced cervix cancer. *Radiotherapy and oncology*, *83*(2), 148-155.

Tishler, R. B., Petit, J., Cormack, R., & Chin, L. (2006). Automatic online adaptive radiation therapy techniques for targets with significant shape change: a feasibility study. *Physics in Medicine & Biology*, *51*(10), 2493.

Velec, M., Moseley, J. L., Eccles, C. L., Craig, T., Sharpe, M. B., Dawson, L. A., & Brock, K. K. (2011). Effect of breathing motion on radiotherapy dose accumulation in the abdomen using deformable registration. *International Journal of Radiation Oncology* Biology* Physics*, *80*(1), 265-272.

Vlachaki, M., Castellon, I., Leite, C., Perkins, T., & Ahmad, S. (2009). Impact of respiratory gating using 4-dimensional computed tomography on the dosimetry of tumor and normal tissues in patients with thoracic malignancies. *American journal of clinical oncology*, *32*(3), 262-268.

Wang, H., Dong, L., O'Daniel, J., Mohan, R., Garden, A. S., Ang, K. K., ... & Cheung, R. (2005). Validation of an accelerated 'demons' algorithm for deformable image registration in radiation therapy. *Physics in Medicine & Biology*, *50*(12), 2887.

Witte, M. G., Sonke, J. J., Siebers, J., Deasy, J. O., & Van Herk, M. (2017). Beyond the margin recipe: the probability of correct target dosage and tumor control in the presence of a dose-limiting structure. *Physics in Medicine & Biology*, *62*(19), 7874.

Wu, C., Jeraj, R., Olivera, G. H., & Mackie, T. R. (2002). Re-optimization in adaptive radiotherapy. *Physics in Medicine & Biology*, *47*(17), 3181.

Wu, Q. J., Li, T., Wu, Q., & Yin, F. F. (2011). Adaptive radiation therapy: technical components and clinical applications. *The cancer journal*, *17*(3), 182-189.

Wu, Q. J., Thongphiew, D., Wang, Z., Mathayomchan, B., Chankong, V., Yoo, S., ... & Yin, F. F. (2008). On-line re-optimization of prostate IMRT plans for adaptive radiation therapy. *Physics in Medicine & Biology*, *53*(3), 673.

Yan, D., Vicini, F., Wong, J., & Martinez, A. (1997). Adaptive radiation therapy. *Physics in Medicine & Biology*, *42*(1), 123.

Yoo, D. S., Wong, T. Z., & Brizel, D. M. (2010, December). The role of adaptive and functional imaging modalities in radiation therapy: approach and application from a radiation oncology perspective. In *Seminars in Ultrasound, CT and MRI* (Vol. 31, No. 6, pp. 444-461). WB Saunders.

Chapter 14

Challenges in IMRT from a Clinician Perspective

Menekşe Turna*

Department of Radiation Oncology, Anadolu Medical Center, Kocaeli, Turkey

Abstract

IMRT is a breakthrough technique in modern radiotherapy with rapid dose fall-off and its ability to modulate the dose on the target organ. Accurate determination and delineation of the target volumes and critical organs are essential for accurate treatment planning. Image registration algorithms play a significant role in many stages of treatment applications, from target volume delineation to response evaluation. Planned treatments with the appropriate IGRT method determined for each region can be applied with high accuracy. There are different IGRT methods that can be used for each treatment system. Strategies that take motion into account should be used in moving targets. It may be appropriate to make an adaptive plan due to the changes in the target volume and patient anatomy during the treatment.

Keywords: IMRT, IGRT, image registration, adaptive radiation

1. Introduction

Intensity-modulated radiation therapy (IMRT) has been an advanced development in radiation oncology and has become routinely available in

---

*Corresponding Author's Email: menekse.turna@gmail.com.

In: Frontiers in Intensity-Modulated Radiotherapy Research
Editor: Sibel Karaca
ISBN: 979-8-88697-252-8

nearly all centers. The success of IMRT has to be evaluated in terms of better survival and reduced toxicity (Beadle et al., 2014; Hummel et al., 2010; Teoh et al., 2011). IMRT outcomes in prostate cancer, lower gastrointestinal, gynecological, head and neck, lung, and breast cancer are superior to 3DCRT and are now accepted in most complex cases (Beadle et al., 2014; Hummel et al., 2010; Teoh et al., 2011). As a result, IMRT has become widespread and is already a standard treatment for many tumor sites.

IMRT is a complex process (Figure 1). Every step has its unique challenges and requires an advanced level of expertise and sophisticated skills.

2. Indications

The Radiation Therapy Oncology Group (RTOG) 0617 study reported worse survival outcomes with dose escalation from 60 Gy to 74 Gy in locally advanced lung cancer and revealed that the volumes hearth doses were independent predictors of survival (Bradley et al., 2020). These findings highlight the importance of minimizing the dose to critical thoracic OARs. Furthermore, a secondary analysis of the study demonstrated that with IMRT, lower heart and lung doses were obtained, and fewer side effects were shown, thus, rationalizing the use of IMRT (Chun et al., 2017).

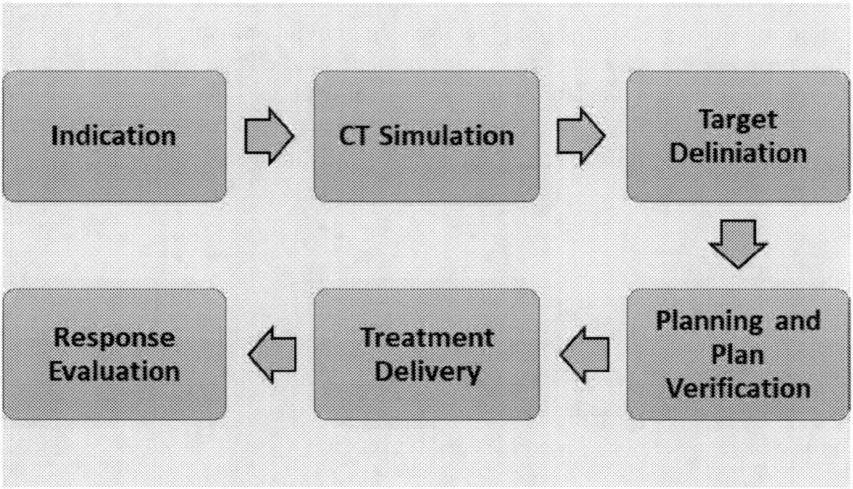

Figure 1. IMRT Workflow.

Systemic treatment options for cancer patients have changed considerably over the past several decades and have significantly improved the survival of many tumor types. However, there is less knowledge regarding the implications of combining radiotherapy with these drugs, as most trials did not prespecify the RT details or exclude patients who received RT. Although this situation is frequently encountered in daily practice, it is not known how it would be safe to administer RT or how we can improve the efficacy in the current era of systemic therapies. The last drug approved for use with radiation was cetuximab in 2004 (Walker et al., 2020). To address this need, the FDA has published an analysis of the use of RT in patients receiving immunotherapy and reported that administration within 90 days following RT does not cause an increase in serious side effects (Anscher et al., 2022). Temporary drug discontinuation, radiation dose modification, and following stricter organ at risk doses can be considered for these situations. There is a need for evidence and multidisciplinary clinical guidelines.

IMRT results in a larger volume of normal tissue receiving lower radiation doses than 3D-CRT and tends to increase the risk of second cancers. These drawbacks are significant in children and patients with an expected prolonged survival (Hall et al., 2003). Another disadvantage of IMRT is the prolonged time for each treatment compared with other treatment techniques, with its unknown biological impact (Wang et al., 2003).

Proton therapy provides a highly conformal and uniform dose to a tumor, especially can be advantageous for some regions, some tumors, and some patients compared to photon beam IMRT (Newhauser et al., 2015) (Figure 2). Especially in childhood cancer, in skull base located chordoma, and in chondrosarcoma tumors is routinely applied in many centers without any randomized data for better oncological results (Hu et al., 2018). In a phase IIB trial, proton beam treatment was found to have a reduced risk of the adverse event than photon IMRT, maintaining similar oncological outcomes for locally advanced esophageal cancer (Lin et al., 2020).

Intensity-modulated proton therapy (IMPT) is a complex, novel form of proton therapy. Several studies demonstrated the dosimetric advantages of IMPT over IMRT (Moreno et al., 2019). However, the delivery of proton therapy is more expensive than the delivery of IMRT (Lievens et al., 2013). Which patients will benefit more from IMPT can be decided by treatment region, dosimetric comparisons with photon IMRT, and artificial intelligence (Kouwenberg et al., 2021).

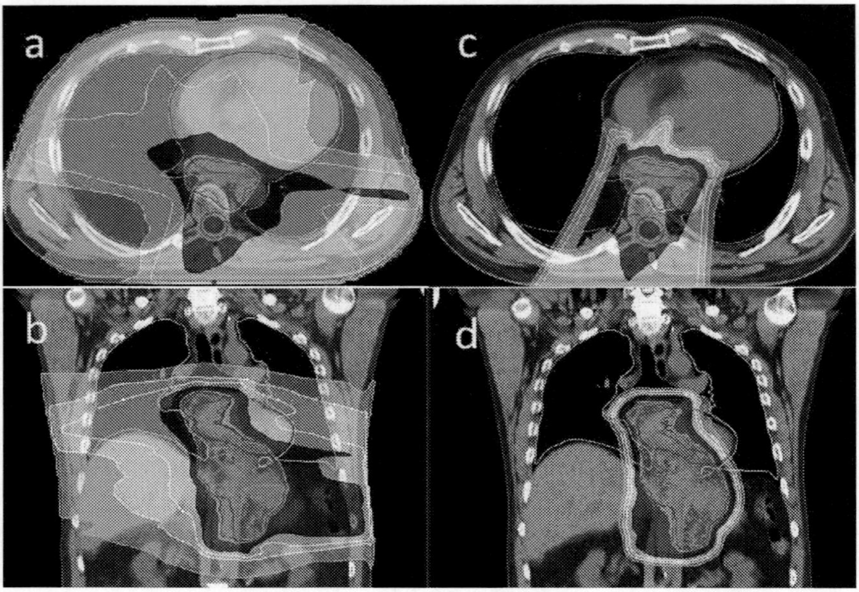

Figure 2. Axial and coronal views of the dose distributions for esophageal cancer. IMRT plans (a, b); proton treatment (c, d). Rapid dose fall-off and heart and lung-sparing with proton plan.

3. Target Delineation and OAR

The highly conformal dose distributions and rapid dose reduction produced by beam intensity modulation require careful delineation of the target and organ at risk. Inadequate delineation of the target volumes can be associated with reduced tumor control in IMRT treatments. (Chen et al., 2017; Peters et al., 2010). Therefore, there are multiple contouring guidelines for target and normal tissue delineation (Niyazi et al., 2016; Lim et al., 2011; Small et al., 2008) Taylor et al., 2005;). This allows uniformity in defining normal tissues and is practical for daily practice and crucial for clinical trial quality assurance.

The first step for correct delineation is planning computed tomography (CT), which should be taken under ideal conditions. Suboptimal images may cause uncertainties and discrepancies in contouring (Chang et al., 2017). Therefore, standardized CT protocols should be established for each tumor site. Parameters such as suitable immobilization devices (thermoplastic masks, vacuum bags), imaging compatible with the IGRT protocol (4D-CT, breath-hold (BH), abdominal compression), use of intravenous, oral, vaginal, or rectal contrast should be indicated in these protocols.

The use of an iodine-based contrast agent is helpful in situations in which contrast is likely to improve the accuracy of the delineations (Williams et al., 2016). The use of intravenous contrast allows us to enhance the visualization of target volumes and adjacent structures, promoting a more accurate delineation of these volumes (Figure 3). Before all contrast administration, risk factors (renal functions, allergic reactions) should be assessed. Although it is known that the contrast agent causes some influence in the plan calculations, these are clinically negligible (Choi et al., 2006; Shibamoto et al., 20071).

Before planning tomography, specific preparations may need to be made according to the anatomical region. For example, an empty stomach with hunger, an empty rectum with enemas or laxatives, and a filled bladder with a certain amount of water can provide optimal anatomy for critical organ doses and tumor doses.

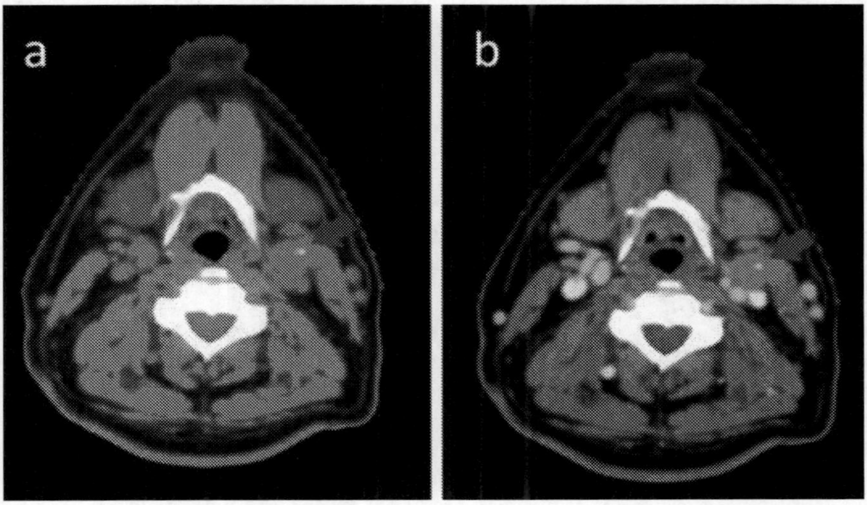

Figure 3. Left neck lymph node (a) without IV contrast and (b) better visualization with IV contrast.

In the presence of metal implants, such as dental fillings or hip replacements, the extreme photon absorption by the metal object generates considerable image artifacts. CT metal artifacts adversely affect RT planning both by creating difficulties in visualization of target and creating uncertainties in RT planning dose calculation (Giantsoudi et al., 2017). Various metal artifact reduction (MAR) methods have been investigated to improve visualization of the organs and dose calculation in RT planning, depending on the location of the metal implant, type of radiation treatment, and treatment site (Li et al., 2013; Brock et al., 2017).

Patients with pacemaker devices may be affected by radiation, and permanent or temporary damage may occur. Therefore, close dialogue with cardiologists is vital during treatment. The dose should be reduced, and deactivation should be planned during the treatment according to the risk situation.

4. Image Registration

The planning tomography alone is often insufficient for accurate contouring due to the low soft tissue resolution. Therefore, registration with secondary imaging methods such as MRI and PET-CT with improved soft-tissue contrast and functional information provides extra information for a better deliniation (Schmidt et al., 2015; Li et al., 2013). The fusions help contour the target volume and patient setup, IGRT, retreatment, replanning, adaptive RT, dose summation, assessment of tumor, and normal organ response during and after RT (Figure 4) (Brock et al., 2017).

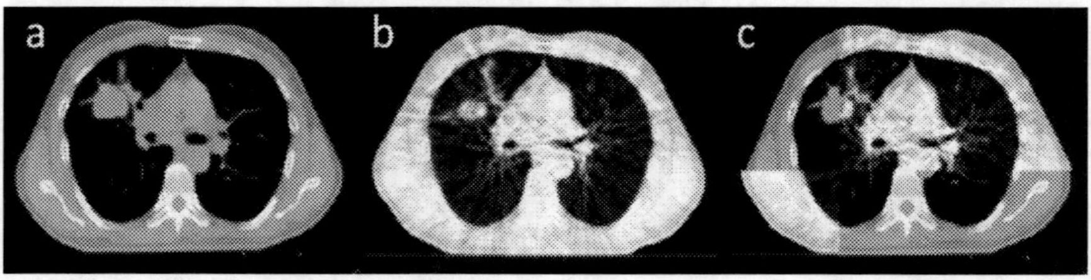

Figure 4. Right lung mass as GTV in planning CT (a), CBCT images of 21st fraction of the treatment for IGRT. Shrinkage of the tumor is seen. (b), daily match, the fusion of both images (c).

In order to use these secondary images in planning, it is necessary to combine them with the planning CT as primary imaging with the help of a fusion algorithm. The image registration algorithms have been classified mainly as rigid (RIR) and deformable (DIR). In rigid registration, only translational and rotational transformation is needed. In deformable registration, volumetric changes and distortion need to be corrected with different algorithms that must be implemented and used with caution (Brock et al., 2017). DIR is commonly used for contour propagation tools online and offline for replanning, atlas auto-segmentation, dose summation, or an adaptive planning.

There is no objective, quantitative parameters that evaluate the fusion quality for individual patient imaging. Professional knowledge and multidisciplinary input are typically needed for evaluation. Education and training are indispensable for the high-quality and effective implementation of image registration. The fact that the secondary images are in the planning position affects the quality of the fusion (Jabbari et al., 2017; Grgic et al., 2009). Fusion quality may be poor due to distortion in peripheral regions in MRI images. It is essential to correct or account for this distortion.

5. IGRT and Motion Management

Image-guided radiation therapy (IGRT) is mainly defined as the use of imaging during or just prior to treatment that verifies the alignment of anatomy between the radiotherapy plan and the patient to verify or improve the accuracy of RT (Sterzing et al., 2011).

It is an indispensable component of IMRT. The prominent role is to maximize accuracy and precision immediately before each radiation treatment fraction and throughout the entire process of treatment delivery (De Los et al., (2013)). There are several different methods for IGRT, as listed below:

- 2D planar - MV, KV, fluoroscopic imaging, or magnetic resonance imaging (MRI)
- 3D volumetric - kV cone-beam CT (CBCT), megavoltage CT (MVCT), MRI or ultrasound
- 4D volumetric - kV-CBCT, MRI, fluoroscopic imaging, or ultrasound
- External anatomy surface based (SGRT)
- Electromagnetic transponders/transmitters.

The planning CT and reference images are matched by hand or with o software for comparison. The analysis and correction process must be fast, simple, and straightforward. IGRT strategy and protocol for specific diseases and types of treatment need to be created in each clinic, considering the patients' characteristics, treatment time, and clinic workload. Effective immobilization reduces the setup and systematic errors (Karaca et al., 2016). In addition, the establishment of departmental PTV margins based on systematic and random uncertainties calculation is required (Stroom et al., 2002).

Respiration, heart beating, peristalsis, organ filling, and emptying are the main reasons for the motion. Different strategies which take into account the motion allow us to treat moving lesions. It is well known that lack of adequate respiratory motion management adversely affects treatment outcomes (Andratschke et al., 2018; Van den et al., 2014). Motion encompassing methods like slow computerized tomography (CT) scanning, inhalation-exhalation breath-hold (BH) CT, four-dimensional (4D) CT, internal target volume (ITV) approach; respiratory gating with an external respiration signal or fiducial; BH with or without active breath controlling and forced shallow breathing with abdominal compression are all valid and acceptable methods (Keall et al., 2006). These methods' reproducibility and consistency during simulation and treatment are critically important. A residual motion may be determined by intra-fractional tracking, even with the breath-hold method (Lens et al., 2016).

Electromagnetic transponders/transmitters can be used for motion tracking of moving targets that cannot be modeled like respiratory motion (Bertholet et al., 2019). These systems can be placed in or near the organ, providing continuous real-time 3D localization without additional ionizing radiation.

6. Adaptive RT and Image Segmentation

Adaptive radiotherapy (ART) is an operation to check for anatomical and functional change throughout the treatment period. It allows modification of the treatment plan to account for variations in target and normal organs and patient contours, ultimately aiming to deliver the dose accurately to minimize normal tissue exposure and maximize the dose to the target (Brock et al., 2019).

These anatomical changes caused by weight loss, tumor regression, variations in organ filling, or other target and organ shape changes are often specific to individual patients and cannot be merely solved with translational and rotational setup corrections (Sonke et al., 2019).

ART implementation is widely varied from a simple process such as making a new plan by taking a new planning tomography to a patient who can lose weight to advanced adaptive RT methods in which auto segmentation, deformable registration, and automated planning are added (Bertholet et al., 2020).

ART implementations can be done at three different timescales: offline between treatment fractions, online immediately before a treatment fraction, and real-time during a fraction (Tunçel, 2021) requires four basic steps: imaging, assessment, replanning, and quality assurance (Green et al., 2019).

The selection of a particular timescale of ART depends on the clinical goal, available technology, and resources. There is a limited consensus on which patients will have the actual benefits, the best time, and the best techniques for adaptation. The staffing burden may outweigh the potential benefits of ART.

Offline adaptation updates the patient's treatment plan after delivering single or multiple treatment fractions, generally following the same clinical workflow as initial treatment planning (Green et al., 2019). However, analyzing interfraction changes from daily IGRT images in an offline adaptive approach is subjective in the current practice. Nevertheless, with the help of software with pre-defined action levels based on in-room imaging, it is possible to identify which replanning might be indicated objectively (Liu et al., 2018). These algorithms make deformable registration with daily imaging and planning CT, deform contours onto daily imaging, calculate the dose, and accumulate and summarise according to the pre-defined dose limits (Glide-Hurst, 2021).

Online adaptation is a procedure that utilizes plan adaptations immediately before the delivery of the fraction while the patient remains in the treatment position. After the imaging, rapid re-contouring, replanning, and plan review are required on an IGRT-derived imaging dataset (Glide-Hurst et al., 2021).

Real-time adaptation automatically adapts the treatment plan during treatment to account for variations within a treatment fraction, such as respiration. It performs adaptation based on real-time imaging to gate the treatment beam or track the target using the multi-leaf collimator (MLC) (Glide-Hurst et al., 2021). Magnetic Resonance-guided radiotherapy (MRgRT) provides real-time information for in-line adaptive protocols to match daily anatomy. Magnetic field strength, real-time auto-segmentation time and accuracy, and latency time between real-time MRI and MR-linac systems are the main challenges in MRgRT (Thorwarth et al., 2021).

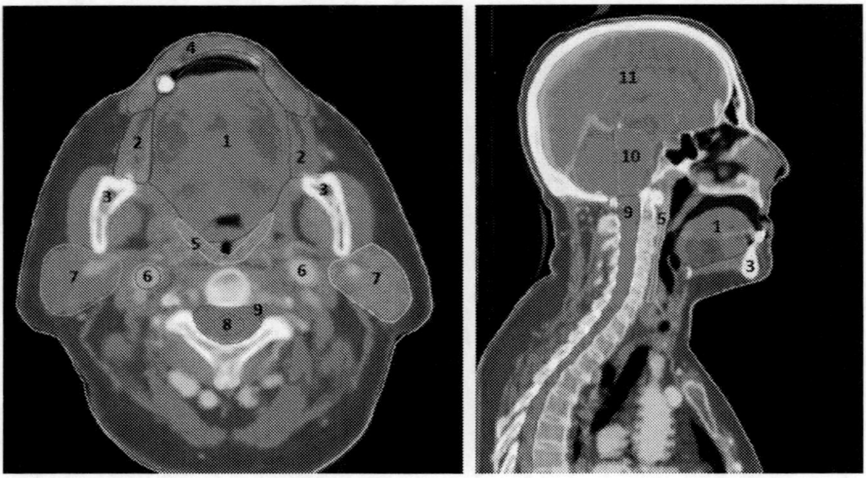

Figure 5. Axial (left) and sagittal (right) view of autosegmentated organ at risk delineations of the head and neck region with Mvision. Oral cavity (1), buccal mucosa (2), mandible (3), lips (4), pharyngeal constrictor muscles (5), carotid arteries (6), parotids (7), spinal cord (8), spinal canal (9), brainstem (10), brain (11).

The manual segmentation of these ROIs is time-consuming for both initial planning, and adaptive RT requires much work. However, with automated segmentation methods and artificial intelligence, it may be possible to reduce these times, provide standardization in contours, and reduce inter-and intra-observer variability. There are several methods for auto segmentation which can be atlas-based or uses machine learning and artificial intelligence (Figure 5).

Conclusion

Standard guidelines in defining the target volume should be used to eliminate inter and intra-observer differences and make objective evaluations. Since contouring of all target volumes and critical organs requires intensive labor and time, automatic contouring algorithms with artificial intelligence or atlas-based can be integrated into daily practice. There is a need for objective methods to evaluate the accuracy of image registration results for each patient. Pre-planned strategies and objective methods are needed in tumors and patients with a high probability of adaptive planning. Proton therapy and IMPT may be advantageous for some patients and diseases. However, objective mechanisms such as intelligent algorithms supported by clinical studies are needed to determine which patient will benefit more from proton treatment than IMRT.

References

Andratschke, N., H. Alheid, M. Allgäuer, G. Becker, O. Blanck, J. Boda-Heggemann, T. Brunner, M. Duma, S. Gerum, M. Guckenberger, G. Hildebrandt, R. J. Klement, V. Lewitzki, C. Ostheimer, A. Papachristofilou, C. Petersen, T. Schneider, R. Semrau, S. Wachter & D. Habermehl. The SBRT Database Initiative of the German Society for Radiation Oncology (DEGRO): Patterns of Care and Outcome Analysis of Stereotactic Body Radiotherapy (SBRT) for Liver Oligometastases in 474 Patients with 623 Metastases. *BMC Cancer* 18, no. 1 (2018). https://doi.org/10.1186/s12885-018-4191-2.

Anscher, M. S., Shaily Arora, Chana Weinstock, Anup Amatya, Pradeep Bandaru, Chad Tang, Andrew T. Girvin, Mallorie H. Fiero, Shenghui Tang, Rachael Lubitz, Laleh Amiri-Kordestani, Marc R. Theoret, Richard Pazdur, Julia A. Beaver. Association of Radiation Therapy with Risk of Adverse Events in Patients Receiving Immunotherapy. *JAMA Oncology* 8, no. 2 (2022): 232. https://doi.org/10.1001/jamaoncol.2021.6439.

Beadle, B. M., Liao, K. P., Elting, L. S., Buchholz, T. A., Ang, K. K., Garden, A. S., Guadagnolo, B. A. Improved Survival Using Intensity-Modulated Radiation Therapy in Head and Neck Cancers: a SEER-Medicare Analysis. *Cancer.* (2014) Mar 1;120(5):702-10. doi: https://doi.org/10.1002/Cncr.28372. Epub 2014 Jan 13. Erratum in: Cancer. (2014) Jun 1;120(11):1754. PMID: 24421077.

Bertholet, J., Antje Knopf, Björn Eiben, Jamie McClelland, Alexander Grimwood, Emma Harris, Martin Menten, Per Poulsen, Doan Trang Nguyen, Paul Keall, Uwe Oelfke. Real-Time Intrafraction Motion Monitoring in External Beam Radiotherapy. *Physics in Medicine & Biology* 64, no. 15 (2019). https://doi.org/10.1088/1361-6560/ab2ba8.

Bertholet, Jenny, Gail Anastasi, David Noble, Arjan Bel, Ruud van Leeuwen, Toon Roggen, Michael Duchateau, Sara Pilskog, Cristina Garibaldi, Nina Tilly, Rafael García-Mollá, Jorge Bonaque, Uwe Oelfke, Marianne C. Aznar and Ben Heijmenr. Patterns of Practice for Adaptive and Real-Time Radiation Therapy (Pop-ART RT) Part II: Offline and Online Plan Adaption for Interfractional Changes. *Radiotherapy and Oncology* 153 (2020): 88-96. https://doi.org/10.1016/j.radonc.2020.06.017.

Bradley, J. D., Chen Hu, Ritsuko R. Komaki, Gregory A. Masters, George R. Blumenschein, Steven E. Schild, Jeffrey A. Bogart, Kenneth M Forster, Anthony M Magliocco, Vivek S Kavadi, Samir Narayan, Puneeth Iyengar, Clifford G Robinson, Raymond B Wynn, Christopher D Koprowski, Michael R Olson, Joanne Meng, Rebecca Paulus, Walter J Curran Jr, Hak Choy. Long-Term Results of NRG Oncology RTOG 0617: Standard- versus High-Dose Chemoradiotherapy with or without Cetuximab for Unresectable Stage III Non-Small-Cell Lung Cancer. *Journal of Clinical Oncology* 38, no. 7 (2020): 706-14. https://doi.org/10.1200/jco.19.01162.

Brock, K. K. Adaptive Radiotherapy: Moving into the Future. *Seminars in Radiation Oncology* 29, no. 3 (2019): 181-84. https://doi.org/10.1016/j.semradonc.2019.02.011.

Brock, K. K., Sasa Mutic, Todd R. McNutt, Hua Li, and Marc L. Kessler. Use of Image Registration and Fusion Algorithms and Techniques in Radiotherapy: Report of the AAPM Radiation Therapy Committee Task Group No. 132. *Medical Physics* 44, no. 7 (2017). https://doi.org/10.1002/mp.12256.

Chang, A. T., Li Tee Tan, Simon Duke, and Wai-Tong Ng. Challenges for Quality Assurance of Target Volume Delineation in Clinical Trials. *Frontiers in Oncology* 7 (2017). https://doi.org/10.3389/fonc.2017.00221.

Chen, A. M., Robert Chin, Philip Beron, Taeko Yoshizaki, Argin G. Mikaeilian, and Minsong Cao. Inadequate Target Volume Delineation and Local–Regional Recurrence after Intensity-Modulated Radiotherapy for Human Papillomavirus-Positive Oropharynx Cancer. *Radiotherapy and Oncology* 123, no. 3 (2017): 412-18. https://doi.org/10.1016/j.radonc.2017.04.015.

Choi, Y., Jeung-Kee Kim, Hyung-Sik Lee, Won-Joo Hur, Young-Seoub Hong, Sungkwang Park, Kijung Ahn, and Heunglae Cho. Influence of Intravenous Contrast Agent on Dose Calculations of Intensity Modulated Radiation Therapy Plans for Head and Neck Cancer. *Radiotherapy and Oncology* 81, no. 2 (2006): 158-62. https://doi.org/10.1016/j.radonc.2006.09.010.

Chun, S. G., Chen Hu, Hak Choy, Ritsuko U. Komaki, Robert D. Timmerman, Steven E. Schild, Jeffrey A. Bogart, Michael C. Dobelbower, Walter Bosch, James M. Galvin, Vivek S. Kavadi, Samir Narayan, Puneeth Iyengar, Clifford G. Robinson, Raymond B. Wynn, Adam Raben, Mark E. Augspurger, Robert M. MacRae, Rebecca Paulus, Jeffrey D. Bradley. Impact of Intensity-Modulated Radiation Therapy Technique for Locally Advanced Non-Small-Cell Lung Cancer: A Secondary Analysis of the NRG Oncology RTOG 0617 Randomized Clinical Trial. *Journal of Clinical Oncology* 35, no. 1 (2017): 56-62. https://doi.org/10.1200/jco.2016.69.1378.

De Los Santos, J., Richard Popple, Nzhde Agazaryan, John E. Bayouth, Jean-Pierre Bissonnette, Mary Kara Bucci, Sonja Dieterich, Lei Dong, Kenneth M Forster, Daniel Indelicato, Katja Langen, Joerg Lehmann, Nina Mayr, Ishmael Parsai, William Salter, Michael Tomblyn, William T. C. Yuh, Indrin J Chetty. Image Guided Radiation Therapy (IGRT) Technologies for Radiation Therapy Localization and Delivery. *International Journal of Radiation Oncology Biology Physics* 87, no. 1 (2013): 33-45. https://doi.org/10.1016/j.ijrobp.2013.02.021.

Giantsoudi, D., Bruno De Man, Joost Verburg, Alexei Trofimov, Yannan Jin, Ge Wang, Lars Gjesteby, and Harald Paganetti. Metal Artifacts in Computed Tomography for Radiation Therapy Planning: Dosimetric Effects and Impact of Metal Artifact Reduction. *Physics in Medicine and Biology* 62, no. 8 (2017). https://doi.org/10.1088/1361-6560/aa5293.

Glide-Hurst, C. K., Percy Lee, Adam D. Yock, Jeffrey R. Olsen, Minsong Cao, Farzan Siddiqui, William Parker, Anthony Doemer, Yi Rong, Amar U Kishan, Stanley H Benedict, X Allen Li, Beth A Erickson, Jason W Sohn, Ying Xiao, Evan Wuthrick. Adaptive Radiation Therapy (ART) Strategies and Technical Considerations: A State of the Art Review from NRG Oncology. *International Journal of Radiation Oncology Biology Physics* 109, no. 4 (2021): 1054-75. https://doi.org/10.1016/j.ijrobp.2020.10.021.

Green, O. L., Lauren E. Henke, and Geoffrey D. Hugo. Practical Clinical Workflows for Online and Offline Adaptive Radiation Therapy. *Seminars in Radiation Oncology* 29, no. 3 (2019): 219-27. https://doi.org/10.1016/j.semradonc.2019.02.004.

Grgic, A., Ursula Nestle, Andrea Schaefer-Schuler, Stephanie Kremp, Carl-Martin Kirsch, and Dirk Hellwig. FDG-PET-Based Radiotherapy Planning in Lung Cancer: Optimum Breathing Protocol and Patient Positioning - an Intraindividual Comparison. *International Journal of Radiation Oncology Biology Physics* 73, no. 1 (2009): 103-11. https://doi.org/10.1016/j.ijrobp.2008.03.063.

Hall, E. J., and Cheng-Shie Wuu. Radiation-Induced Second Cancers: The Impact of 3D-CRT and IMRT. *International Journal of Radiation Oncology Biology Physics* 56, no. 1 (2003): 83-88. https://doi.org/10.1016/s0360-3016(03)00073-7.

Hu, M., Liyang Jiang, Xiangli Cui, Jianguang Zhang, and Jinming Yu. Proton Beam Therapy for Cancer in the Era of Precision Medicine. *Journal of Hematology & Oncology* 11, no. 1 (2018). https://doi.org/10.1186/s13045-018-0683-4.

Hummel, S., E. L. Simpson, P. Hemingway, M. D. Stevenson, and A. Rees. Intensity-Modulated Radiotherapy for the Treatment of Prostate Cancer: A Systematic Review and Economic Evaluation. *Health Technology Assessment* 14, no. 47 (2010). https://doi.org/10.3310/hta14470.

Jabbari, K., Atefeh Shirvani, and Alireza Amouheidari. Evaluation of Effective Parameters on Quality of Magnetic Resonance Imaging-Computed Tomography Image Fusion in Head and Neck Tumors for Application in Treatment Planning. *Advanced Biomedical Research* 6, no. 1 (2017): 161. https://doi.org/10.4103/abr.abr_182_16.

Karaca, S., Hamit Başaran, Timur Koca, and Ferhat Özbayrak. An Evaluation of Inter-Fractional Set-up Errors in Patients Treated with Distinct Immobilization Equipment for Varying Anatomical Regions. International Journal of Medical Physics, *Clinical Engineering and Radiation Oncology* 05, no. 02 (2016): 121-29. https://doi.org/10.4236/ijmpcero.2016.52013.

Keall, P. J., Gig S. Mageras, James M. Balter, Richard S. Emery, Kenneth M. Forster, Steve B. Jiang, Jeffrey M. Kapatoes, Daniel A. Low, Martin J. Murphy, Brad R. Murray, Chester R. Ramsey, Marcel B. Van Herk, S. Sastry Vedam, John W. Wong, Ellen Yorke. The Management of Respiratory Motion in Radiation Oncology Report of Aapm Task Group 76A). *Medical Physics* 33, no. 10 (2006): 3874-3900. https://doi.org/10.1118/1.2349696.

Kouwenberg, J., Joan Penninkhof, Steven Habraken, Jaap Zindler, Mischa Hoogeman, and Ben Heijmen. Model Based Patient Pre-Selection for Intensity-Modulated Proton Therapy (IMPT) Using Automated Treatment Planning and Machine Learning. *Radiotherapy and Oncology* 158 (2021): 224-29. https://doi.org/10.1016/j.radonc.2021.02.034.

Lens, E., Oliver J. Gurney-Champion, Daniël R. Tekelenburg, Zdenko van Kesteren, Michael J. Parkes, Geertjan van Tienhoven, Aart J. Nederveen, Astrid van der Horst, and Arjan Bel. Abdominal Organ Motion during Inhalation and Exhalation Breath-Holds: Pancreatic Motion at Different Lung Volumes Compared. *Radiotherapy and Oncology* 121, no. 2 (2016): 268-75. https://doi.org/10.1016/j.radonc.2016.09.012.

Li, H., Camille Noel, Haijian Chen, H. Harold Li, Daniel Low, Kevin Moore, Paul Klahr, Jeff Michalski, Hiram A Gay, Wade Thorstad, Sasa Mutic. Clinical Evaluation of a Commercial Orthopedic Metal Artifact Reduction Tool for CT Simulations in Radiation Therapy. *Medical Physics* 39, no. 12 (2012): 7507-17. https://doi.org/10.1118/1.4762814.

Li, J., and Ying Xiao. Application of FDG-PET/CT in Radiation Oncology. *Frontiers in Oncology* 3 (2013). https://doi.org/10.3389/fonc.2013.00080.

Lievens, Y., and Madelon Pijls-Johannesma. Health Economic Controversy and Cost-Effectiveness of Proton Therapy. *Seminars in Radiation Oncology* 23, no. 2 (2013): 134-41. https://doi.org/10.1016/j.semradonc.2012.11.005.

Lim, K., William Small, Lorraine Portelance, Carien Creutzberg, Ina M. Jürgenliemk-Schulz, Arno Mundt, Loren K. Mell, Nina Mayr, Akila Viswanathan, Anuja Jhingran, Beth Erickson, Jennifer De los Santos, David Gaffney, Catheryn Yashar, Sushil Beriwal, Aaron Wolfson, Alexandra Taylor, Walter Bosch, Issam El Naqa, Anthony Fyles, Gyn IMRT Consortium. Consensus Guidelines for Delineation of Clinical Target Volume for Intensity-Modulated Pelvic Radiotherapy for the Definitive Treatment of Cervix Cancer. *International Journal of Radiation Oncology Biology Physics* 79, no. 2 (2011): 348-55. https://doi.org/10.1016/j.ijrobp.2009.10.075.

Lin, S. H., Brian P. Hobbs, Vivek Verma, Rebecca S. Tidwell, Grace L. Smith, Xiudong Lei, Erin M. Corsini, Isabel Mok, Xiong Wei, Luyang Yao, Xin Wang, Ritsuko U. Komaki, Joe Y. Chang, Stephen G. Chun, Melenda D. Jeter, Stephen G. Swisher, Jaffer A. Ajani, Mariela Blum-Murphy, Ara A. Vaporciyan, Reza J. Mehran, Albert C. Koong, Saumil J. Gandhi, Wayne L. Hofstetter, Theodore S. Hong, Thomas F. Delaney, Zhongxing Liao, Radhe Mohan. Randomized Phase IIB Trial of Proton Beam Therapy versus Intensity-Modulated Radiation Therapy for Locally Advanced Esophageal Cancer. *Journal of Clinical Oncology* 38, no. 14 (2020): 1569-79. https://doi.org/10.1200/jco.19.02503.

Liu, C., Jinkoo Kim, Akila Kumarasiri, Essa Mayyas, Stephen L. Brown, Ning Wen, Farzan Siddiqui, and Indrin J. Chetty. An Automated Dose Tracking System for Adaptive Radiation Therapy. *Computer Methods and Programs in Biomedicine* 154 (2018): 1-8. https://doi.org/10.1016/j.cmpb.2017.11.001.

Moreno, A. C., Steven J. Frank, Adam S. Garden, David I. Rosenthal, Clifton D. Fuller, Gary B. Gunn, Jay P. Reddy, William H. Morrison, Tyler D. Williamson, Emma B. Holliday, Jack Phan, Pierre Blanchard. Intensity Modulated Proton Therapy (IMPT) - the Future of IMRT for Head and Neck Cancer. *Oral Oncology* 88 (2019): 66-74. https://doi.org/10.1016/j.oraloncology.2018.11.015.

Newhauser, W. D., and Rui Zhang. The Physics of Proton Therapy. *Physics in Medicine and Biology* 60, no. 8 (2015). https://doi.org/10.1088/0031-9155/60/8/r155.

Niyazi, M., Michael Brada, Anthony J. Chalmers, Stephanie E. Combs, Sara C. Erridge, Alba Fiorentino, Anca L. Grosu, Frank J Lagerwaard, Giuseppe Minniti, René-Olivier Mirimanoff, Umberto Ricardi, Susan C. Short, Damien C. Weber, Claus Belka. Estro-ACROP Guideline 'Target Delineation of Glioblastomas. *Radiotherapy and Oncology* 118, no. 1 (2016): 35-42. https://doi.org/10.1016/j.radonc.2015.12.003.

Peters, L. J., Brian O'Sullivan, Jordi Giralt, Thomas J. Fitzgerald, Andy Trotti, Jacques Bernier, Jean Bourhis, Kally Yuen, Richard Fisher, and Danny Rischin. Critical Impact of Radiotherapy Protocol Compliance and Quality in the Treatment of Advanced Head and Neck Cancer: Results from Trog 02.02. *Journal of Clinical Oncology* 28, no. 18 (2010): 2996-3001. https://doi.org/10.1200/jco.2009.27.4498.

Schmidt, M. A., and Geoffrey S. Payne. Radiotherapy Planning Using MRI. *Physics in Medicine and Biology* 60, no. 22 (2015). https://doi.org/10.1088/0031-9155/60/22/r323.

Shibamoto, Y., Asaka Naruse, Hiroshi Fukuma, Shiho Ayakawa, Chikao Sugie, and Natsuo Tomita. Influence of Contrast Materials on Dose Calculation in Radiotherapy Planning Using Computed Tomography for Tumors at Various Anatomical Regions: A Prospective Study. *Radiotherapy and Oncology* 84, no. 1 (2007): 52-55. https://doi.org/10.1016/j.radonc.2007.05.015.

Small, W., Loren K. Mell, Penny Anderson, Carien Creutzberg, Jennifer De Los Santos, David Gaffney, Anuja Jhingran, Lorraine Portelance, Tracey Schefter, Revathy Iyer, Mahesh Varia, Kathryn Winter, Arno J Mundt. Consensus Guidelines for Delineation of Clinical Target Volume for Intensity-Modulated Pelvic Radiotherapy in Postoperative Treatment of Endometrial and Cervical Cancer. *International Journal of Radiation Oncology Biology Physics* 71, no. 2 (2008): 428-34. https://doi.org/10.1016/j.ijrobp.2007.09.042.

Sonke, J. J., Marianne Aznar, and Coen Rasch. Adaptive Radiotherapy for Anatomical Changes. *Seminars in Radiation Oncology* 29, no. 3 (2019): 245-57. https://doi.org/10.1016/j.semradonc.2019.02.007.

Sterzing, F., Rita Engenhart-Cabillic, Michael Flentje, and Jürgen Debus. Image-Guided Radiotherapy. *Deutsches Ärzteblatt international*, 2011. https://doi.org/10.3238/arztebl.2011.0274.

Stroom, J. C., and Ben J. M. Heijmen. Geometrical Uncertainties, Radiotherapy Planning Margins, and the ICRU-62 Report. *Radiotherapy and Oncology* 64, no. 1 (2002): 75-83. https://doi.org/10.1016/s0167-8140(02)00140-8.

Taylor, A., Andrea G. Rockall, Rodney H. Reznek, and Melanie E. B. Powell. Mapping Pelvic Lymph Nodes: Guidelines for Delineation in Intensity-Modulated Radiotherapy. *International Journal of Radiation Oncology Biology Physics* 63, no. 5 (2005): 1604-12. https://doi.org/10.1016/j.ijrobp.2005.05.062.

Teoh, M., C. H. Clark, K. Wood, S. Whitaker, and A. Nisbet. Volumetric Modulated Arc Therapy: A Review of Current Literature and Clinical Use in Practice. *The British Journal of Radiology* 84, no. 1007 (2011): 967-96. https://doi.org/10.1259/bjr/22373346.

Thorwarth, D., and Daniel A. Low. Technical Challenges of Real-Time Adaptive MR-Guided Radiotherapy. *Frontiers in Oncology* 11 (2021). https://doi.org/10.3389/fonc.2021.634507.

Tunçel, N. Adaptive Radiotherapy from Past to Future Frontiers. *International Journal of Radiology & Radiation Therapy* 8, no. 2 (2021): 81-84. https://doi.org/10.15406/ijrrt.2021.08.00298.

Van den Begin, R., Benedikt Engels, Thierry Gevaert, Michaël Duchateau, Koen Tournel, Dirk Verellen, Guy Storme, and Mark De Ridder. Impact of Inadequate Respiratory Motion Management in SBRT for Oligometastatic Colorectal Cancer. *Radiotherapy and Oncology* 113, no. 2 (2014): 235-39. https://doi.org/10.1016/j.radonc.2014.11.005.

Walker, A. J., Theodore L. DeWeese, and Akila N. Viswanathan. Drug-Radiotherapy Combinations in 2020 - a Landmark Year? *JAMA Oncology* 7, no. 3 (2021): 349. https://doi.org/10.1001/jamaoncol.2020.6139.

Wang, J. Z., X. Allen Li, Warren D D'Souza, and Robert D Stewart. Impact of Prolonged Fraction Delivery Times on Tumor Control: A Note of Caution for Intensity-Modulated Radiation Therapy (IMRT). *International Journal of Radiation Oncology Biology Physics* 57, no. 2 (2003): 543-52. https://doi.org/10.1016/s0360-3016(03)00499-1.

Williams, K., and H. Probst. Use of IV Contrast Media in Radiotherapy Planning CT Scans: A UK Audit. *Radiography* 22 (2016). https://doi.org/10.1016/j.radi.2016.06.006.

Chapter 15

Secondary Cancer Risk and Intensity Modulated Radiotherapy

Emel Haciislamoglu*
Department of Radiation Oncology, Karadeniz Technical University, Trabzon, Turkey

Abstract

Radiotherapy (RT) is an essential therapeutic modality in therapy for cancer, and one of its most significant recent advancements is intensity-modulated radiotherapy (IMRT). It is distinguished by extremely conformal dose distribution to the tumour and thus greater normal tissue sparing. This necessitates an extended beam-on time, resulting in bigger low dose volumes and higher out-of-field ionising radiation to peripheral healthy tissue located far away from the target (Hall and Wuu, 2003; Kry et al., 2005). As a consequence, it is becoming progressively clear that current RT, such as IMRT, might be the reason for higher risk of secondary cancer compared to prior three-dimensional conformal radiotherapy (3DCRT), particularly in teenage with good survival (Grant et al., 2017; Piotrowski et al., 2017; Xiang et al., 2020). It is uncertain what causes radiation-induced secondary malignancy. Nevertheless, due to the large number of cancer survivors, it is now a major issue in oncology, and attempts are being undertaken to avoid or reduce the occurrence of radiation-induced secondary malignancy. There are several models available for theoretically determining the risk associated with RT. These models range in complexity, and they might be used to extrapolate epidemiological knowledge acquired from conventional treatment approaches to new RT techniques, as well as to compare the

*Corresponding Author's Email: emel.haciislamoglu@ktu.edu.tr.

In: Frontiers in Intensity-Modulated Radiotherapy Research
Editor: Sibel Karaca
ISBN: 979-8-88697-252-8

risks related to different treatment techniques. The influence of IMRT dose distributions on secondary cancer risks is a hot issue in study, with numerous recent model studies assessing risks for different age groups and IMRT characteristics. Furthermore, the risk of secondary cancer is affected by a number of variables, including immunosuppression, age at irradiation, hormonal and psychosocial impacts, and genetic predisposition.

Keywords: intensity-modulated radiotherapy, secondary cancer risk

1. Introduction

RT is an integral part of cancer treatment, and more than half of all patients with cancer require it at some moment. The proportion of long-term cancer survivors has increased dramatically as treatment approaches have advanced. The increasing survivability of patients with cancer has resulted in a new and expanding group at risk for adverse effects. The adverse effects of RT on healthy tissue can be classified as early (or acute) or late (or chronic) (Bentzen, 2006). Acute adverse effects occur during or shortly after RT (De Ruysscher et al., 2019). When the dose is restricted and tissue turnover is rapid, including in the oral mucosa and gut, acute adverse effects are frequently curable. Chronic adverse effects are those that appear many months or even years after RT (De Ruysscher et al., 2019). Late adverse effects are typically persistent and progressive, resulting in a decrease in patients' standard of living following therapy. Unlike early adverse effects, the duration to response of late-responding tissues is dose-dependent and influenced by factors including cellular senescence, chronic inflammation, hypoxia, and fibrosis.

Secondary cancer induction is an extremely severe late adverse consequence of cancer therapy. Long-term cancer survivors, in particular, are at an elevated risk of acquiring secondary cancer. Currently, after overcoming an initial cancer, 17–19% of people acquire radiation-induced secondary cancer (Morton et al., 2014). This is attributable to three factors: continuing lifestyle, genetic predisposition, and treatment modalities like radiation therapy and chemotherapy. Only around 5% of all treatment-related second malignancies are caused by radiation therapy. Nevertheless, estimating the frequency of solely radiation on second malignancies is challenging since there are other variables that predispose people to second malignancies.

Data on radiation-induced cancers derive from atomic bomb victims and medically exposed people, notably secondary tumours in RT patients. Victims of atomic bombs have an increased incidence of carcinomas in organs like the gastrointestinal tract, breast, thyroid, and bladder, which increases linearly with radiation up to roughly 2.5 Sv. At higher exposures, the dose-response association for radiation-induced carcinogenesis is quite ambiguous. Certain human and animal analyses show a reduction at higher doses, which is commonly ascribed to cell death; other data indicate a dose plateau. RT patients also have an increased incidence of carcinomas, typically in locations far from the therapy fields; there is also an increased frequency of sarcomas in the extensively irradiated in-field tissues.

Numerous large investigations of atomic bomb victims' statistics have calculated the dose-response relation for radiation carcinogenesis up to 1 or 2 Gy (Preston et al., 2004; Walsh et al., 2004). This dose range is critical for radiation safety, as lower doses are of special relevance. Nevertheless, knowing the form of the dose-response curve for radiation-induced cancer at doses greater than 1 Gy is equally significant. Portions of the client volume may get high doses in RT patients, and it is thus critical to understanding the patient's risk of developing cancer as a consequence of the RT. The form of the dose-response curve for radiation-induced cancer is now being debated (Daşu et al., 2005; Schneider et al., 2010; Schneider and Kaser Hotz, 2005; Shuryak et al., 2009).

The transition from conventional RT to 3DCRT entails decreasing the number of normal tissues getting a high dose while increasing the dose to the target volume, which comprises the tumour and a small portion of normal tissue. On the contrary, the shift from 3DCRT to IMRT includes additional fields, and the dose-volume histograms reveal that a wider amount of normal tissue is subjected to lower doses as a result. Furthermore, the amount of monitor units is multiplied by a ratio of two to three, increasing total body exposure owing to leaking radiation. Both of these variables raise the chance of subsequent malignancies. Furthermore, various variables influence the occurrence of secondary cancer risk.

2. Radiation and Malignant Transformation

Ionising radiation is utilized for cancer treatment since it produces ions (electrically charged particles) in the cells of the tissues it passes into. Ions are formed by withdrawing electrons from atoms and molecules. This might harm cells or modify their deoxyribonucleic acid (DNA), causing them to cease developing.

Ionising radiation can be strong electromagnetic radiation or subatomic particles like alpha, beta, and neutrons. Even though the processes by which X and gamma rays interact with matter and tissue vary, they always create positively and/or negatively charged ions, which subsequently react with the absorbing matter to produce physicochemical alterations. The strength of these electromagnetic radiations also will impact how far they penetrate, with greater energy photons penetrating deeper than low energy photons. Energy is deposited inside the tissue when they interact with tissues and cells. These physicochemical alterations result in malignant cell modifications via mutations.

It is generally known that radiation may induce malignant transformation. Since the earliest discoveries of cancer within scientists exposed to x-rays in the early twentieth century, radiation has been recognised to cause cancer. Information has been acquired through observational studies of Japanese atomic bomb victims, industrial radiation exposure, and the use of RT in medicine (Suit et al., 2007).

Normal cells undergo a multistep transition into cancerous cells. Over the last few centuries, the unique aspects of tumour cells have been thoroughly assessed and recognised as cancer hallmarks, which also include dysregulation of cellular procedures of that kind as cell proliferation and cellular energetics, as well as the acquirement of genome instability and eternal life (Hanahan and Weinberg, 2011). Many in vitro transition models have been investigated in order to further explain the processes implicated in the development of tumour cells.

The molecular basis of the significant relationship among ionising radiation and carcinogenesis is studied in normal cells that have adequate DNA-repair machinery (Mavragani et al., 2017). Nevertheless, little is understood about the consequences of radiation on cells which have already developed oncogenic properties. Ionising radiation is the reason for DNA damage in cycling cells, which, if not corrected or treated incorrectly, can result in cell inactivation or heritable, viable mutations. The latter can result in cell transition, which is regarded to be the first stage in the creation of cancer.

3. Radiation-Induced Secondary Cancer Risk

Due to the obvious rising amount of cancer people who survived, radiation-induced secondary cancer is getting a significant problem in oncology, and steps are being taken to avoid or mitigate the occurrence of secondary cancer. According to epidemiological research, conventional RT is associated with a little but considerable risk of radiation-induced secondary cancer (Brenner et al., 2000; Grantzau et al., 2013).

Because of the extended latency of carcinogenesis, results for contemporary treatments such as IMRT are not yet accessible. However, the influence of numerous of the factors under consideration for IMRT has been studied theoretically, and the results demonstrate the complexities of the risk problem for modern treatment approaches (Followill et al., 1997; Ruben et al., 2011).

Radiation-induced secondary cancer is one of the most serious late side effects of RT, and it has an effect on ideal treatment decision-making. Numerous components contribute to the advancement of secondary cancer, including the patient's age at the time of radiation, the radiation dose obtained and the quantity of normal tissue irradiated, the type of irradiated organ and tissue, the type of radiation, the radiation methodology, and the patient's family and individual background of cancer, as well as external exposures (Ng and Shuryak, 2014) (Figure1).

3.1. Age at Radiation

The age at which a person is exposed to radiation has a major influence on the formation of radiation-induced secondary cancer. While the cancer risks associated with childhood radiation exposure have been well reported in the literature (Kleinerman, 2006; Little, 2008), the link between the radiation-induced cancer risk and age of exposure in adults is less obvious.

When compared to the elder population, childhood radiation exposure dramatically raises the risk of subsequent cancer (Hall, 2006). Numerous variables can affect why children have a greater impact on secondary cancer risk than grown-ups: larger responsiveness to ionising therapies, an increased rate of genetic receptivity, a longer time of follow-up, and simply because a radiation field has a greater impact due to the differentiation in height and weight.

Grown-ups' bone marrow, colon, mammary gland, lungs, and stomach easily acquire cancer as a consequence of exposure to radiation, whereas children's chances of acquiring thyroid cancer and skin cancer are very great.

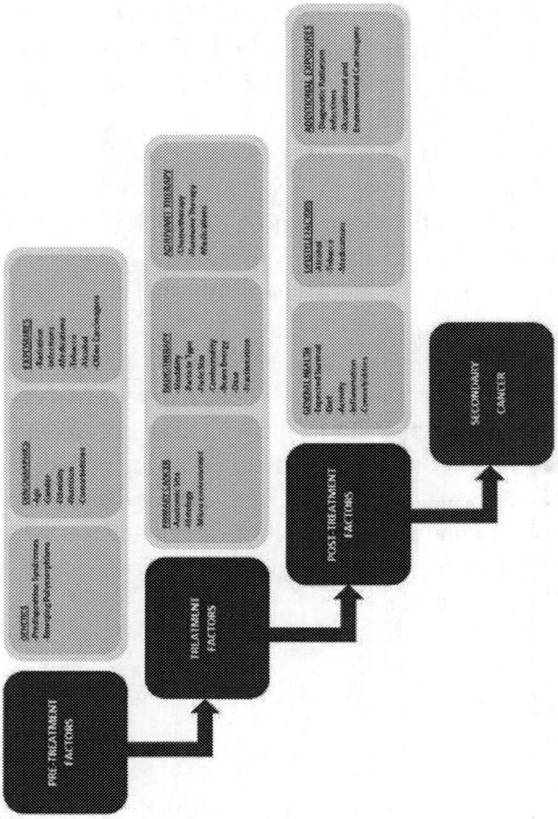

Figure 1. Schematic representation of the multiple factors' secondary cancer development.

3.2. Volume of Irradiated Area

In RT, it is well understood that the isodose effect of normal tissue reduces with increasing area or quantity of tissue irradiated, resulting in a significant shift in therapeutic ratio when a big tumour is cured. This link is known as the "volume effect," and numerous models, such as the dose volume histogram and integral probability, have been devised to measure it. Even though the distribution of these models is built on clinical evidence, there is significant difference across models, and every model can only be used in certain circumstances.

Volume-related effects are a crucial factor to consider in clinical RT. The initial argument for considering irradiated volume has become obscured by an absence of clarity and a misreading of certain early clinical data. There is a specific requirement to distinguish our understanding of physiologically iso-effective radiation responses from the clinical idea of normal tissue tolerance as they apply to variations in treatment dose.

3.3. Type of Irradiated Organ and Tissue

Radiation does not have an identical effect on all biological cells. Cells which are continually replicating are more sensitive than non-reproducing cells. This is because proliferating cells require precise DNA information in order for their offspring to survive. The proportionate responsiveness of the cells that comprise the living organism's multiple organs corresponds with their responsiveness. As a consequence, living cells might well be classified according to their frequency of multiplication, which also indicates their radiation responsiveness. This demonstrates that various cell systems are responsive in distinct manners.

Because lymphocytes and blood-producing cells are regenerating all the time, they are the most vulnerable. Reproductive and gastrointestinal cells renew more slowly and with less sensitivity. Nerve and muscle cells regenerate the slowest.

3.4. Type of Radiation

The energy density delivered by radiation varies depending on the kind of radiation. In comparison to -particles and -rays, -particles and protons offer greater energy to substances in a much smaller area. Even for the same absorbed dose, cell damage varies due to differences in ionisation intensity.

As compared to traditional photon RT, proton therapy is an enhanced particle treatment with distinct dosimetric features that result in a lower entry dose and a lower departure dose. Several dosimetric investigations have shown that proton treatment can provide appropriate target volume coverage while delivering a lower integral dose to adjacent tissues (Lomax et al., 1999). Clinical evidence shows a decreased risk of secondary malignancy following proton treatment when compared to historical photon data (Yock and Caruso, 2012), while longer follow-up in proton-treated cohorts is required.

3.5. Radiation Technique

The evolution of current external beam radiation therapy, marked by a technical shift from rectangular portals to irregular forms with stiff collimation, to computer-controlled multileaf collimators, has permitted progressively accurate dose distribution to specific tumour areas.

New radiation approaches like as IMRT and Volumetric Modulated Arc Therapy (VMAT) have been developed to allow dose escalation while minimising toxicity. Fears have been made that current IMRT may be linked to higher secondary primary cancer risks than earlier 3DCRT, owing to greater small dose quantities and more out-of-field ionising exposure reaching peripheral tissue farther away from the focus.

Conceptual worries have been expressed about a possible significant rise in secondary cancer risk when employing contemporary RT procedures vs 3D-CRT (Kry et al., 2007; Stathakis et al., 2007). Nevertheless, direct clinical evidence of higher secondary malignancies from IMRT over 3DCRT is still missing because IMRT is a relatively young technique in clinics, with just around 20 years of widespread usage (Huang et al., 2011; Zelefsky et al., 2012).

3.6. Estimates of Radiotherapy-Related Risk of Secondary Cancer

Radiation-induced secondary cancers are an uncommon but substantial late impact of radiation therapy in cancer victims. Assessments of secondary cancer risk following RT are getting increasingly significant, particularly for newer RT techniques such as IMRT, which irradiates relatively high quantities of healthy tissues with modest doses of radiation (Hall and Wuu, 2003; Hall, 2004). There is currently inadequate clinical evidence to form solid conclusions concerning the influence of IMRT on secondary cancer risks.

The majority of knowledge on the dose-response of radiation-induced cancer comes from information on atomic bomb survivors. Because the dose span of significant importance for radiation safety reasons is between 0 and 1 Gy, the examination of atomic bomb survivors is mainly cantered on this range. Assessments of secondary cancer danger for dose more than 1 Gy, on the other hand, are being increasingly significant for RT patients. Linear dose–response curves adequately explain the risks of subsequent cancer following radiation exposure. Nevertheless, epidemiology does not give the required information for secondary cancer danger in RT sufferers, because a tiny amount of the body is exposed to large doses while the remainder of the body is subjected to small dose. Models are used to quantify secondary cancer risk: at small doses, the linear-no-threshold (LNT) assumption is commonly used (Mullenders et al., 2009). Thus, the majority of current models are only applicable for small doses and cannot be readily expanded to RT. Transfer issues may stem from radiation therapy characteristics like large doses and dose rates, fragmented therapies, significant non-uniformity of the dose over the treated organ, and the employment of multiple radiation modalities.

There are several models available for theoretically determining the danger associated with RT. These models range in functionality, and they might be utilised to extrapolate epidemiological data acquired from traditional therapy approaches to novel RT techniques, as well as to compare the hazards related to alternative therapy strategies. The BEIR VII Committee had two rival risk models at its fingertips: the excess relative risk (ERR) model and the excess actual risk (EAR) model. The ERR is calculated by dividing the rate of disease in an affected group by the rate of illness in an unexposed group, minus 1.0. The EAR is calculated by subtracting the incidence of illness in an exposed individual from the incidence of illness in a non - exposed group. These models calculate the cancer risk at a specific period after exposure, and their worth is dependent on the subject's age and gender at the exposure time. A third model, known as the lifetime attributable chance, is used to quantify the lifelong cancer risk from that exposure. The lifetime attributable risk (LAR) is the change in the rate of a disease among the exposed and unexposed populations.

Numerous epidemiological researches have been conducted to explore the initiation of secondary cancers after RT (Bhatia et al., 1996; Verellen and Vanhavere, 1999), but handful of them connect the incidence of secondary cancers to the exact doses obtained by the irradiated part of the body or raise the matter of the shape of the dose response curve. Moreover, the consequences of dose heterogeneity all through the irradiated organ have received even less consideration. Nevertheless, published research suggest that dose inhomogeneity plays a key role in forecasting the risk of subsequent cancer, and hence it must be taken into consideration by the usage of dose volume histograms for forecasting reasons Because of the uneven dose distribution throughout the organ, numerous approaches for assessing the secondary cancer risk following RT have been established. To explain radiation-induced cancer following RT in the irradiated organs, the dose distributions can be transformed into organ equivalent dose (OED). The OED idea holds that if two dose distributions in an organ create the very same radiation-induced cancer risk, they are comparable (Schneider et al., 2005).

Including the traditional technique of evaluating the likely deterministic effects, theoretical predictions of cancer danger from RT may be utilised as an additional criterion for the selection of effective therapeutic strategies. The findings also imply that the conflict among the cell death and the production of carcinogenic mutations should be considered for more accurate risk calculations. Moreover, if this rivalry is already included in studies of epidemiologic studies from RT applications, more realistic parameters may be derived.

Conclusion

Cancer survivor statistics are increasing as a result of significant advancements in current treatment choices, while late-occurring consequences including such radiation-induced secondary cancer are becoming increasingly relevant. An overview of therapies, including specific screening suggestions and lifestyle counselling, is required for every young and old people received with RT in order to properly organise long-term follow-up. Secondary cancers are complicated, with initial cancer therapies and genetic predisposition playing important roles, not to mention lifestyle variables and environmental exposures. To resolve this concern further, substantial cohort investigations with clinical evidence and adequate follow-up are required.

References

Bentzen, S. M. (2006). Preventing or reducing late side effects of radiation therapy: radiobiology meets molecular pathology. *Nature Reviews Cancer*, *6*(9), 702-713.

Bhatia, S., Robison, L. L., Oberlin, O., Greenberg, M., Bunin, G., Fossati-Bellani, F., & Meadows, A. T. (1996). Breast cancer and other second neoplasms after childhood Hodgkin's disease. *New England Journal of Medicine*, *334*(12), 745-751.

Brenner, D. J., Curtis, R. E., Hall, E. J., & Ron, E. (2000). Second malignancies in prostate carcinoma patients after radiotherapy compared with surgery. *Cancer: Interdisciplinary International Journal of the American Cancer Society*, *88*(2), 398-406.

Daşu, A., Toma-Daşu, I., Olofsson, J., & Karlsson, M. (2005). The use of risk estimation models for the induction of secondary cancers following radiotherapy. *Acta Oncologica*, *44*(4), 339-347.

De Ruysscher, D., Niedermann, G., Burnet, N. G., Siva, S., Lee, A. W., & Hegi-Johnson, F. (2019). Radiotherapy toxicity. *Nature Reviews Disease Primers*, *5*(1), 1-20.

Followill, D., Geis, P., & Boyer, A. (1997). Estimates of whole-body dose equivalent produced by beam intensity modulated conformal therapy. *International journal of radiation oncology, biology, physics*, *38*(3), 667-672.

Grant, E. J., Brenner, A., Sugiyama, H., Sakata, R., Sadakane, A., Utada, M., ... & Ozasa, K. (2017). Solid cancer incidence among the life span study of atomic bomb survivors: 1958–2009. *Radiation research*, *187*(5), 513-537.

Grantzau, T., Mellemkjær, L., & Overgaard, J. (2013). Second primary cancers after adjuvant radiotherapy in early breast cancer patients: a national population based study under the Danish Breast Cancer Cooperative Group (DBCG). *Radiotherapy and Oncology*, *106*(1), 42-49.

Hall, E. J. (2004). Henry S. Kaplan Distinguished Scientist Award 2003 The crooked shall be made straight; dose–response relationships for carcinogenesis. *International journal of radiation biology*, *80*(5), 327-337.

Hall, E. J. (2006). Intensity-modulated radiation therapy, protons, and the risk of second cancers. *International Journal of Radiation Oncology* Biology* Physics*, *65*(1), 1-7.

Hall, E. J., & Wuu, C. S. (2003). Radiation-induced second cancers: the impact of 3D-CRT and IMRT. *International Journal of Radiation Oncology* Biology* Physics*, *56*(1), 83-88.

Hanahan, D., & Weinberg, R. A. (2011). Hallmarks of cancer: the next generation. *cell*, *144*(5), 646-674.

Huang, J., Kestin, L. L., Ye, H., Wallace, M., Martinez, A. A., & Vicini, F. A. (2011). Analysis of second malignancies after modern radiotherapy versus prostatectomy for localized prostate cancer. *Radiotherapy and Oncology*, *98*(1), 81-86.

Kleinerman, R. A. (2006). Cancer risks following diagnostic and therapeutic radiation exposure in children. *Pediatric radiology*, *36*(2), 121-125.

Kry, S. F., Followill, D., White, R. A., Stovall, M., Kuban, D. A., & Salehpour, M. (2007). Uncertainty of calculated risk estimates for secondary malignancies after radiotherapy. *International Journal of Radiation Oncology* Biology* Physics*, *68*(4), 1265-1271.

Kry, S. F., Salehpour, M., Followill, D. S., Stovall, M., Kuban, D. A., White, R. A., & Rosen, I. I. (2005). The calculated risk of fatal secondary malignancies from intensity-modulated radiation therapy. *International Journal of Radiation Oncology* Biology* Physics*, *62*(4), 1195-1203.

Little, M. P. (2008). Leukaemia following childhood radiation exposure in the Japanese atomic bomb survivors and in medically exposed groups. *Radiation protection dosimetry*, *132*(2), 156-165.

Lomax, A. J., Bortfeld, T., Goitein, G., Debus, J., Dykstra, C., Tercier, P. A., ... & Mirimanoff, R. O. (1999). A treatment planning inter-comparison of proton and intensity modulated photon radiotherapy. *Radiotherapy and Oncology*, *51*(3), 257-271.

Mavragani, I. V., Nikitaki, Z., Souli, M. P., Aziz, A., Nowsheen, S., Aziz, K., ... & Georgakilas, A. G. (2017). Complex DNA damage: a route to radiation-induced genomic instability and carcinogenesis. *Cancers*, *9*(7), 91.

Morton, L. M., Onel, K., Curtis, R. E., Hungate, E. A., & Armstrong, G. T. (2014). The rising incidence of second cancers: patterns of occurrence and identification of risk factors for children and adults. *American Society of Clinical Oncology Educational Book*, *34*(1), e57-e67.

Mullenders, L., Atkinson, M., Paretzke, H., Sabatier, L., & Bouffler, S. (2009). Assessing cancer risks of low-dose radiation. *Nature Reviews Cancer*, *9*(8), 596-604.

Ng, J., & Shuryak, I. (2015). Minimizing second cancer risk following radiotherapy: current perspectives. *Cancer management and research*, *7*, 1.

Piotrowski, I., Kulcenty, K., Suchorska, W. M., Skrobała, A., Skórska, M., Kruszyna-Mochalska, M., ... & Malicki, J. (2017). Carcinogenesis induced by low-dose radiation. *Radiology and oncology*, *51*(4), 369-377.

Preston, D. L., Pierce, D. A., Shimizu, Y., Cullings, H. M., Fujita, S., Funamoto, S., & Kodama, K. (2004). Effect of recent changes in atomic bomb survivor dosimetry on cancer mortality risk estimates. *Radiation research*, *162*(4), 377-389.

Ruben, J. D., Lancaster, C. M., Jones, P., & Smith, R. L. (2011). A comparison of out-of-field dose and its constituent components for intensity-modulated radiation therapy versus conformal radiation therapy: implications for carcinogenesis. *International Journal of Radiation Oncology* Biology* Physics*, *81*(5), 1458-1464.

Schneider, U., & Kaser-Hotz, B. (2005). Radiation risk estimates after radiotherapy: application of the organ equivalent dose concept to plateau dose–response relationships. *Radiation and environmental biophysics*, *44*(3), 235-239.

Schneider, U., Besserer, J., & Hartmann, M. (2013, December). Hypofractionated radiotherapy has the potential for second cancer reduction. In *STRAHLENTHERAPIE UND ONKOLOGIE* (Vol. 189, No. 12, pp. 1078-1078). NEUMARKTER STRASSE 43, D-81673 MUNICH, GERMANY: URBAN & VOGEL.

Schneider, U., Zwahlen, D., Ross, D., & Kaser-Hotz, B. (2005). Estimation of radiation-induced cancer from three-dimensional dose distributions: Concept of organ equivalent dose. *International Journal of Radiation Oncology* Biology* Physics*, *61*(5), 1510-1515.

Shuryak, I., Hahnfeldt, P., Hlatky, L., Sachs, R. K., & Brenner, D. J. (2009). A new view of radiation-induced cancer: integrating short-and long-term processes. Part I: approach. *Radiation and environmental biophysics*, *48*(3), 263-274.

Stathakis, S., Li, J., & Ma, C. C. (2007). Monte Carlo determination of radiation-induced cancer risks for prostate patients undergoing intensity-modulated radiation therapy. *Journal of applied clinical medical physics*, *8*(4), 14-27.

Suit, H., Goldberg, S., Niemierko, A., Ancukiewicz, M., Hall, E., Goitein, M., ... & Paganetti, H. (2007). Secondary carcinogenesis in patients treated with radiation: a review of data on radiation-induced cancers in human, non-human primate, canine and rodent subjects. *Radiation research*, *167*(1), 12-42.

Verellen, D., & Vanhavere, F. (1999). Risk assessment of radiation-induced malignancies based on whole-body equivalent dose estimates for IMRT treatment in the head and neck region. *Radiotherapy and Oncology*, *53*(3), 199-203.

Walsh, L., Rühm, W., & Kellerer, A. M. (2004). Cancer risk estimates for gamma-rays with regard to organ-specific doses. *Radiation and environmental biophysics*, *43*(3), 145-151.

Xiang, M., Chang, D. T., & Pollom, E. L. (2020). Second cancer risk after primary cancer treatment with three-dimensional conformal, intensity-modulated, or proton beam radiation therapy. *Cancer*, *126*(15), 3560-3568.

Yock, T. I., & Caruso, P. A. (2012). Risk of second cancers after photon and proton radiotherapy: a review of the data. *Health physics*, *103*(5), 577-585.

Zelefsky, M. J., Housman, D. M., Pei, X., Alicikus, Z., Magsanoc, J. M., Dauer, L. T., ... & Zhang, Z. (2012). Incidence of secondary cancer development after high-dose intensity-modulated radiotherapy and image-guided brachytherapy for the treatment of localized prostate cancer. *International Journal of Radiation Oncology* Biology* Physics*, *83*(3), 953-959.

Chapter 16

Reirradiation

Hamit Basaran[*]
Department of Radiation Oncology, Selcuk University, Konya, Turkey

Abstract

Reirradiation is an important treatment option for the development of relapse or secondary cancers in patients in long-term follow-up who received radiotherapy (RT) due to the diagnosis of malignancy. Although recent reviews and writings on reirradiation are mostly based on past clinical and experimental data, it has become imperative with the technological advances in today's diagnostic imaging, treatment planning, and radiation therapy systems. The tolerance of normal tissues seems to decrease significantly in the reirradiation phase, thus making it one of the most difficult situations in the decision and application phase of radiation oncology. In this chapter, we will mention the evidence-based technical recommendations for the second serial irradiation of patients with brain malignant tumours, head and neck cancer (HNC), lung cancer, and brain metastases, which are the most common indications for reirradiation and current advances.

Keywords: brain malignant tumours, brain metastases, head and neck cancer, lung cancer, reirradiation

---

[*]Corresponding Author's Email: drhbasaran@gmail.com.

In: Frontiers in Intensity-Modulated Radiotherapy Research
Editor: Sibel Karaca
ISBN: 979-8-88697-252-8

1. Introduction

Recent research on reirradiation mostly focuses on clinical and experimental data from the past two decades. The first cases of reirradiation are based on Desjardins' reporting of reirradiation of thoracic Hodgkin's lymphoma in the 1920s (Desjardins et al. 1930). Lee et al. (1926) reported their experience with more than 300 patients treated for recurrent inoperable breast cancer at Memorial Hospital. Garland et al. (1950) reported the results of patients with HNC treated with RT from 1932–1948. They observed that some of the patients with relapse could be treated with reirradiation as a result of the study. According to the final result, three of 105 patients with lip cancer and three of 71 patients with tongue cancer developed marginal recurrence. They were reirradiated after previous RT and growth were arrested. No details were reported about doses, time intervals, efficacy, or toxicity.

Murphy et al. (1956) published a report on patients who developed local recurrence in the follow-up of patients who received curative RT for cervical cancer. According to this report, curative or palliative treatment with reirradiation should be performed in these patients if a second surgical approach has a high risk of permanent side effects and death in these patients, and they report that previous RT is not contraindicated. Despite the historical significance of reirradiation studies in the twentieth century, advanced imaging systems, 3-D treatment planning, image-guided radiation therapy (IGRT), stereotactic radiosurgery (SRS), intensity-modulated radiation therapy (IMRT), and volumetric modulated arc therapy (VMAT) have made reirradiation mandatory in the treatment of recurrences or secondary cancers in the area previously treated with RT. There are an increasing number of cases and publications about reirradiation in the literature. This shows that experienced clinicians take seriously selected patients with an appropriate risk/benefit ratio.

The concept of reirradiation appears in two ways in the clinic,

1. Recurrent tumors in previously irradiated areas
2. Secondary cancers due to benign or malignant causes, which is a devastating complication of previous RT (Kleinerman et al., 2006).

RT is used as a definitive or adjuvant treatment in many cancer diseases. Especially as a result of multimodal treatment and advanced technological methods, longer life spans are achieved in most patients. Prolonged survival may increase the risk of regional recurrence in previously irradiated malignant patients. There is a need for additional therapeutic measures, such as reirradiation, which provides local control or symptom palliation after enhanced multimodal therapy. Therefore, previously irradiated anatomical volumes may require a second or sometimes a third radiation therapy. Rescue surgery is the main treatment for recurrences in the follow-up period of malignant diseases, but surgery may not be possible in most cases due to the high risk of complications and morbidity. In this case, the second preferred treatment method is chemotherapy. In many studies, it is said that the response rate is up to 40% with this treatment, and chemotherapy is generally preferred in the treatment of systemic recurrences. In these cases, reirradiation becomes an important salvage treatment with acceptable side effects. However, to achieve this success, the total dose to be administered must be limited to normal tissue tolerance. It is a difficult and complex process for physicians to decide to reirradiate for patients (Embring et al., 2020). Factors to be considered in this process include the type of organ at risk in and around the irradiated area, total dose, fraction dose, normal tissue changes due to radiation, and patient performance. Although malignancies secondary to RT are rare in patients who have received radiation therapy before, they are a devastating complication due to the widespread use of RT, the increase in the number of patients, and the positive effects of effective treatments (Mazonakis et al., 2017; Ron et al., 2003). According to the Berrington et al. (2011) study, Surveillance, Epidemiology, and End Results (SEER) data from the US Surveillance suggest that the risk of a second solid tumour 15 years after RT in adult patients is 0.005%. As result, the Bassal et al. (2006) study reported that the incidence of second malignancy was much higher in paediatric patients. This is probably due to a greater frequency of underlying genetic syndromes in children and increased radio sensitivity in children compared to adult patients.

2. Improve the Probability of Reirradiation with Advanced Techniques

Reirradiation in radiation oncology is one of the most difficult issues to decide on since the radiation resistance of normal tissues is significantly reduced in secondary RT compared to the primary RT series. In this chapter, modern radiation therapy planning and delivery techniques that enable better preservation of normal tissues for re-treatment of patients who have previously been treated with RT in the event of relapse will be discussed. As mentioned earlier, mediastinal reirradiation of Hodgkin's disease was first reported in the 1920s (Desjardins et al. 1930). However, in the last 100 years, significant progress has been made in the field of radiation oncology. Especially in the last decade, the results of studies comparing IMRT, IGRT, SRS, and stereotactic body radiation therapy (SBRT) with conventional and conformal approaches have been published. With the application of advanced methods, it has been possible to apply a larger total dose, achieve better protection of organs at risk, and at the same time achieve a better dose homogeneity index (HI), and conformity index (CI) in the concept of reirradiation. In palliative reirradiation applications, it has been shown to give more effective doses to the relapse area with new planning and application methods using advanced technology. If all the developments in reirradiation are discussed, it is known for sure that in 2D or 3D conformal treatments, organs at risk are above the required normal tissue constraint. Therefore, it is possible to apply more effective doses with curative reirradiation using reirradiation with IMRT, SBRT, SRS, high-dose-rate brachytherapy (HDR-BRT), and proton beam RT (PBRT) techniques. Reirradiation is probably one of the most difficult treatment decisions in the field of RT because the tolerance of normal tissue in the second irradiation series decreases significantly compared to before primary RT. If there is sufficient time for the normal tissue to heal between the patient's primary treatment and reirradiation, tissue repair will occur and radiation tolerance will increase significantly. If the radiation damage is not fully repaired in this short time due to early local recurrence, the tolerance of the surrounding tissues decreases and it becomes difficult to decide to reirradiate. In this case, therapy should be administered by minimising the irradiated volume and maximising the dose to meet the acceptable risk of toxicity.

3. Technical Guidance in Reirradiation

In reirradiation biology, it is very important to reach the appropriate balance targets between tumour regression and toxicity. Reirradiation treatment plans need to be tailored to the patient, depending on the site of relapse, treated volume, the normal tissue pattern, and the dose-volume histogram of previous treatment. Appropriate treatment device selection, photon energies, gamma rays, electrons, or protons should be preferred for each patient. In cases of superficial recurrence, kilovoltage X-rays or electrons should be preferred. If it is possible to place the catheters in an appropriate geometry, intraoperative brachytherapy can be applied. Intensity-modulated arc techniques such as tomotherapy or VMAT may be considered for recurrences requiring photon therapy (Tieler et al., 2011). Another preferred method in the second series of irradiations is stereotactic treatments. These treatments are defined as stereotactic SBRT and SRS. In the SBRT method, very high doses of radiation are directed to the planned target with millimetre precision using beams of various intensities. In this method, beams sent from different angles create a high dose on the target while providing a minimum dose and side effects to the organs at risk. The SRS method was first defined by Swedish neurosurgeon Lars Leksell in 1951 as a treatment method with a single stereo tactically directed high-dose radiation fraction in the treatment of malignant masses in the brain using the gamma knife device. This non-invasive method, as a RT technique, has been preferred in the treatment of brain lesions for years. After the 1990s, developments in computer technology and imaging techniques allowed the application of these treatments outside the brain. The CyberKnife device was developed by neurosurgeon Dr. John Adler in 1990 and has been used since 2000. Today, CyberKnife is used in 10-20% of all cancer treatments and is preferred for reirradiation. With Cyber Knife technology, it is planned to obtain the best dose homogeneity and conformity index for the target tumour tissue while minimising damage to the organs at risk around the tumour.

Proton Beam therapy is an RT method that reveals excellent physical potential compared to photon therapy. The proton beam has a very low input and output radiation dose and leaves the maximum radiation dose on the target. Compared to photon treatments, homogeneous treatment plans can be developed by generating lower entry and exit doses with fewer proton beams but high doses on the target tissue, significantly reducing the radiation exposure of non-target tissues. The thin therapeutic index in the second series of irradiation is of great interest because it significantly reduces the toxicities of reirradiation by reducing the dose taken by the organs at risk with proton therapy. Protons have a known energy range in tissues. As the speed of protons decreases, the rate of energy accumulation increases, with the dosimetric accumulation in the terminal range of the beam an explosive peak, followed by a sudden drop with no radiation dose. This is called the Bragg peak of proton therapy (Paganetti et al., 2012). As a result, with the recent increase in proton treatment centres, clinical experience of reirradiation using these treatments is increasing. The main rationale for this therapy is to prevent the toxic effect of reirradiation by decreasing the volume of surrounding organs while delivering a maximum dose to the target.

4. Feasibility of Reirradiation in Brain Tumours

The main treatment for high-grade brain tumours is surgical resection. Concomitant postoperative RT with adjuvant temozolomide is a standard adjuvant approach, but according to the results of the Stup et al. study, the 5-year overall survival (OS) of these patients is increased to 9.8% with the addition of temozolomide to postoperative RT (Stup et al., 2009). These low OS rates indicate that most of the patients relapse within 1-2 years due to the infiltrating nature of the tumour. Because of the high morbidity risk associated with repeated surgical interventions, additional neurosurgical intervention is generally not possible. On the other hand, resistance due to repeated CT protocols limits the chance of systemic treatment. Reirradiation remains a standard treatment at this stage of the disease. Generally, radiation oncologists are not willing to reirradiate relapsed brain tumours to avoid the clinical consequences of radio necrosis, which occurs as a late side effect, especially in these patients, due to normal tissue damage and late toxicity. However, there appears to be a lack of prospective data on reirradiation. Moreover, there is no standard treatment method supported by phase III randomised trials, except for small clinical series. Wong et al. (1999) reported that many of the recurrent diffuse gliomas were within 2 cm of the surgically resected area. In the event of relapse, treatment options include surgical resection, systemic therapy, and reirradiation, but no agreed standard treatment consensus has been established. According to the results of Brem et al.'s (1995) study, salvage surgery has a survival advantage of up to 8 weeks when compared only surgery with a placebo. In Huncharek et al. (1998), a systematic review was published on the treatment of relapsed diffuse gliomas. This review included 36 randomised uncontrolled and 4 randomised controlled trials, consisting of 40 studies. According to the results of 32 studies evaluating survival after CT, nitrosoureas and platinum were the most effective drugs for improving OS. Based on the analysis of this review, the median OS of patients treated with reirradiation was 44.7 weeks. Wick et al. (2007) Phase II study investigating the effects of systemic agents on recurrent gliomas showed that the use of temozolomide in relapses was associated with OS. Future systemic therapies will focus on monotherapy with CT or targeted agents without systemic toxic effects. In studies evaluating the history of patients with second series irradiation, it may limit these treatments that cause neurological toxicity such as radio necrosis. However, re-irradiation has attracted more attention due to the recently developed RT devices, techniques and imaging, and its ability to reduce late neurological toxic effects. There are many retrospective clinical studies on the reirradiation of central nervous system tumours (CNS) in the literature. Although various techniques such as fractionated stereotactic RT, SRS, and conformal RT are preferred in these studies, a wide variety of doses and target volumes are used, emphasising that there is no standard approach (Nieder et al., 2008). In recent years, 3D conformal RT has provided new and important gains for the patient and the radiation oncologist thanks to the magnetic resonance imaging added to the linear accelerator devices used in RT. In comparison to traditional RT, this device allows for the protection of normal tissues and the reduction of late neurological toxicity by targeting with special images and measurements, destroying the definition of recurrent tumour. On the other hand, with IMRT, which is the sophisticated form of conformal RT, it is possible to improve the target compliance and further improve the dose distribution by using multi-modulated beams.

Two important studies in the treatment of recurrences in brain tumours with reirradiation will be reviewed. Kazmi et al. (2019) conducted a meta-analysis investigating the efficacy and toxicity of reirradiation in patients with recurrent glioblastoma. This research created a biomedical database of 2095 patients with recurrent glioblastoma from 50 studies from 1998 to 2018. According to meta-analysis results, 6- and 12-month OS were 73% and 36%, respectively. 6- and 12-month progression-free survival (PFS) was 43% and 17%, and grade > 3 adverse events were reported at 7% (4-10%). The subgroup analysis showed that prospective studies reported higher rates of toxicity, and studies using brachytherapy had longer OS. When the dose-response relationship was sought in external RT, no statistically significant difference was found between the groups above and below 36 Gy at the 2 Gy equivalent dose (EQD2), but 6-month PFS was found to be superior to the short fractionation scheme (5 fractions). Another important study, in a systematic review and meta-analysis by Kulinich et al. (2021), analysed OS, PFS, and radio necrosis of patients treated with reirradiation with or without bevacizumab in the treatment of patients with relapsed high-grade glioma. A total of 1399 patients who received standard treatment for their first treatment were included in the study. Of these, 954 patients received reirradiation alone and 445 patients who received reirradiation plus bevacizumab were compared. In multivariate analysis, adding Bevacizumab to reirradiation significantly improved OS from 2.51 to 4.92 months (P = 0.041), but there was no significant difference in PFS (P = 0.099). In patients receiving bevacizumab, rates of radionecrosis were significantly lower at 2.2% versus 6.5% (P 0.001). Eventually, the combination of reirradiation and Bevacizumab may improve survival and reduce the risk of necrosis in recurrent gliomas.

5. Reirradiation in Head and Neck Cancer (HNC): Is It Possible?

Concurrent chemoradiotherapy (CRT) has an important role in the definitive treatment of HNC, specifically squamous cell carcinomas. Most of these patients are diagnosed at the localized stage and are treated with surgery or RT with or without CT. Despite advances in the primary treatment of HNCs, 30–50% of all patients receiving curative therapy may still develop local relapse (Blanchard et al., 2015). Treatment of regional recurrence of HNC or second primary malignancies after primary RT is always a difficult decision for specialists. Although salvage surgery is the standard treatment, only 20% of cases can be performed, and CT has not been proven as a curative treatment option. Therefore, reirradiation is a problem frequently encountered by radiation oncologists in this patient group. Because of the severe acute and late toxicity associated with the treatment in these patients, it can be safely applied in combination with reirradiation and sometimes CRT in well-selected cases. Serious treatment-related morbidity remains an important side-effect of concurrent reirradiation with CT. In general, the previously administered radiation dose is below the tolerance dose of normal tissues, and the dose of organs at risk decreases with the time elapsed from primary treatment, but the precise additional RT dose in the case of reirradiation has not yet been determined. Therefore, radiation oncologists are reluctant to reirradiate normal tissues, especially critical structures such as the brain, brain stem, optic nerves, chiasma, and larynx. Furthermore, the administered dose to a high-risk target should be effective, enabling them to control recurrent tumours. On the other hand, RT treatment of second primary cancers in previously irradiated areas remains one of the most difficult issues for radiation oncologists. In recent years, with the publication of the results of the addition of cetuximab to radiation by Bonner et al. (2010), significant improvements have emerged in local-regional tumour control and OS. In addition, with the introduction of modified fractionation programs by Blanchard et al. (2011), significant advances were made in the second series of HNC irradiation. These reirradiation regimens are considered standard in both organ preservation and unresectable conditions.

Deciding to apply a single modality or combined treatment options in reirradiated patients is important in terms of predicted serious toxicity, and appropriateness of patient selection is advised for the improvement of the therapeutic index. In the retrospective study of Tanvetyanon et al. (2009), patients with relapsed HNC were treated with curative intent reirradiation. According to the results of this study, the probability of death 24 months after reirradiation was correlated with the combination of patients' comorbidity and prognostic factors, including organ dysfunction, isolated neck recurrence, tumour size, and time from the first treatment. In a retrospective study, Choe et al. compared the survival outcomes of 166 relapsed patients who received salvage surgery followed by adjuvant concomitant CT plus reirradiation and definitive reirradiation. Salvage surgery before reirradiation, the sum of the second serial irradiation dose, and the time from the first RT were defined as the prognostic factors affecting the final OS (Choe et al., 2011). After the decision to reirradiate, increasing the dose or adding CT to RT is used as a treatment sensitisation strategy. Patients included in these studies were treated in standard fractionation with conventional techniques and occasionally with brachytherapy. In the Skolyszewski et al. (1980) study, local control rates for recurrent tumours were reported as 27% and the 5-year OS rate as 17%. Dawson et al. (2001) treated 34 relapsed patients using more advanced techniques such as 3D-CRT and IMRT, with a total reirradiation dose of 60 Gy. At follow-up, the 2-year local control rate and 3-year OS were reported as 27% and 22%, respectively.

According to Salama et al. (2006), the effect of total dose on tumour control and survival was investigated in a post-reirradiation survival analysis of 115 head and neck recurrent disease cases at the University of Chicago. In the group treated with a total dose of 58 Gy, 3-year local control rates, PFS and OS were reported as 56%, 38% and 30%, respectively, and these rates were statistically significant compared to the group treated. This study revealed that total dose is an independent prognostic factor in multivariate analysis. In recent years have shown that reirradiation and concurrent chemotherapy agents, especially taxanes, are effective in survival (Langer et al., 2007). But the results of Bonner's (2010) phase III randomised study showed that cetuximab concomitantly with RT compared to RT alone in locally advanced HNCs significantly increases locoregional and OS. This indicates that the use of cetuximab alone is effective in chemotherapy-resistant head and neck cancer patients (Baselga et al., 2005). In a multicentre phase II study, Lartigau et al. (2013) investigated the efficacy and safety of hypofractionated SBRT with 5 weeks of cetuximab in 60 relapsed head and neck cancer patients who had received a previous dose of curative RT. While the response rate was 58% and the 1-year OS rate was 48% during the 3-month follow-up period, it was reported that acute toxicity, especially skin toxicity, was low. As with all solid tumours, in patients with relapsed HNC or in cases considered the second primary due to radiation, patients eligible for surgery, salvage surgery with acceptable morbidity is considered the treatment of choice. Although salvage surgery alone is successful in a select proportion of relapsed cases, postoperative reirradiation is preferred in advanced cases with the presence of risk factors for local-regional relapses such as positive surgical margins and lymph node metastases with extranodal spread (Jonkman et al., 2007). In a prospective phase III GORTEC/GETTEC study, 130 patients who had previously been treated with RT were diagnosed with recurrent or second primary HNC and were given 60Gy of adjuvant treatment with 5-FU concurrently after salvage surgery. Locoregional tumour control (p 0.0010) and disease -free survival (p = 0.01) were statistically significant in the group that received post-operative CRT (Janot et al., 2008).

The primary treatment-related morbidity and adverse effects such as the dry mouth and swallowing disorders depend on the total dose and irradiated volume have been demonstrated in numerous reports with normal tissue complication probability (NTCP) models, but at the reirradiation stage, the NTCP model is not available. Therefore, if reirradiation is to be performed, the initial treatment modality (RT or CRT) should be considered. Clinical target volume (CTV) may be limited to the gross tumour volume (GTV) in primary RT or to postoperative high-risk areas when considering sole or concomitant reirradiation in these patients. Using advanced radiation techniques such as IMRT and SRS, limiting the target volume to high-risk areas and using high doses per fraction seems to be extremely important to reduce radiation-related morbidity. The results of locoregional control and survival with advanced methods such as IMRT or SBRT are very promising. Cengiz et al. (2011) published the results of fractionated reirradiation with CyberKnife in 37 patients with recurrent HNC. According to the results of these studies, 27% of patients (n = 10) had complete tumour regression, 29.8% of patients (n = 11) had partial response, and 27% of patients (n = 10) had stable disease. Local control was achieved in 83.8% of patients. OS and PFS were 11.93 and 10.5 months, respectively. One-year PFS and OS were reported as 41% and 46%, respectively. Grade II or higher complication rates were observed in 13.3% of patients. In the follow-up, it was reported that 7 patients (15.2%) died from carotid artery bleeding. This study demonstrated a promising treatment modality for achieving local control in patients who were previously treated with high doses of radiation, despite the relatively high morbidity and mortality with SBRT. In their retrospective study, Ozyigit et al. (2011) compared the reirradiation results of 51 locally recurrent nasopharyngeal patients. 24 patients were included in the reirradiation programme with SBRT and 27 patients with 3D conformal methods. Patients in the SBRT arm were given 30Gy in 5 fractions consecutively. A total of 57 Gy was administered at 2Gy/day in the conventional arm. At the end of 24 months of follow-up, 2-year local control rates were reported as 82% and 80% for the SBRT and CRT arms, respectively ($p = 0.6$). For the SBRT and CRT arms, 2-year cancer-specific survival was reported as 64% and 47%, respectively ($p = 0.4$). Severe late toxicities in the SBRT and CRT arms occurred in 21% and 48% of patients, respectively ($p = 0.04$). Fatal complications occurred in 12.5% of patients in the SBRT arm and in 14.8% of patients in the CRT arm. According to the results of this study, SBRT can be applied and seems less toxic than conventional methods for reirradiation of patients with local relapse nasopharynx.

6. Feasibility of Reirradiation in Lung Cancer

According to the World Health Organisation (WHO) report, lung cancer is the biggest health problem that has challenged health systems worldwide in the past and in the coming years. According to the 2020 data of GLOBCAN Estimated Incidence, Mortality, and Prevalence Worldwide, it is the most common cancer with 2.2 million new cases. Among all cancer types, it is the cancer type that causes the most deaths, with approximately 1.8 million deaths constituting 16.7% of all male cancers (Sung et al., 2020). Although surgery is the usual treatment of early or localised disease, many are treated with concomitant chemoradiotherapy, which remains the standard of treatment because most of them are diagnosed at a locally advanced stage (Sibley et al., 1998).

Locoregional recurrence and distant metastases are frequently encountered concepts in the follow-up period of lung cancer. These recurrences can be divided into three categories,

1. Local recurrences originating from the lung parenchyma, bronchial stump, and chest wall

2. Local-regional recurrences such as mediastinal lymph nodes
3. Distant metastases such as bone, brain, liver, or contralateral lung.

However, the possible scenario may occur in any combination of these, so a special treatment plan is required for each patient, and when necessary, patients should be presented in multidisciplinary councils and the best treatment decision should be made.

Biological and technological developments that have emerged in recent years give hope for the diagnosis and treatment of recurrent lung cancer. With SBRT and SRS methods, successful dose escalation and thus reirradiation of regional recurrences can be denied. In addition to technological developments such as CyberKnife, the successful use of protons and carbon ions in therapy has been a source of hope for the future. Conventional RT has been used for many years in the treatment of locoregional recurrences of lung cancer after primary RT (Green et al., 1982; Tetar et al., 2015). But an adequate dose and timing of RT for curative or palliative treatments over these 30 years are still not well known. There is also no obvious data on the toxic effects that can be caused by reirradiation, especially when the patient receives a high dose of primary radical RT and when a recurrence develops.

Despite these challenging aspects, studies have been published showing that reirradiation is a viable method in the treatment of recurrent lung cancer (Okamoto et al., 2009). The presence of parenchymal recurrence, postoperative recurrence, postoperative irradiation patients, and secondary cancer should be considered in the evaluation of these recurrent patients for reirradiation. The stage of the relapsed disease, the time elapsed between the development of relapse and primary RT, and the total biological effective dose of the primary and reirradiation courses appear to be factors that affect the success of the relapse treatment. Therefore, for recurrences with distant metastases that are not suitable for more ablative therapy, palliative RT and best-care support can be recommended. On the other hand, brachytherapy can be performed with the chest disease team through tubes placed in the main airways in patients who do not have a postoperative external beam RT (EBRT) indication but are thought to have positive surgical margins on the stump. Apart from this indication, brachytherapy can be applied in selected cases that relapse after primary RT. Hauswald et al. treated 41 symptomatic recurrent bronchial carcinomas with HDR brachytherapy between 1987 and 2005 and published their results. All patients had previously received radiation with a median dose of 56Gy. The median dose administered by reirradiation in this study was reported as 15Gy. The time between primary EBRT and reirradiation has been reported as 9 months (Hauswald et al., 2010). After a median follow-up of 6.7 months, 6, 12, and 24 months of OS were reported as 58%, 18%, and 7%, respectively. The median OS time was 6.7 and local control was 73%. The Karnofsky performance score of 80% (p = 0.0012) and total dose of 15Gy (p = 0.029) were found to be good prognostic factors. Beavis et al. (2005) published the first report on the use of IMRT in the retreatment of a patient with lung cancer. When the conventional techniques are compared with the IMRT plan, the target coverage is quite superior to the IMRT plan. It has been reported that IMRT can provide a significant advantage in cases of reirradiation and play an important role in reirradiation. The results of previous studies have shown that it is difficult to achieve a cure in radiation therapy with reirradiation doses of 60Gy and fear of excessive toxicity in local recurrence of lung cancer. The study by Vyfhuis et al. (2018) showed that with the latest advances in the field of radiation, it is possible to increase the radiation dose above 60Gy by reirradiation, and the results are encouraging. Several studies in recent years have shown that the higher cumulative dose of reirradiation with 3D, 4D, or IMRT techniques allows for consistent use. In the McAvoy study, a total of 102 patients underwent reirradiation for intrathoracic recurrence of lung cancer. All patients received an EQD2 mean of 70Gy RT for primary treatment. The median EQD2 dose was 60.48Gy and the median time to reirradiated dose was 17 months. After a median follow-up of 6.5 months, local disease-free survival, distant metastasis-free survival, and OS were reported as 11.43, 11.43, and 14.71 months, respectively. Serious toxicity of oesophageal and pulmonary origin has been reported as 7% and 10%, respectively. Several parameters that predict low local control, such as T4 disease, squamous histology, and Eastern Cooperative Oncology Group (ECOG) performance status, were reported as > 1 (McAvoy et al., 2014). The results of this study show that IMRT and proton therapy may be good options in the treatment of recurrent lung cancer, but patients should be carefully selected to increase the survival rate and minimise the risk of death due to serious side effects (Rulach et al., 2018). When we investigate the content and diversity of studies in the literature, we see that there are very sophisticated RT plans, dose per fraction, total dose, and different techniques and algorithms used for the treatment of relapsed lung cancer or second primary. The issue of the dose to be administered will not be discussed, but the common view of radiation oncologists in reirradiation applications of relapse cases has been tried to be revealed. It can be said that there is a tendency towards more radical and definitive approaches than palliative ones.

7. Feasibility of Reirradiation in Brain Metastasis (BM)

Brain metastasis (BM) is the most common intracranial malignancy (Rulach et al., 2018). In cancer patients, BM may develop at some stage in 30–40% of patients (Kotecha et al., 2018). BM is mostly caused by lung cancer, breast cancer, colon cancer, and malignant melanoma. In patients who develop BM, the primary goal of treatment is to provide symptom palliation and increase neurological symptom-free survival rather than OS, but long-term survival and even cure are aimed at a selected small group of patients that have known oligometastatic cancer. The recommended treatment for BM is whole-brain RT (WBRT). The first-line approaches commonly used are surgical metastasectomy and SRS. Treatment of metastases in a single fraction with short-term WBRT and SRS, or a combination of these treatments, results in improved neurologic symptom-free survival and local control. The Radiation Therapy Oncology Group (RTOG) 69-01 study (Borgelt et al., 1980) reported that the median OS of patients treated with WBRT compared with steroids without RT was 3-6 months and 1-2 months, respectively. This study investigates the prognostic predictions of patients who develop BM with underlying cancer-causing metastases. According to the data of the study, the presence of comorbid disease, patient performance status, number, size, and location of BM, and size and pattern of extracranial parenchymal metastases are considered important factors in determining patient prognosis. RTOG recursive partitioning analysis (RPA) classes first defined by Gaspar et al. (1997) and then graded prognostic assessment (GPA) scores developed by Sperduto et al. (2008) were used as prognostic indexes, especially for metastatic breast and non-small cell lung cancer (NSCLC). In this GPA system, age, Karnofsky Performance Status (KPS), number of BM, and presence of extracranial metastases are prognostic and are used as parameters. For each of these parameters, 3 different scores (0, 0.5, or 1) are used and patients are classified. The scoring system takes into account age (60; 50-59; 50), KPS (70; 70-80; 90-100), and the number of BM (> 3; 2-3; 1). While patients in class I had the best survival with 3.5–4 points, the class II group had 3 points, the class III group 1.5–2.5 points, and class IV showed lower survival with 0–1 point. A phase III study by the European Organisation for Research and Treatment of Cancer (EORTC) 22952–26001 conducted in Germany evaluated whether administering adjuvant WBRT increases the time to functional independence after surgery or radiosurgery of BM. 359 cancer patients with stable systemic disease or primary tumour under control, 1-3 BM, and performance status 0 to 2 were treated with either complete surgery or radiosurgery and randomly assigned to the adjuvant WBRT or observation arm. Radiosurgery was performed on 199 patients, and surgery on 160 patients. From the radiosurgery group, 100 patients were included in the observation arm and 99 patients were included in the WBRT arm. After surgery, 79 patients were assigned to the follow-up arm and 81 patients to the adjuvant WBRT arm. WBRT at sites with metastases (surgery: 59% to 27%, P 0.001) (SRS: 31% to 19%, P 0.040) and non-metastasis (surgery: 42% to 23%, P 0.008). The 2-year recurrence rate was reduced (SRS: 48% to 33%, P 0.023). It has been reported that after SRS or surgery of BM, adjuvant WBRT reduces cranial relapses and neurologic symptoms but fails to improve OS (Kocher et al., 2011). Other groups exploring this important issue include the 2006 study of the Japanese Working Group on Radiation Oncology (JROSG) and the Secondary Analysis of the JOSH 99-1 Randomised Study. In the first phase, 3 randomised clinical trials of this group, the WBRT plus SRS arm and the SRS alone arm were compared for patients with BM 1 to 4. It was reported that the addition of WBRT to SRS significantly reduced its recurrence in both the initial metastatic region and other brain regions, but it did not improve OS significantly (Aoyama et al., 2006).

In a Japanese study, a total of 132 patients, 88 of whom had NSCLC, with a BM of 1 to 4, were included using the GPA classification model, and the RT administered was reanalysed. The median follow-up was 8.05 months and the mean SRS dose was 21.9Gy in SRS alone and 16.6Gy in WBRT + SRS (WBRT 30Gy in 10 fractions in 2–2.5 weeks). The median OS was 16.7 vs. 10.6 months, respectively (P = 0.04). As a result, a total of forty-seven patients with 26 SRS and 21 WBRT plus SRS treatment in GPA 2.5 groups and 41 patients with GPA 2 (19 patients only SRS and 22 patients WBRT plus SRS) had a favourable prognosis. Overall survival was significantly better in WBRT plus SRS in the GPA 2.5-4 group compared to SRS alone (Aoyama et al., 2015).

The Preferred Reporting Items for Systematic Reviews and Meta-Analyses (PRISMA) study evaluated its therapeutic effect for studies comparing SRS alone with WBRT plus SRS and using the GPA classification in patients with NSCLC with a maximum of 4 BM. Based on this meta-analysis, SRS plus WBRT in both GPA classes did not significantly improve OS (GPA2: P = 0.71; GPA2: P = 0.54) but significantly prolonged brain recurrence in the group receiving SRS plus WBRT (GPA2: P = 0.005; GPA2: P .00001). Eventually, reirradiation performed with only the SRS method as a salvage treatment was found to be statistically as significant as the frequently used method in 2 subgroups (GPA2: P = 0.01) and (GPA2: P = 0.006). The rate of Grade 3 or 4 late side effects from RT was similar in the 2 subgroups between SRS and SRS+WBRT. The most important result of the study showed that the combined treatment did not have an OS advantage over SRS alone (Qie et al., 2018). However, appropriate treatment options remain important for patients who relapse after brain irradiation, especially in the patient group with GPA2 after these combined treatments. Several prospective clinical studies have been published investigating the role of reirradiation of BM.

While evaluating all these studies, some factors require choosing among different treatment options: Is primary extracranial disease under control, and is control expected to continue? Will systemic therapy be recommended? Does brain control affect patient survival or is a treatment focused on symptom palliation? Does the operation provide local control for the patient? Is local control possible without surgery? Could the total dose of radiation delivered to critical structures cause serious side effects in patients with long-term life expectancy? Does the dose of RT to be given have functional consequences? How long was the initial RT response of the lesions?

Cooper et al. (1990) planned a second cranial radiation therapy of 2,500cGy in 10 fractions in 52 patients to alleviate symptoms caused by recurrent BM. The most important criterion among the selection criteria of the study was that the general condition of the patient was good for at least 4 months after the first radiation therapy, and then the neurological symptoms worsened again. They had received 30Gy RT of 300cGy/10 Fraction from the first treatment. At the end of the treatment, 22 patients (42%) responded to reirradiation, and at least one level of improvement in their neurological function status was noted. After the second treatment, survival was reported as a mean of 5 months. At the end of the study, they say that reirradiation should be considered in patients who are in good general condition but experience worsening neurological symptoms for 4 months or more after the first palliative WBRT. In a review of 49 whole-brain reirradiation trials, the median time between two treatments was 11.5, with a median starting dose of 30Gy and a median reirradiation dose of 20Gy. The median KPS was 70 and the median OS was 3 months (Guo et al., 2016). Along with technological developments, progress was observed in the field of reirradiation after WBRT. Sterzing et al. (2009) reported that they applied WBRT with helical tomotherapy, reirradiation for multiple recurrent or newly developing BM despite the previous WBRT, and simultaneous integrated boost (SIB) for metastases and reported acute side effects. The number of patients in this study was low, but the new technique and dose applications are inspiring. Radiation plans with excellent homogeneity index (HI) and conformity index (CI) and low max doses in normal brain tissue were promising. In this study, the mean radiation time was 13 minutes and the observed acute side effect was a mild headache. A recent study by the Cleveland Clinic examined GS and local control after reirradiation with SRS in 1789 recurrent BM. The median OS of patients from the development of first brain metastasis was 17.7 months and the median survival after salvage SRS was 9.9 months. Median OS after rescue SRS was analysed in two groups. Patients with a first recurrence > 6 months after WBRT had a median follow-up of 12.3 months, compared to 6.8 months for patients with a first recurrence less than 6 months after WBRT (P = 0.0061). The primary tumour site did not affect OS after SRS. Twenty-five percent of patients (n = 28) developed recurrence after the first SRS, with a mean duration time of 5.2 months. According to the results of this study, it was emphasised that patients who developed relapse after WBRT and were treated with SRS had good local control and survival after SRS, while the results were promising (Chao et al., 2008).

Conclusion

Reirradiation in the treatment of recurrences or secondary cancers due to RT in the area previously treated with RT is a good option to control local-regional progression and reduce symptoms. Based on the analysis presented in this chapter, satisfactory results can be obtained for the local recurrence of many cancer types when carefully selected by experienced centres with the help of advanced technical treatment devices, taking into account the possible dangers of reirradiation. With patients preferring modern and advanced RT techniques such as IMRT for reirradiation of local recurrences after primary treatment, interest in second-serial irradiation has grown.

References

Aoyama, H., Shirato, H., Tago, M., Nakagawa, K., Toyoda, T., Hatano, K., ... & Kobashi, G. (2006). Stereotactic radiosurgery plus whole-brain radiation therapy vs stereotactic radiosurgery alone for treatment of brain metastases: a randomized controlled trial. *Jama*, *295*(21), 2483-2491.

Aoyama, H., Tago, M., & Shirato, H. (2015). Stereotactic radiosurgery with or without whole-brain radiotherapy for brain metastases: secondary analysis of the JROSG 99-1 randomized clinical trial. *JAMA oncology*, *1*(4), 457-464.

Baselga, J., Trigo, J. M., Bourhis, J., Tortochaux, J., Cortés-Funes, H., Hitt, R., ... & Eckardt, A. (2005). Phase II multicenter study of the antiepidermal growth factor receptor monoclonal antibody cetuximab in combination with platinum-based chemotherapy in patients with platinum-refractory metastatic and/or recurrent squamous cell carcinoma of the head and neck. *Journal of clinical oncology*, *23*(24), 5568-5577.

Bassal, M., Mertens, A. C., Taylor, L., Neglia, J. P., Greffe, B. S., Hammond, S., ... & Kadan-Lottick, N. S. (2006). Risk of selected subsequent carcinomas in survivors of childhood cancer: a report from the Childhood Cancer Survivor Study. *Journal of Clinical Oncology*, *24*(3).

Bassal, M., Mertens, A. C., Taylor, L., Neglia, J. P., Greffe, B. S., Hammond, S., ... & Kadan-Lottick, N. S. (2006). Risk of selected subsequent carcinomas in survivors of childhood cancer: a report from the Childhood Cancer Survivor Study. *Journal of Clinical Oncology*, *24*(3).

Berrington de Gonzalez A., Curtis R. E., Kry S. F., Gilbert E., Lamart S., Berg C. D., Stovall M., Ron E. (2011). Proportion of second cancers attributable to radiotherapy treatment in adults: a cohort study in the US SEER cancer registries. *Lancet Oncol,* 12(4):353–36.

Blanchard, P., Hill, C., Guihenneuc-Jouyaux, C., Baey, C., Bourhis, J., & Pignon, J. P. (2011). Mixed treatment comparison meta-analysis of altered fractionated radiotherapy and chemotherapy in head and neck cancer. *Journal of clinical epidemiology*, *64*(9), 985-992.

Blanchard, P., Lee, A., Marguet, S., Leclercq, J., Ng, W. T., Ma, J., ... & Group, M. N. C. (2015). Chemotherapy and radiotherapy in nasopharyngeal carcinoma: an update of the MAC-NPC meta-analysis. *The lancet oncology*, *16*(6), 645-655.

Blanchard, P., Lee, A., Marguet, S., Leclercq, J., Ng, W. T., Ma, J., ... & Group, M. N. C. (2015). Chemotherapy and radiotherapy in nasopharyngeal carcinoma: an update of the MAC-NPC meta-analysis. *The lancet oncology*, *16*(6), 645-655.

Borgelt, B., Gelber, R., Kramer, S., Brady, L. W., Chang, C. H., Davis, L. W., ... & Hendrickson, F. R. (1980). The palliation of brain metastases: final results of the first two studies by the Radiation Therapy Oncology Group. *International Journal of Radiation Oncology* Biology* Physics*, *6*(1), 1-9.

Brem, H., Piantadosi, S., Burger, P. C., Walker, M., Selker, R., Vick, N. A., ... & Schold, S. C. (1995). Placebo-controlled trial of safety and efficacy of intraoperative controlled delivery by biodegradable polymers of chemotherapy for recurrent gliomas. *The Lancet*, *345*(8956), 1008-1012.

Cengiz, M., Özyiğit, G., Yazici, G., Doğan, A., Yildiz, F., Zorlu, F., ... & Akyol, F. (2011). Salvage reirradiaton with stereotactic body radiotherapy for locally recurrent head-and-neck tumors. *International Journal of Radiation Oncology* Biology* Physics*, *81*(1), 104-109.

Chao, S. T., Barnett, G. H., Vogelbaum, M. A., Angelov, L., Weil, R. J., Neyman, G., ... & Suh, J. H. (2008). Salvage stereotactic radiosurgery effectively treats recurrences from whole-brain radiation therapy. *Cancer*, *113*(8), 2198-2204.

Choe, K. S., Haraf, D. J., Solanki, A., Cohen, E. E., Seiwert, T. Y., Stenson, K. M., ... & Salama, J. K. (2011). Prior chemoradiotherapy adversely impacts outcomes of recurrent and second primary head and neck cancer treated with concurrent chemotherapy and reirradiation. *Cancer*, *117*(20), 4671-4678.

Cooper, J. S., Steinfeld, A. D., & Lerch, I. A. (1990). Cerebral metastases: value of reirradiation in selected patients. *Radiology*, *174*(3), 883-885.

Dawson, L. A., Myers, L. L., Bradford, C. R., Chepeha, D. B., Hogikyan, N. D., Teknos, T. N., ... & Eisbruch, A. (2001). Conformal re-irradiation of recurrent and new primary head-and-neck cancer. *International Journal of Radiation Oncology* Biology* Physics*, *50*(2), 377-385.

Desjardins, A. U. (1930). The value of radiotherapy in mediastinal tumors. *California and Western Medicine*, *32*(6), 377.

Embring, A., Onjukka, E., Mercke, C., Lax, I., Berglund, A., Bornedal, S., ... & Friesland, S. (2020). Overlapping volumes in re-irradiation for head and neck cancer–an important factor for patient selection. Radiation Oncology, 15(1), 1-10.

Garland, L. H., & Sisson, M. (1950). Results of irradiation in cancer of the lip, tongue and ear. *California Medicine*, *73*(4), 312.

Gaspar, L., Scott, C., Rotman, M., Asbell, S., Phillips, T., Wasserman, T., ... & Byhardt, R. (1997). Recursive partitioning analysis (RPA) of prognostic factors in three Radiation Therapy Oncology Group (RTOG) brain metastases trials. *International journal of radiation oncology, biology, physics*, *37*(4), 745-751.

Green, N., & Melbye, R. W. (1982). Lung cancer: retreatment of local recurrence after definitive irradiation. *Cancer*, *49*(5), 865-868.

Guo, S., Balagamwala, E. H., Reddy, C., Elson, P., Suh, J. H., & Chao, S. T. (2016). Clinical and radiographic outcomes from repeat whole-brain radiation therapy for brain metastases in the age of stereotactic radiosurgery. *American Journal of Clinical Oncology*, *39*(3), 288-293.

Hauswald, H., Stoiber, E., Rochet, N., Lindel, K., Grehn, C., Becker, H. D., ... & Harms, W. (2010). Treatment of recurrent bronchial carcinoma: the role of high-dose-rate endoluminal brachytherapy. *International Journal of Radiation Oncology* Biology* Physics*, *77*(2), 373-377.

Huncharek, M., & Muscat, J. (1998). Treatment of recurrent high grade astrocytoma; results of a systematic review of 1,415 patients. *Anticancer Research*, *18*(2B), 1303-1311.

Janot, F., de Raucourt, D., Benhamou, E., Ferron, C., Dolivet, G., Bensadoun, R. J., ... & Bourhis, J. (2008). Randomized trial of postoperative reirradiation combined with chemotherapy after salvage surgery compared with salvage surgery alone in head and neck carcinoma. *J Clin Oncol*, *26*(34), 5518-5523.

Jonkman, A., Kaanders, J. H., Terhaard, C. H., Hoebers, F. J., van den Ende, P. L., Wijers, O. B., ... & Langendijk, J. A. (2007). Multicenter validation of recursive partitioning analysis classification for patients with squamous cell head and neck carcinoma treated with surgery and postoperative radiotherapy. *International Journal of Radiation Oncology* Biology* Physics*, *68*(1), 119-125.

Kazmi, F., Soon, Y. Y., Leong, Y. H., Koh, W. Y., & Vellayappan, B. (2019). Re-irradiation for recurrent glioblastoma (GBM): a systematic review and meta-analysis. *Journal of Neuro-oncology*, *142*(1), 79-90.

Kleinerman, R. A. (2006). Cancer risks following diagnostic and therapeutic radiation exposure in children. *Pediatric radiology*, *36*(2), 121-125.

Kocher, M., Soffietti, R., Abacioglu, U., Villa, S., Fauchon, F., Baumert, B. G., ... & Mueller, R. P. (2011). Adjuvant whole-brain radiotherapy versus observation after radiosurgery or surgical resection of one to three cerebral metastases: results of the EORTC 22952-26001 study. *Journal of Clinical Oncology*, *29*(2), 134.

Kotecha, R., Gondi, V., Ahluwalia, M. S., Brastianos, P. K., & Mehta, M. P. (2018). Recent advances in managing brain metastasis. *F1000Research*, *7*.

Kulinich, D. P., Sheppard, J. P., Nguyen, T., Kondajji, A. M., Unterberger, A., Duong, C., ... & Yang, I. (2021). Radiotherapy versus combination radiotherapy-bevacizumab for the treatment of recurrent high-grade glioma: a systematic review. *Acta Neurochirurgica*, *163*(7), 1921-1934.

Langer, C. J., Harris, J., Horwitz, E. M., Nicolaou, N., Kies, M., Curran, W., ... & Ang, K. (2007). Phase II study of low-dose paclitaxel and cisplatin in combination with split-course concomitant twice-daily reirradiation in recurrent squamous cell carcinoma of the head and neck: results of Radiation Therapy Oncology Group Protocol 9911. *Journal of clinical oncology*, *25*(30), 4800-4805.

Lartigau, E. F., Tresch, E., Thariat, J., Graff, P., Coche-Dequeant, B., Benezery, K., ... & Kramar, A. (2013). Multi institutional phase II study of concomitant stereotactic reirradiation and cetuximab for recurrent head and neck cancer. *Radiotherapy and Oncology*, *109*(2), 281-285.

Lee, B. J. Tannenbaum N. E. (1926). Recurrent inoperable carcinoma of the breast. JAMA; 86:250-6.

Mantovani, C., Gastino, A., Cerrato, M., Badellino, S., Ricardi, U., Levis, M. (2021). Modern Radiation Therapy for the Management of Brain Metastases From Non-Small Cell Lung Cancer: Current Approaches and Future Directions. *Front Oncol*. 2;11: 772-789.

Mazonakis, M., & Damilakis, J. (2017). Cancer risk after radiotherapy for benign diseases. *Physica Medica*, *42*, 285-291.

McAvoy, S., Ciura, K., Wei, C., Rineer, J., Liao, Z., Chang, J. Y., ... & Gomez, D. R. (2014). Definitive reirradiation for locoregionally recurrent non-small cell lung cancer with proton beam therapy or intensity modulated radiation therapy: predictors of high-grade toxicity and survival outcomes. *International Journal of Radiation Oncology* Biology* Physics*, *90*(4), 819-827.

Murphy, W. T., & Schmitz, A. (1956). The results of re-irradiation in cancer of the cervix. *Radiology*, *67*(3), 378-385.

Nieder, C., Astner, S. T., Mehta, M. P., Grosu, A. L., & Molls, M. (2008). Improvement, clinical course, and quality of life after palliative radiotherapy for recurrent glioblastoma. *American journal of clinical oncology*, *31*(3), 300-305.

Okamoto, Y., Murakami, M., Yoden, E., Sasaki, R., Okuno, Y., Nakajima, T., & Kuroda, Y. (2002). Reirradiation for locally recurrent lung cancer previously treated with radiation therapy. *International Journal of Radiation Oncology* Biology* Physics*, *52*(2), 390-396.

Ozyigit, G., Cengiz, M., Yazici, G., Yildiz, F., Gurkaynak, M., Zorlu, F., ... & Akyol, F. (2011). A retrospective comparison of robotic stereotactic body radiotherapy and three-dimensional conformal radiotherapy for the reirradiation of locally recurrent nasopharyngeal carcinoma. *International Journal of Radiation Oncology* Biology* Physics*, *81*(4), e263-e268.

Paganetti, H. (2012). *Proton therapy physics, Series in medical physics and biomedical engineering.* CRC Press, Boca Raton.

Qie, S., Li, Y., Shi, H. Y., Yuan, L., Su, L., & Zhang, X. (2018). Stereotactic radiosurgery (SRS) alone versus whole brain radiotherapy plus SRS in patients with 1 to 4 brain metastases from non-small cell lung cancer stratified by the graded prognostic assessment: A meta-analysis (PRISMA) of randomized control trials. *Medicine*, *97*(33).

Ron, E. (2003). Cancer risks from medical radiation. *Health physics*, *85*(1), 47-59.

Rulach, R., Hanna, G. G., Franks, K., McAleese, J., & Harrow, S. (2018). Re-irradiation for locally recurrent lung cancer: Evidence, risks and benefits. *Clinical Oncology*, *30*(2), 101-109.

Salama, J. K., Vokes, E. E., Chmura, S. J., Milano, M. T., Kao, J., Stenson, K. M., ... & Haraf, D. J. (2006). Long-term outcome of concurrent chemotherapy and reirradiation for recurrent and second primary head-and-neck squamous cell carcinoma. *International Journal of Radiation Oncology* Biology* Physics*, *64*(2), 382-391.

Sibley, G. S., Jamieson, T. A., Marks, L. B., Anscher, M. S., & Prosnitz, L. R. (1998). Radiotherapy alone for medically inoperable stage I non-small–cell lung cancer: the duke experience. *International Journal of Radiation Oncology* Biology* Physics*, *40*(1), 149-154.

Skołyszewski, J., Korzeniowski, S., & Reinfuss, M. (1980). The reirradiation of recurrences of head and neck cancer. *The British Journal of Radiology*, *53*(629), 462-465.

Sperduto, P. W., Berkey, B., Gaspar, L. E., Mehta, M., & Curran, W. (2008). A new prognostic index and comparison to three other indices for patients with brain metastases: an analysis of 1,960 patients in the RTOG database. *International Journal of Radiation Oncology* Biology* Physics*, *70*(2), 510-514.

Sterzing, F., Welzel, T., Sroka-Perez, G., Schubert, K., Debus, J., & Herfarth, K. K. (2009). Reirradiation of multiple brain metastases with helical tomotherapy. *Strahlentherapie und Onkologie*, *185*(2), 89-93.

Stieler, F., Wolff, D., Bauer, L., Wertz, H. J., Wenz, F., & Lohr, F. (2011). Reirradiation of spinal column metastases. *Strahlentherapie und Onkologie*, *187*(7), 406-415.

Stupp, R., Hegi, M. E., Mason, W. P., Van Den Bent, M. J., Taphoorn, M. J., Janzer, R. C., ... & National Cancer Institute of Canada Clinical Trials Group. (2009). Effects of radiotherapy with concomitant and adjuvant temozolomide versus radiotherapy alone on survival in glioblastoma in a randomised phase III study: 5-year analysis of the EORTC-NCIC trial. *The lancet oncology*, *10*(5), 459-466.

Sung, H., Ferlay, J., Siegel, R. L., Laversanne, M., Soerjomataram, I., Jemal, A., & Bray, F. (2021). Global cancer statistics 2020: GLOBOCAN estimates of incidence and mortality worldwide for 36 cancers in 185 countries. *CA: a cancer journal for clinicians*, *71*(3), 209-249.

Tanvetyanon, T., Qin, D., Padhya, T., Kapoor, R., McCaffrey, J., & Trotti, A. (2009). Survival outcomes of squamous cell carcinoma arising from sinonasal inverted papilloma: report of 6 cases with systematic review and pooled analysis. *American journal of otolaryngology*, *30*(1), 38-43.

Tetar, S., Dahele, M., Griffioen, G., Slotman, B., Senan, S. (2015). High-dose conventional thoracic re-irradiation for lung cancer: updated results. *Lung cancer*, 88:235–236.

Vyfhuis, M. A., Rice, S., Remick, J., Mossahebi, S., Badiyan, S., Mohindra, P., & Simone, C. B. (2018). Reirradiation for locoregionally recurrent non-small cell lung cancer. *Journal of thoracic disease*, *10*(Suppl 21), S2522.

Wick, A., Felsberg, J., Steinbach, J. P., Herrlinger, U., Platten, M., Blaschke, B., ... & Wick, W. (2007). Efficacy and tolerability of temozolomide in an alternating weekly regimen in patients with recurrent glioma. *Journal of Clinical Oncology*, *25*(22), 3357-3361.

Wong, E. T., Hess, K. R., Gleason, M. J., Jaeckle, K. A., Kyritsis, A. P., Prados, M. D., ... & Yung, W. A. (1999). Outcomes and prognostic factors in recurrent glioma patients enrolled onto phase II clinical trials. *Journal of Clinical Oncology*, *17*(8), 2572-2572.

Chapter 17

Radiation Protection Aspects of IMRT

Hakan Eren*

Ege University, Faculty of Medicine, Department of Radiation Oncology, Izmir, Turkey

Abstract

The rapid increase in the application of new therapeutic techniques such as intensity-modulated radiotherapy (IMRT) motivates research into radiation safety management and shielding designs of facilities using medical linear accelerators. To this end, it becomes important to gather information about linear accelerator facilities and treatments workload, shielding design, shielding management and the way to obtain shielding information. However, the need to establish standardised armor design information and to clarify uncertain pathways for knowledge acquisition is also highlighted. Conventional assumptions used in room shielding calculations are reevaluated for IMRT. For the same single fraction tumour dose administered, the total monitor units (MUs) for IMRT are much higher than for conventional therapy. Therefore, the exposure contribution from linear accelerator (LINAC) head leakage would be significantly larger than with conventional treatments. For conventional multileaf collimator (MLC) IMRT treatments, the workload for primary barrier calculations is determined by patient tumour doses. The same calculation for accelerator-based tomotherapy IMRT requires scaling by the mean number of treatment slices. However, rotational therapy provides a minor usability factor that compensates for this increase. Traditional primary barriers have been reported to be sufficient for both dynamic MLC and tomotherapy IMRT. However, the excessive head leakage produced by these modalities requires an increase in secondary

---

*Corresponding Author's Email:hakan.eren@ege.edu.tr.

In: Frontiers in Intensity-Modulated Radiotherapy Research
Editor: Sibel Karaca
ISBN: 979-8-88697-252-8

barrier protection. When designing protection for an IMRT facility, increases in accelerator head leakage should be considered for secondary protection. The adequacy of secondary prevention will depend on the number of IMRT patients. For traditional facilities being evaluated for IMRT, existing primary barriers will typically be sufficient. IMRT represents a significant technological advance in its ability to deliver highly conformal radiation therapy. With increased accessibility, general clinical practice has become increasingly common. However, there are a few precautions worth commenting on regarding the clinical application of IMRT. In theory, the increased irradiated volume and the leakage radiation that sometimes accompanies IMRT can contribute to unexpected complications and safety concerns. The extended delivery time of IMRT with the associated incremental LINAC MUs may result in photoactivation of elements within the linear accelerator collimator, thus increasing accidental radiation exposure to patients and personnel when high-energy photons are used. Increased volumes of normal tissues exposed to lower doses of radiation via IMRT could theoretically promote carcinogenesis and complications due to the "bystander" effect, low dose hyper-radiosensitivity and reduced repair of double-stranded DNA breaks at very low doses.

Keywords: intensity modulated radiotherapy, linear accelerator, tomotherapy, radiation protection, shielding, leakage, IMRT factor, workload in IMRT

1. Introduction

Intensity-modulated radiation therapy (IMRT) is a treatment technique in which the radiation intensity is modulated to increase treatment effectiveness. High photon energies of 4 to 15 MV are often used by IMRT to deliver powerful doses to the tumour (Bucci, Bevan, and Roach, 2005). The delivery of radiation to the tumour with IMRT is more compatible than conformal radiation therapy as a three-dimensional (3DCRT). Therefore, IMRT treatment technique is more efficacious in protecting organs at risk than 3DCRT (Arbea et al., 2010). In IMRT, unlike 3DCRT, the beam is collimated by the continuous application of a locally beam shielding multileaf collimator (MLC). This treatment technique contains a relatively long period and a higher number of (MUs) to give the same prescription dose to tumour of the patient (Jeraj and Robar, 2004). So, more conservative protection conditions are preferred in IMRT requiring a longer irradiation time than 3DCRT. Consideration should be given to the leaked radiation dose rather than the predicted dose, as it is a measure of the actual amount of MU transmitted (Rohrig, 2006). The increasing use of IMRT makes radiation protection designs more critical in sections containing linear accelerator (LINAC) devices.

Clinically, it has recently issued warnings in opposition to exceeding workload values and recommended workload reassessment. A few concerns have been raised against evaluating shielding where instantaneous dose rate (IDR) is taken into account without considering utilisation, occupancy factor and workload. If standardised detailed safety regulatory procedures have not been established or there are no standards for LINAC installations, differences can arise among licensing authorities' interpretations of organised provisions. In this context, studies on innovations in radiotherapy shielding design are limited. With the above limitations, a detailed review of the state of shielding design for IMRT in radiation oncology departments is presented.

2. Workload and IMRT Factor

In report 151 of the National Radiation Protection Council (NCRP 151) (Rohrig, 2006), the workload is identified as the radiation dose maximum delivered from LINAC throughout the study. In this study, the weekly workload (W) is the sum of (Gy/week), the mean absorbed prescribed radiation dose per delivery to the patient (D_f), the mean number of patients treated in a day (N) and the number of working days per week of the clinic. It also includes week-long and device and patient-based quality assurance (QA) processes that are carried out periodically. The relationship of all the components of the above-mentioned workload is given in Equation (1).

$$W\left(\frac{Gy}{week}\right) = \left(D_f\left(\frac{Gy}{treatment}\right) \times N\left(\frac{treatments}{day}\right) \times 5\left(work\frac{days}{week}\right)\right) + W_{QA} \quad (1)$$

An equivalent dose of the neutron was calculated in primary barrier protection for photon beams having energies greater than 10 MV with increased photoneutron production. Equations 1 and 2 are used to calculate the weekly equivalent of neutron dose on the other side of the laminated barrier at the maximum collimator field size aperture.

$$H_n\left[\frac{\mu Sv}{week}\right]=\frac{D_0\times R\times F_{max}}{\left(\frac{t_m}{2}+t_2+0.3\right)}\times\left[10^{-\left(\frac{t_1}{TVL_x}\right)}\right]\left[10^{-\left(\frac{t_2}{TVL_n}\right)}\right] \quad (2)$$

H_n is the weekly neutron dose equivalent, D_0 is the photon beam dose absorbed weekly at the concentric, R is the neutron generation coefficient for F_{max} which is the maximum field width at the concentric, t_m is the thickness of metal plate, t_1 and t_2 are the thickness of the first and second plates of concrete of respectively, for the primary photon beam TVL_x is the tenth value layer thickness in concrete, for neutrons TVL_n is the tenth half value layer thickness in concrete and the distance between the external plane of barrier and the seating point is 0.3. With the use of MLC, IMRT allows the radiation dose to be given at high intensity on the tumour by controlling the beam intensity. IMRT or volumetric modulated arc therapy (VMAT) involves much more irradiation time and radiation MUs than should be delivered to the tumour in 3DCRT. In IMRT and 3DCRT, the desired radiation dose to the tumour per fraction is the same. But with increasing MUs in IMRT, the leakage radiation increases from the accelerator head; therefore, the leakage radiation increased by IMRT applications in radiotherapy departments is calculated by the IMRT (IF) factor.

In NCRP 151 (Rohrig, 2006), the IMRT Factor (IF) indicates that it is calculated by Equation (3).

$$IF=\frac{MU_{(IMRT)}}{MU_{3D-CRT}};\ MU_{IMRT}=\sum_{i=1}^{n}\frac{MU_i}{Prescribeddose_i} \quad (3)$$

The ratio of MU per unit given by IMRT to MU provided by 3DCRT is called the IMRT factor. The range recommended by the NCRP 151 is 2-10. The p in Equation (4) is the cure rate of IMRT/VMAT excluding 3DCRT from the total number of treatments.

$$f=(1-p)+p\times IF(4)$$

The workload in Equation (5) describing the IMRT factor includes the dose W_L from the leak radiation. It is obtained by multiplying f and W. (Kwon et al., 2022).

$$W_L=f\times W(5)$$

Conventional radiotherapy is gradually being replaced by IMRT. In IMRT, the LINAC and the MLC in its head modulate the radiation beam through computer and software control. Basically, the overall dose delivery to the tumour is achieved through many small segments. Treatment delivery methods in IMRT are not efficient in terms of the use of MUs contrasted to traditional treatment. As a result, increased irradiation MUs with IMRT cause leakage in the LINAC head. The additional MUs required for IMRT compared to conventional treatment were estimated by Followill, Geis, and Boyer (1997) to be about two to five factors. Currently, the prescribed dose and fraction schemes for IMRT are equal to traditional therapy despite recommended dose increases (Mohan et al., 2000). In delivery technique, these changes may render parts of the existing NCRP radiation protection formalism unsuitable for the plan of linear accelerator rooms primarily planned for IMRT.

The formalism of new room protection is proposed in IMRT installations by Mutic et al. (Mutic et al., 2001). For reducing the intricacy of the transition, the recently developed model builds on the current formalism and applies suitable corrections for the data factors according to the unique characteristics of IMRT. As described below, irradiation on the barrier of primary is in proportion to the dose given to the tumour. However, exposure reaching the secondary barrier is commensurate to the number of MUs, largely due to leakage of the linear accelerator head. So, the suggested protection calculation model separates the workload concepts, MUs and tumour dose by describing separate workloads for thickness calculations at the primary and secondary barriers.

Two density modulated distribution methods will be explored which are called MLC in dynamic (known as DMLC) or static MLC (known as SMLC) modes within tomotherapy. In the technique of DMLC, the leaves of MLC move during the delivery of the beam. The SMLC technique stops the leaves throughout irradiation and stops the irradiation throughout leaf movement (A. L. Boyer et al., 1997; A. Boyer et al., 1999). While the occurring dose distributions may have measurable differences, they will be considered equivalent for room shielding design purposes. Linear accelerator-induced tomotherapy treatments are carried out using a commercial third-generation DMLC attached to a traditional linear accelerator (Verellen et al., 1997).

Calculation of protecting barrier thickness is conventionally divided into primary beam-intercepting barriers (called primary barriers) and barriers intended to reduce radiation emitted from the head of the linear accelerator and scattered from the body of the patient (called secondary barriers). The requirements at the secondary barrier for radiation of leakage and scattered are accounted for individually. The formalism of IMRT protection does not eliminate the distinction between primary and secondary barriers. The P, d, and T factors in Equation (6) apply in the same way as with traditional therapy setups in all cases examined and would not be mentioned anymore in the next sections.

To determine the necessary barrier thickness for a traditional megavoltage therapy room, the conventional Equation (6) is given by:

$$B = \frac{Pd^2}{WUT} m \quad (6)$$

in this formula, B is the factor of transmission, P is the allowable rate of exposure ($Sv.wk^{-1}$), d is the interval between the source of radiation and the estimation point (m), the factor of utilisation is U, T is the factor of occupancy, the workload is called W ($Sv.wk^{-1}$) and m is the result of the correction factors in the secondary barrier calculations which finding in the NCRP 49 (NCRP Report No 049). In photon beams with high energy, the factor of quality is assumed to be 1. The formalism of installations of conventional therapy has been defined in NCRP 49.

3. Primary Barriers

3.1. DMLC Technique

The traditional workload definition for primary DMLC barriers has been changed. The workload ($W_{p,c}$) is used for calculations in (c) traditional (p) primary barrier. It was reputed to be the equivalence of the total dose (TD) weekly administered to patients.

$$W_{p,c} = TD = E_c MU_c \cong MU_c \quad (7)$$

In this formula, E_c is the efficiency which defining as the proportion of MUs for dose in tumour in a week and MU_c is the MUs delivered over the week. In this assumption, the LINAC is calibrated at d_{max} and if it is calibrated at another depth an appropriate factor must be used to change the monitor unit (MU). While the equivalence between MUs and dose is not entirely accurate (actually assuming E_c=1), Equation (7) provides a conservative prediction of fluency for primary protection calculations.

Because of the relatively insufficient delivery of DMLC, ED<<1, where D denotes DMLC. Using MUs as workloads may overestimate the unattenuated dose rate up to 10 with 1/ED. A model is proposed that separates MUs and provides dose weekly, using the predicted total tumour dose weekly for calculations primary barrier and the total MUs given in a week for secondary barrier leak calculations and workload.

$$W_{p,D} = TD \quad (8)$$

In this formula, $W_{p,D}$ is the workload of primary barrier for a room of DMLC. It is same to expressing that the out-of-room exposure with time-integrated for a fraction of treatment with DMLC is the equal as for fraction of an open treatment portal for the same total area of cross-section. In model, the total flux which passing through the tumour is assumed being the same in IMRT like for conformal radiotherapy, with the primary difference as a result of the redistribution of fluency to avoid organs at risk. Equivalence so assuming the number of beams and therefore the average flux in every beam doesn't differ significantly.

One of the theories found in traditional conservation calculations is that the rate of protection is configured to cover the maximum field size, specifically the field size 40x40 cm^2 at the isocenter. Traditional radiotherapy and especially IMRT fields are in most cases significantly less than the largest field size. So, the use factor for conformal radiotherapy and IMRT is:

$$U_{p,D} = \eta(f_s)U_c \qquad (9)$$

in this formula,

$$\eta(f_s) = \frac{D(f_s)}{D(40\times40)}, \qquad (10)$$

η(fs) is a defined proportion of exposure rates except for the primary barrier to the 40x40 cm^2 field size for mean field size f_s and U_c is the conventional utilisation factor (eg, for lateral beams is 0,25). The term $\eta(f_s)$ is similar to conventional S_{cp} (Khan, 2014), but is mainly driven by scattering in the primary barrier. $\eta(f_s)$ value depends on the factors which are affecting the scattered radiation, which means the barrier thickness and its placement relative to the LINAC, the beam energy, and the distance from the barrier to the measuring point.

3.2. Technique of Tomotherapy

With the identical reasons that the workload of the primary barrier for DMLC setups is equivalent to TD (Equation (8)), the workload of tomotherapy is,

$$W_{p,t} = TD \quad (11)$$

In this formula, tomotherapy is denoted by the subscript t.

In tomotherapy, the use factor includes more than one component. Tomotherapy gives radiation to successive indexes by sliding the patient relative to the beam therefore same part of the primary barrier is the beam on during each index treated while the accelerator rotates. So, the use factor for the primary barrier contains the mean number of indexes (indicated with I) used for treating patients.

Since treatment is delivered by arcs, κ, a geometric ingredient of the use factor, is determined as a fraction of the total turning angle of the gantry at which the beam comes to the primary barrier and as a direct target point of interest.

$$\kappa = \frac{\theta_i}{\theta_t} \qquad (12)$$

where, θ_i is the angle seen by the collimator (for example, 11.4° in order to a 20 cm long collimator placed on the linear accelerator central axis from a 100 cm source) and θ_t is the rotation angle of gantry which irradiated totally. As a typical, θ_t varies between 180° and 320°, is concluded respectively κ=0,063 and κ=0,034. The κ describes the range of gantry angle at that the primary barrier irradiating by the beam of the tomotherapy. Due to significant scattering at the primary barrier and the addition of leakage radiation to conducted radiation when the head of the gantry rotates close to the barrier, κ factor is expected to undervalue exposure except for the primary barrier. To account for these effects, the correction factor (λ) is contained in the use factor. $U_{p,t}$ is called the factor used for tomotherapy. So, it is given as:

$$U_{p,t=}\eta(f_s = 3.8 \times 20)I\kappa\lambda \qquad (13)$$

4. Secondary Barriers

4.1. Leakage

4.1.1. Techniques of DMLC and Tomotherapy

For secondary barriers, E_c=1 assumption in Equation (7) underestimates head leakage. Since the load leakage is commensurate with the number of MUs which is emitted from the LINAC, the leakage of the head for the workload is calibrated equally to the total MUs delivered in a week.

$$W_{l,D} = MU \quad (14)$$

$$W_{l,t} = MU \quad (15)$$

In these formulas, $W_{l,D}$ for DMLC delivery and $W_{l,t}$ for tomotherapy delivery are barrier workloads for leakage (l)(given in Equation (6)).

For a particular population of the patient, the total number of MUs irradiated in the week is a function of irradiation efficiency; the E_D/E_c or E_t/E_c ratio would be determined by the potential increment in leakage barrier protection components in IMRT facilities compared to conventional radiotherapy setups. Appropriate values for E_D/E_c and E_t/E_c ratios haven't been established, but are probably bigger than 2 in DMLC and up to 10 in tomotherapy (Followill, Geis, and Boyer, 1997; Mutic and Low, 1998). Like with conventional radiotherapy, for both modalities the factor of use (U) setting to one.

4.2. Scatter

4.2.1. Techniques of DMLC and Tomotherapy

In the formula, the workload in the radiation of scattered is based on the whole given tumour dose in the week.

$$W_{s,D} = TD \quad (16)$$

$$W_{s,t} = TD \quad (17)$$

In the above formulas, containing the scattering radiation called (s), $W_{s,D}$, and $W_{s,t}$ are barrier workloads in DMLC and tomotherapy application, respectively. The intensity of scattering radiation is in proportion to the energy involved in the patient. The delivery of IMRT is not anticipated to significantly change the absorbed total energy. Therefore, the formalism of calculating the scattered radiation for the barrier in workload is like the primary protection calculations for the DMLC.

Khan briefly summarised the conventional assumption of the relative importance of scattering radiation and leakage of the head: For megavoltage radiotherapy installations, the barrier to leakage is usually much greater than is necessary for deflected radiation as leakage radiation penetrates more than scattered radiation. This explanation has been made with traditional therapy in mind, nevertheless applies even more for IMRT facilities because of the increased head-leak component. It is assumed that scattering-radiation protection can be neglected for IMRT facilities (Mutic et al. 2001).

5. Radiation Safety Concerns in IMRT Applications

In the delivery of IMRT, LINAC collimator leaves can enter and exit the main photon beam in a complex version over and over during a treatment to get the prescribed dose intensity for tumour in the body of the patient. This complex version of radiation delivery is frequently accompanied by an increment in necessary linear accelerator MUs. As a result, the collimator leaves are exposed to the primary photon beam for a long time. If the incident photons have sufficient energy, a result of prolonged exposure may have photoactivation of elements inside the collimator. This causes the formation of by-products that are radioactive and can increase the radiation exposure of patients as well as technical and therapy personnel. Elements in collimators involved in such reactions include ^{28}Al, ^{56}Mn, and ^{24}Na. There is an energy of threshold that photonuclear activation may be formed, which differs for each sensitive element and generally exceeds 8 MeV. So, using high-energy photons in IMRT can, in principle, induce activity in the collimator which depends on its compound. Rawlinson et al. (2002) estimated that with a LINAC workload of 18 MV photons and 60,000 MUs per week, radiotherapy staff would get about 60 μSv with traditional treatments, but perhaps up to 330 μSv per week if using IMRT. Thus, with IMRT and high-energy photons, the doses of therapy personnel can be increased approximately 6 times. Other studies have shown differences in exciting activity from a LINAC brand to the other (Perrin, Walker, and Mackay, 2003; D. S. Followill, 2003). Ways to alleviate this concern contain avoiding IMRT of high energy whenever feasible and scheduling these patients with IMRT as the end of the day as possible (scheduling treatment appointments) when the requirement for high-energy X-rays is inevitable. Even though IMRT with high energy some groups have preferred, research has shown that photon energies bigger than 6 MV aren't ordinarily necessary when using multi-field IMRT. Some recommendations have been given for Linear accelerator manufacturers' attempt to design collimators at reduced sensitivity to activation of photonuclear.

5.1. Considerations Concerning Intensity Profile and Dose Distribution of Radiation

5.1.1. Carcinogenesis of Radiation

IMRT produces the very optimal dose distribution of radiation currently possible by photon irradiation. In some situations, there is an increment within integral dose and volume of irradiation accompanying increased conformity. As stated earlier, the increment of LINAC MUs required for IMRT may increase leakage of radiation and extra exposure because of photoactivation of the collimator. In patients of head and neck treated with IMRT using 6 MV high-energy X-ray, the estimated total dose of the body is approximately eight times higher than with conventional radiation therapy: 242 mSv versus 1969 mSv (Verellen and Vanhavere, 1999). There are potential concerns about the theoretical conclusions of this increment of low-dose exposure via IMRT, especially in terms of radiation carcinogenesis (Verellen and Vanhavere, 1999; Hall and Wuu, 2003). Hall and Wuu (2003) have calculated that in patients living 10 years, IMRT would almost dual the incidence of secondary malignancies compared with traditional radiotherapy, approximately from %1,00 to %1,75, and the absolute numbers could be greater for patients having longer survival and younger.

The most widely accepted model for the carcinogenesis of radiation is the linear unthreshold (LNT) model, in which high-dose exposures are extrapolated to low doses. However, this is a highly contentious topic and there is data either for or opposite the fundamental model of LNT. Data getting from irradiation of single-cell microbeam experiments using alpha particles have shown as the nucleus isn't the only target that can cause the conversion or death of a cell. Related experiments have shown that irradiation of neighboring cells can induce transformation and apoptosis in cells of non-irradiated, the so-named "bystander" effect (Sawant et al., 2022), which will be discussed in more detail in the following section. Such findings recommend that the LNT hypothesis may greatly underestimate the potential for radiation exposure in low doses. Otherwise, microbeam irradiation experiments with alpha particles have also shown that accurately an alpha particle transition per cell has significantly less oncogenic potential compared to the Poisson distribution average of exactly one alpha particle transition per cell (Miller et al., 1999). In these experiments, accurately an alpha particle per cell was found not to differ in oncogenic potential from non-irradiated controls. These data suggest that the LNT model overrates the risk of radiation exposure of low-level and raises suspicion about the validity of the extrapolation from high doses to exposure of an alpha particle for a cell. Recent in vitro proof that human fibroblasts are surprisingly incapable of repairing double-stranded deoxyribonucleic (DNA) breaks following photon radiation with a low dose, but show effective repair at high dose levels or repeated exposures of low-dose levels (Rothkamm and Löbrich, 2003). The survival ratios of these cells are reduced following doses low, consistent with doses in low hyper radiosensitivity. However, from an organism perspective, removal of damaged cells using irradiation in a low-dose may be a way to reduce the danger of carcinogenesis.

Although there are varied estimates of the potential of carcinogenic in IMRT, the simple way to assess it is through a careful getting analysis of real data. The complex process in IMRT allows for the reconfiguration of integral dose and irradiating volume that could be analysed retrospectively. It will be important for the department of radiation oncology to gather data on these factors prospectively in patients who have undergone definitive treatment with IMRT techniques like tomotherapy with serial and helical (Tomé and Fowler, 2002). In this way, data can be collected that will allow researchers to assess the correct impact of increased exposure to low-dose related to IMRT.

5.1.2. Acute Effects in Adverse

The bigger volume of organs at risk occasionally irradiated to doses low while using IMRT has resulted in some speculation regarding possible complications. A mechanism by which this can occur is using low-dose hypersensitivity. At doses below 0,1 Gy, several cell lines showed a paradoxical reduction in survival in vitro, deviating from estimates made by extrapolation of cell-survival lines at bigger doses. In doses above about 0,3 Gy, there is an increment in radiation resistance up to approximately 1,0 Gy, beyond that the cell survival curve accepts the characteristics downward bending pattern. Related to this is, for example, a counterintuitive "reverse fractionation effect" where three times a minimal 0,4 Gy per day for more than five days may verify more cytocidal dose than 1,2 Gy per day in total. Joiner initially suggested that DNA repair mechanisms are not activated in very low doses, concluding in reduced cell survival (Joiner et al., 2001). This seems consistent with Rothkamm and Löbrich's (2003) observation that low-dose radiation inducing double-stranded DNA repair is inefficient a surprise. Cell cycle studies by Marples et al. (2004) showed low dose hyper-sensitivity in asynchronous and G2 phase enriched cell populations, however, did not find hyper-sensitivity in populations of G1 and S phases. They conclude that hypersensitivity in low-dose may be the result of early entrance into mitosis of radiation-damaged cells in the G2 phase.

Another theoretical concern regarding bigger volumes of organs at risk exposed to low dose radiation via IMRT relates to the "bystander" effect. Conventional thinking accepts which nuclear DNA is the single or primary target for the fatal effects of radiation. The data now show that the target of radiation effects extends far away from the confines of the cell nucleus and especially the irradiated cell. Cell irradiation may, in certain cases, cause death and damage to adjacent "bystander" cells that are non-irradiated. During only a few fractions (< 1%) of the cell, the nucleus was hit, and up to 40% of the cells had increased sister chromatid exchange frequency. Subsequent experiments approved DNA mutations in "bystander" cells (Nagasawa and Little, 2010). As an interesting, further analysis found out which mutations in cells of "bystander" generally pointed mutations, whereas cells that were directly hit showed more frequent deletions (Huo, Nagasawa, and Little, 2001). As anecdotal, many physicians noted unexpected complications during the initial clinical implementation of IMRT in the head and neck, like increased erythema of skin and lip irritation with pain in unexpected places. While some thought it might be a result of the "bystander" effect or low dose hypersensitivity, it now appears that these effects have a more mundane explanation, sometimes lying in the unusual dose distributions created by IMRT planning (Welsh et al., 2005).

6. Radiation Protection and Dose Limits

In diagnostic and therapeutic irradiation, it is the personnel, patients, and society affected by radiation. Basic principles of radiation protection while making dose limitations in community and occupational irradiation; the justification or justification of the applications in diagnostic and therapeutic irradiation, the exposure of the personnel to the lowest possible radiation doses (optimisation), ALARA the reference dose levels for radiation officers and the society are taken into consideration (IAEA Safety Standards, 2014).

The statement "Exposure to radiation produces biological damage and there is no dose limit at which radiation damage will not occur" is an accepted principle of radiation protection. However, in 1956, the International Commission on Radiation Protection (ICRP) stated "The largest radiation dose allowed to be received by a person is the dose that will not cause somatic effects in that person and is the lowest in genetic damage that will occur" (Report on Amendments during 1956 to the Recommendations of the International Commission on Radiological Protection, 1957).

The work of the ICRP helps protect the environment and prevent the effects of cancer and other diseases related to exposure to radiation ionise.

Since 1928, the ICRP has published over a hundred reports on all aspects of radiological protection. Most of them deal with a specific field in radiological protection, but a few publications, called basic recommendations, describe the general system of radiation protection. The ICRP is not an official organisation, but a scientific commission that prepares recommendations on radiation protection. The ICRP set the first of its recommendations in 1928 and declared the limit to be an estimated 1000 mSv per year. Later, it has brought the following limits as recommendations over the years:

- 5 mSv per week in 1934
- 3 mSv per week in 1951
- In 1956 it was 50 mSv per year for workers and 5 mSv per year for the public
- ALARA in 1973
- In 1990, 20 mSv/year for employees 1 mSv per year for the public (5 years average) (ICRP 60) (Sowby, 1981)
- In 2007, 20 mSv/year for employees, 1 mSv/year for the public (5 years average) (Recommendations of the International Commission on Radiological Protection. ICRP Publication 103, 2007).

Conclusion

IMRT is more compatible with the delivery of radiation than 3DCRT. The more conservative protection conditions are preferred in IMRT requiring a longer irradiation time than 3DCRT. Tomotherapy primary protection barriers won't be bigger than traditional installations and primary protection will be defined by traditional requirements if the room of linear accelerator will be used according to both treatments of traditional and tomotherapy. The minor cross-section combined with the use of rotational beam in therapy gives a relatively small effective utilisation factor as the beam repeatedly hits the same place on the walls for every slice treated. Due to the large increase in monitor units per patient, the secondary protective thickness of the barrier will increase markedly. The output of IMRT in delivery systems would precisely improve and perhaps even exceed traditional therapy. For conservative calculation purposes, a conservative prediction of patient load with IMRT will equal current or anticipated patient numbers of traditional therapy (Mutic et al., 2001).

The protective designs and management of medical LINAC rooms are becoming more important for organisations that use IMRT than 3DCRT. First, it is important to assess the status of a conservation plan, management and standards of safety among different departments using IMRT or another treatment technique, as appropriate containment management must take into account the increase in leakage dose. It is seen that most facilities follow the standard advice specified by the related international organisations, containing the guidelines of NCRP 151, in their protective designs. However, it is important the requirements of improving and publishing as standard protective design information and clarification of indefinite acquisition ways to obtain protection information. These data may be used as a basis for setting up a safety check system for departments using medical linear accelerators, thereby enabling the development of sufficiently secure protective designs. Studies in the future will make guidance on the development of suitable protection (Kwon et al., 2022).

Because of the relatively bigger treatment time and increasing linear accelerator MUs required with IMRT, the radioactivity induced in the collimator may become a radiation safety issue. IMRT with <18 MV photon energy may minimise this concern. In nearly all cases, 6 MV photon IMRT provides adequate dose distribution and reduces potential photoactivation. When photons with high energy are needed, it might be best to apply these treatments towards the end of the day for reducing unneeded exposure to other patients and staff. Manufacturers of linear accelerators must take this potential concern into account when designing collimators. For maximising tumour control, every IMRT plan of treatment ought to be attentively reviewed to ensure that the low dose in DVH isn't significant. A way to achieve this is to need the EUD to exceed or equal the treatment dose. As IMRT may get the higher irradiated volume of the patient, there is potential in theory for an increment in secondary malignancies and systematic studies ought to be conducted to formally investigate this. Studies ought to explore the probability of complications related to a bigger number of organs at risk of getting low-dose radiation with IMRT because of the effect of "bystander" and low-dose hyper-radiosensitivity (Welsh et al., 2005). When reviewing IMRT plans, care should also be taken to avoid negative effects by paying attention to hotspots in unusual locations. In IMRT plans, it is cautious to review each CT slice to approve that there are no hotspots in unusual locations of patient anatomy that could cause unexpected acute reactions.

References

Arbea, Leire, Luis I. Ramos, Rafael Martínez-Monge, Marta Moreno, and Javier Aristu. (2010). Intensity-Modulated Radiation Therapy (IMRT) vs. 3D Conformal Radiotherapy (3DCRT) in Locally Advanced Rectal Cancer (LARC): Dosimetric Comparison and Clinical Implications. *Radiation Oncology* 5 (1): 1–9.

Boyer, A., L. Xing, C. M. Ma, B. Curran, R. Hill, A. Kania, and A. Bleier. (1999). Theoretical Considerations of Monitor Unit Calculations for Intensity Modulated Beam Treatment Planning. *Medical Physics* 26 (2): 187–95.

Boyer, Arthur L., Paul Geis, Walter Grant, and Mark Carol M. (1997). *Physics Contribution* 3016.

Bucci, M. K., A. Bevan, and M. Roach. (2005). Advances in Radiation Therapy: Conventional to 3D, to IMRT, to 4D, and Beyond. *CA: A Cancer Journal for Clinicians* 55 (2): 117–34.

Followill, David, Paul Geis, and Arthur Boyer. (1997). Estimates of Whole-Body Dose Equivalent Produced by Beam Intensity Modulated Conformal Therapy. *International Journal of Radiation Oncology Biology Physics* 38 (3): 667–72.

Followill, David S. (2003). Neutron Source Strength Measurements for Varian, Siemens, Elekta, and General Electric Linear Accelerators. *Journal of Applied Clinical Medical Physics* 4 (3): 189.

Huo, L., H. Nagasawa, and J. B. Little. (2001). HPRT Mutants Induced in Bystander Cells by Very Low Fluences of Alpha Particles Result Primarily from Point Mutations. *Radiation Research* 156 (5 I): 521–25.

IAEA Safety Standards. (2014). Radiation Protection and Safety of Radiation Sources: International Basic Safety Standards General Safety Requirements Part 3.

Jeraj, M., and V. Robar. (2004). 2004_Multilead Collimator in Radiotherapy. *Radiology and Oncology* 38 (3): 235–40.

Joiner, Michael C., Brian Marples, Philippe Lambin, Susan C. Short, and Ingela Turesson. (2001). Low-Dose Hypersensitivity: Current Status and Possible Mechanisms. *International Journal of Radiation Oncology Biology Physics* 49 (2): 379–89.

Khan, Faiz M. (2014). *The Physics of Radiation Therapy*. 5th Ed.

Kwon, Na Hye, Dong Oh Shin, So Hyun Ann, Jin Sung Kim, Sang Hyoun Choi, and Dong Wook Kim. (2022). Analysis of Radiation Safety Management Status of Medical Linear Accelerator Facilities in Korea. *Nuclear Engineering and Technology* 54 (2): 449–55.

Marples, B., B. G. Wouters, S. J. Collis, A. J. Chalmers, and M. C. Joiner. (2004). Low-Dose Hyper-Radiosensitivity: A Consequence of Ineffective Cell Cycle Arrest of Radiation-Damaged G2-Phase Cells. *Radiation Research* 161 (3): 247–55.

Miller, Richard C., Gerhard Randers-Pehrson, Charles R. Geard, Eric J. Hall, and David J. Brenner. (1999). The Oncogenic Transforming Potential of the Passage of Single α Particles through Mammalian Cell Nuclei. *Proceedings of the National Academy of Sciences of the United States of America* 96 (1): 19–22.

Mohan, Radhe, Qiuwen Wu, Matthew Manning, and Rupert Schmidt-Ullrich. (2000). Radiobiological Considerations in the Design of Fractionation Strategies for Intensity-Modulated Radiation Therapy of Head and Neck Cancers. *International Journal of Radiation Oncology Biology Physics* 46 (3): 619–30.

Mutic, Sasa, and Daniel A. Low. (1998). Whole-Body Dose from Tomotherapy Delivery. *International Journal of Radiation Oncology Biology Physics* 42 (1): 229–32.

Mutic, Sasa, Daniel A. Low, Eric E. Klein, James F. Dempsey, and James A. Purfy. (2001). Room Shielding for Intensity-Modulated Radiation Therapy Treatment Facilities. *International Journal of Radiation Oncology Biology Physics* 50 (1): 239–46.

Nagasawa, Hatsumi, and John B. Little. (2010). Radation-Research-Bystander-Effect-Paper-J-Little-1999.Pdf 152 (5): 552–57.

NCRP Report No 049. n.d.

Perrin, Bruce, Anne Walker, and Ranald Mackay. (2003). A Model to Calculate the Induced Dose Rate around an 18 MV ELEKTA Linear Accelerator. *Physics in Medicine and Biology* 48 (5).

Rawlinson, J. Alan, Mohammad K. Islam, and Duncan M. Galbraith. (2002). Dose to Radiation Therapists from Activation at High-Energy Accelerators Used for Conventional and Intensity-Modulated Radiation Therapy. *Medical Physics* 29 (4): 598–608.

Report on Amendments during 1956 to the Recommendations of the International Commission on Radiological Protection. (1957). *Acta Radiologica* 48 (6): 493–95.

Rohrig, Norman. (2006). *Structural Shielding Design and Evaluation for Megavoltage X- and Gamma-Ray Radiotherapy Facilities, NCRP Report No. 151. Health Physics*. Vol. 91.

Rothkamm, Kai, and Markus Löbrich. (2003). Evidence for a Lack of DNA Double-Strand Break Repair in Human Cells Exposed to Very Low x-Ray Doses. *Proceedings of the National Academy of Sciences of the United States of America* 100 (9): 5057–62.

Sawant, Author S. G., C. R. Geard, D. J. Brenner, E. J. Hall, No Mar, S. G. Sawant, C. R. Geard, D. J. Brenner, and E. J. Hall. (2022). The Bystander Effect in Radiation Oncogenesis: I. Transformation in C3H 10T 1/2 Cells In Vitro Can Be Initiated in the Unirradiated Neighbors of Irradiated Cells. *Radiation Research,* 155 (3): 397–401.

Sowby, F. D. (1981). Annals of the ICRP. *Annals of the ICRP* 6 (1): 1.

The 2007 Recommendations of the International Commission on Radiological Protection. ICRP Publication 103. (2007). *Annals of the ICRP* 37 (2–4): 1–332.

Tomé, Wolfgang A., and Jack F. Fowler. (2002). On Cold Spots in Tumor Subvolumes. *Medical Physics* 29 (7): 1590–98.

Verellen, Dirk, Nadine Linthout, Dirk Van Den Berge, Arjan Bel, and Guy Storme. (1997). Clinical Investigation With Intensity-Modulated Head and Neck Region. *Radiation Oncology* 39 (April): 99–114.

Verellen, Dirk, and Filip Vanhavere. (1999). Risk Assessment of Radiation-Induced Malignancies Based on Whole-Body Equivalent Dose Estimates for IMRT Treatment in the Head and Neck Region. *Radiotherapy and Oncology* 53 (3): 199–203.

Welsh, James S., Jeffery P. Limmer, Steven P. Howard, David Diamond, Paul M. Harari, and Wolfgang Tomé. (2005). Precautions in the Use of Intensity-Modulated Radiation Therapy. *Technology in Cancer Research and Treatment* 4 (2): 203–10.

Chapter 18

Quality of Life after IMRT

Zumrut Arda Kaymak*
Department of Radiation Oncology, Medical Faculty,
Suleyman Demirel University, Isparta, Turkey

Abstract

Radiotherapy has been a hesitant treatment because of its severe acute and late side effects. For the possibility of a cure, the patients had to risk permanent sequels that would seriously affect their quality of life. As conventional radiotherapy techniques begin to disappear and intensity-modulated radiotherapy (IMRT) becomes common, IMRT has been a hope for reducing these side effects. In dose-volume studies, the superiority of IMRT over conventional methods and its reduction in critical organ doses have been shown in literature for almost every cancer site. However, extended follow-up periods and randomised trials were required to demonstrate with evidence-based medicine whether these dose distribution advantages are reflected in the clinic and whether they contribute to the patients' quality of life.

Keywords: head and neck cancers, intensity-modulated radiotherapy, late side effects, prostate cancer, quality of life

---

*Corresponding Author's Email: ardakaymak84@yahoo.com.

In: Frontiers in Intensity-Modulated Radiotherapy Research
Editor: Sibel Karaca
ISBN: 979-8-88697-252-8

1. Introduction

Through the medical developments in the last 20 years, cancer has become a disease detected at earlier stages and treated much more effectively. As a result of the improvements in surgery, the use of novel systemic agents, and advanced radiotherapy technology, the overall survival rates of most cancer types have been prolonged (Tong et al., 2019). While the overall 5-year survival rate was 49% in 1979, this rate increased to 70% in 2015 (Noone et al., 2018). Apart from the acute side effects of cancer treatment methods, long-term chronic side effects are also an essential issue that the patients and clinicians should deal with. When treating cancer, the primary goal of the surgical and radiation oncologist is maximum tumour control as well as minimal loss of organs, tissues and their functions. The effects of cancer and cancer treatments can be such that they will completely change a cancer survivor's life (Firkins et al., 2020). According to the cancer site, eating-swallowing, cognitive, sexual, respiration, urinary and gastrointestinal dysfunctions, fibrosis and chronic muscle pains, and psychosocial changes affect the quality of life (QoL) of patients after radiotherapy according to cancer site (Bian et al., 2015; Ge et al., 2020; Klopp et al., 2018; Schover et al., 2014).

With the widespread use of intensity-modulated radiotherapy (IMRT), a significant decrease in the acute and late toxicity of radiotherapy has been compared with conventional radiotherapy techniques in many studies, and the contribution of IMRT to the QoL of cancer patients has been demonstrated (Alterio et al., 2019; Alterio et al., 2021; Bauman et al., 2012; Bittner et al., 2015; Xu et al., 2017;). Although all the frequent cancer sites have been occasionally evaluated in terms of QoL after IMRT, the QoL has been a more prominent topic in some cancer types. The QoL has come to the fore, especially in cancers with extended survival, such as prostate cancer (Forster et al., 2021; Hamstra et al., 2018; Murthy et al., 2020; Nakai et al., 2018;). In addition, the head and neck cancers mainly treated with IMRT have also been the subject of many studies in terms of late toxicity and QoL (Davy and Heathcote, 2021; Nguyen and Ringash, 2018).

In this chapter, the methods of assessing the QoL after IMRT will be described firstly, and secondly, the post-IMRT QoL will be discussed in terms of different cancer sites in the light of the recent literature.

2. Measurement Tools for QoL

QoL consists of three main components based on the definition of health by the World Health Organisation. These main components, defined as physical, social and mental health, are evaluated with indicators that affect one or more of them, and their related role limitations are also revealed (Ware and Sherbourne, 1992). In cancer patients, physical symptoms related to cancer-specific and cancer treatment side effects are also included in QoL evaluation. The need for questionnaire development for the objective assessment of QoL in international clinical trials was recognised in the 1980s, and several questionnaires were introduced. The most commonly used ones for cancer patients can be listed as the European Organisation for Research and Treatment of Cancer quality of life questionnaire (EORTC QLQ-C30), the Short-Form 36 (SF-36) and the Functional Assessment of Cancer Therapy (FACT) (Firkins et al., 2020).

2.1. European Organisation for Research and Treatment of Cancer Quality of Life questionnaire (EORTC QLQ-C30)

The first version of the scale was developed in 1987, later revised in 1995, and defined as EORTC QLQ-C30. It is a 30-item core-cancer-specific questionnaire consisting of five functional scales (physical, role, cognitive, social, and emotional); three symptom scales (pain, fatigue, and nausea and vomiting); and a global health and quality-of-life scale. There are also other single-item measures that include symptoms commonly reported by cancer patients (dyspnoea, appetite loss, sleep disturbance, constipation, and diarrhoea) and the perceived financial impact of the disease and treatment (Aaronson et al., 1993).

2.2. The Functional Assessment of Cancer Therapy (FACT)

It was developed by Cella et al. in 1993 (Cella et al., 1993). It consists of 33 items and has been used to evaluate the general QoL of cancer patients. There are subscales such as FACT-Breast, FACT-bone marrow transplant, FACT-Bladder, FACT-Cognitive function, FACT-Prostate.

2.3. The Medical Outcomes Study 36-Item Short-Form (SF-36)

A health screening form is widely utilised to evaluate QoL in clinical practice and research (Ware et al., 1992). The form consists of eight health concepts: physical functioning (10 items), bodily pain (2 items), role limitations due to physical health problems (4 items), role limitations due to personal or emotional problems (4 items), emotional well-being (5 items), social functioning (2 items), energy/fatigue (4 items), and general health perceptions (5 items). Scores for each domain range from 0 to 100; the lowest score represents the worst health condition.

3. QoL after Prostate Cancer IMRT

In treating prostate cancer, IMRT is a prominent treatment option for high, intermediate and even low-risk patients considering the patient's life expectancy (Scherr et al., 2003). The prevalence of IMRT and image-guided radiotherapy improved the therapeutic ratio with more accurate dose delivery and reduced early and late side effects (Bruner et al., 2015; Ferreira et al., 2019). However, IMRT can still cause long-term complications such as urinary, sexual and intestinal dysfunctions (Donovan et al., 2016; Lardas et al., 2017). The most commonly used recent questionnaires to evaluate QoL of prostate cancer patients are the Expanded Prostate Cancer Index Composite (EPIC), University of California—Los Angeles Prostate Cancer Index (UCLA-PCI), European Organisation for Research and Treatment of Cancer Quality of Life Questionnaire—Prostate-specific 25-item (EORTC QLQ-PR 25 Functional Assessment of Cancer Therapy-Prostate (FACT-P), Patient-Oriented Prostate Utility Scale (PORPUS), and Prostate Cancer Quality of Life Instrument (PC-QoL) (Schmidt et al., 2014).

In the preliminary report of the RTOG 0126 trial, the authors compared patient-reported outcomes in patients with intermediate-risk prostate cancer treated with 3-dimensional conformal radiotherapy (3DCRT) or IMRT. In this randomised study, in the 3DCRT arm, only a 23.4Gy boost was applied to the prostate after 55,8Gy to the prostate and seminal vesicle, while 79.2Gy was applied to the prostate and proximal seminal vesicle in the IMRT arm. Bowel and bladder functions of the patients were evaluated with the Functional Alterations due to Changes in Elimination (FACE), and erectile function was evaluated with the International Index of Erectile Function (IIEF) pre-treatment and post-treatment 3, 6, 12 and 24 months. Despite the significant decrease in normal tissue doses with IMRT, no significant difference was found between FACE and IIEF scores in both arms (Bruner et al., 2015).

In high-risk cases, after prostate-only irradiation, urinary incontinence, dysuria, urgency, nocturia, erectile dysfunction, late rectal bleeding, faecal incontinence are post-IMRT side effects that affect the patient's QoL (Bruner et al., 2015; Ferreira et al., 2019). After demonstrating the benefits of prophylactic pelvic lymph node irradiation (Delouya and Taussky, 2018; Dirix et al., 2006; Kaidar-Person et al., 2013), the question arose whether bowel dysfunction would be one of the late side effects. In a randomised trial, high-risk prostate cancer patients were randomised to prostate-only or whole pelvic irradiation arms and evaluated in terms of QoL and acute acute-late gastrointestinal and genitourinary toxicity. In the trial, QoL was assessed using EORTC QLQ-C30 and PR-25 questionnaire pre-treatment and every 3–6 months post-IMRT. After a median follow-up period of 44.5 months, no RTOG grade 4 toxicity was observed in both arms, while gastrointestinal side effects of grade 2 and above were similar (6.8% for the whole pelvis and 3.8% for the prostate-only groups, $p = 0.39$). Nevertheless, the genitourinary toxicity was higher in the whole pelvic-IMRT arm (17.7% vs. 7.5%, $p = 0.03$). However, since there was no significant difference in QoL scores between the two arms, the authors concluded that whole pelvis IMRT increased genitourinary toxicity compared to prostate-only IMRT, but this was not reflected in patient-reported QoL (Murthy et al., 2020).

In a recent study, physician-reported and patient-reported acute and late toxicity were compared in high-risk prostate cancer patients who underwent whole pelvic IMRT. Physician-reported toxicity was assessed by Common Terminology Criteria for Adverse Events (CTCAE) version 4.0. The patients-reported gastrointestinal toxicities through RT-ARD score, genitourinary through DAN-PSS, sexual and hormonal through EPIC-26, and QoL through EORTC QLQ-C30. As a result of the study, patient-reported gastrointestinal toxicity and related QoL were affected at the 60th month following IMRT, and also it was found to be significantly different from physician-reported toxicity. However, sexual, hormonal and general QoL were not different from baseline (Petersen et al., 2022).

For 70-80Gy conventionally fractionated IMRT, the Quantec rectal dose constraints recommendations are V60Gy < 35–45%, V70Gy < 15–25%, V75Gy < 5–10% in order to limit the rates of grade 2 and 3 late rectal bleeding below 15% and 10% Michalski et al., 2019). Evidence from long-time follow-up trials shows that compliance with dose limits reduces late rectal bleeding

(Ebert et al., 2015; Fonteyne et al., 2015). As a result of a 5-year follow-up study, strict dose limitations in prostate patients undergoing both postoperative and definitive IMRT significantly reduced ≥grade 2 rectal toxicity (16% vs 5%, $p < 0.001$). However, the same result was not obtained for urinary toxicity. The grade 2 and 3 rectal toxicity rates were reported as %11 and %1 for all patients, and grade 2 and 3 urinary toxicity rates as %22 and %23 for definitive and postoperative groups, respectively (Fonteyne et al., 2015).

In a systemic review, QoL results of IMRT were compared with other treatment options (active surveillance and surgery). Eighteen studies were assessed, and it was concluded that the QoL of patients who underwent active surveillance was better than IMRT and surgery, while urinary and sexual dysfunctions were more common with surgery, and bowel functions with IMRT than others (Lardas et al., 2017).

Erectile function can be preserved in 45-70% of patients in the 2nd year after prostate radiotherapy (Alemozaffar et al., 2012; Roach et al., 2004; Siglin et al., 2010). The higher the dose of the penile bulb exposed during RT, the greater the risk of erectile dysfunction (Roach et al., 2010). Although the use of phosphodiesterase type 5 inhibitors after radiotherapy has been shown to improve erectile function, its benefit during radiotherapy is controversial (Pisansky et al., 2014; Weber et al., 1999; Zelefsky et al., 2014). When assessing post-IMRT erectile function, it is essential to consider whether the patient is on androgen deprivation therapy and whether he has any pre-treatment dysfunction (Benedict et al., 2014; Daly et al., 2012). A randomised controlled trial demonstrated the benefit of a hydrogel spacer placed between the prostate and rectum to reduce the penile bulb dose during prostate IMRT and thus erectile dysfunction. In the study, the baseline and post-IMRT sexual QoL of the patients were evaluated with EPIC, and at the end of the median 37-month follow-up period, the patient reported sexual QoL was found to be better in the group using the hydrogel spacer (Hamstra et al., 2018). The benefits of hydrogel spacer for rectal and urinary toxicity were represented for the same study population. Both ≥grade 1-2 rectal toxicity and ≥grade 1 urinary toxicity were lower in the spacer arm (9.2% vs 2.0%; $p = 0.028$; 5.7% vs 0%; $p = 0.012$; 15% vs 4%; $p = 0.046$, respectively). The percentage of patients who experienced a decrease in bowel QoL (41% vs 14%; $p = 0.002$) and urinary QoL (30% vs 17%; $p = 0.04$) at three years after IMRT was significantly higher in the group without spacer (Hamstra et al., 2017).

4. QoL after Head and Neck Cancers IMRT

Head and neck cancer treatment is a multidisciplinary process that requires combined approaches, including surgery, radiotherapy and chemotherapy (Marta et al., 2014). 5-year survival rates after treatment with radiotherapy are reported to be more than 80% in stage 1-2 disease and 60-70% in stage 3-4 disease (Pignon et al., 2009). Xerostomia is the most common side effect of head and neck radiotherapy that can cause several other consequences (chewing, swallowing, taste dysfunctions, deterioration of dental and oral mucosal health) that will affect patients' QoL (Wijers et al., 2002). Compared to conventional RT techniques, IMRT has been a saviour for radiation oncologists in the head and neck region where the target volume and critical organs are nearby. By IMRT, not only the major salivary glands but also the spinal cord, brain stem, lens, optic nerves, inner ear, oral cavity and larynx (in case of not being the primary tumour site) are exposed to lower doses (Lee et al., 2007). There are many clinical trials, reviews and meta-analyses in the literature comparing the QoL of head and neck cancer patients after IMRT with those treated with conventional techniques. The QoL and RT-related side effects of patients have been assessed by EORTC QLQ-C30, EORTC QLQ Module for Head and Neck Cancer (EORTC QLQ H&N35), Head and Neck Quality of Life instrument (HNQOL), University of Washington Quality of Life Questionnaire (UWQOL), SF36, and xerostomia questionnaire (XQ) in different studies. As a result of a recent meta-analysis involving seven studies and a total number of 761 patients, it was indicated that IMRT resulted in better global health status and cognitive functions when the QoL of patients with head and neck cancer treated with IMRT and conventional radiotherapy were compared ($p = 0.004$). In addition, the xerostomia scores were lower in IMRT-treated patients ($p = 0.001$). However, no difference was found between the two groups regarding emotional and social functions ($p = 0.531$ and $p = 348$, respectively) (Ge et al., 2020).

In another systematic review, IMRT and conventional radiotherapy were compared in terms of not only side effects but also loco-regional control and overall survival. In the review, which included five studies, the total number of patients was 434 in the IMRT arm and 437 in the conventional radiotherapy arm. The primary tumour site was the nasopharynx in the majority of patients (82%), and stage 3-4 disease was present in 62.1% of the patients. The xerostomia was graded by the RTOG/EORTC or the Common Toxicity Criteria (CTC) version 3.0 scoring systems. In comparison, the grade 2-4 xerostomia rate was 57.4-82.1% in the conventional radiotherapy arm and 15-

39.3% in the IMRT arm at six months-1-year post-radiotherapy. Three of the five studies provided local control and overall survival results, with a not statistically significant advantage in the IMRT arm (Marta et al., 2014).

Radioprotector agents for salivary glands have been used and investigated for many years, but their effectiveness is insufficient. Recently, detection and selectively sparing of salivary gland stem cells, new lubricants and salivary stimulating agents or submandibular gland transplantation have been investigated. Among all these approaches, IMRT seems to play the most fundamental role in maintaining salivary gland functions (Jensen et al., 2019).

Swallowing dysfunction is another side effect that impairs QoL after head and neck radiotherapy. After concurrent chemoradiotherapy, which is applied for organ preservation in laryngeal cancer, swallowing dysfunction rates have been reported as 17-24% (Ward et al., 2016). Impaired swallowing can lead to consequences such as malnutrition and aspiration pneumonia (Rosenthal et al., 2006). Swallowing function can be evaluated with patient-reported questionnaires such as M.D. Anderson Dysphagia Inventory (MDADI)-the sole questionnaire validated to specifically assess oropharyngeal dysphagia (OPD) (Chen et al., 2001), as well as with objective methods such as the video fluoroscopic swallowing study (VFSS) and fiberoptic endoscopic evaluation of swallowing (FEES) (Speyer, 2013). A review of 22 studies argued that there is evidence that patients treated with IMRT have better swallowing functions than those treated with 3D conformal radiotherapy (Ursino et al., 2017).

A German study consisting of 111 patients with head and neck cancer planned to reveal QoL progression within one year after IMRT; patients were evaluated by EORTC QLQ-C30 and QLQ HN35 at the beginning of IMRT, end of IMRT, at 6-8th weeks, sixth months, and 1st-year post-IMRT. The domains that increased over 30 points at the end of IMRT compared to baseline scores were swallowing, smelling, tasting, social eating, dry mouth and sticky saliva. The scores of smelling, tasting, dry mouth and sticky saliva were remained significantly higher than baseline, although they were in better condition after one year. At one-year post-IMRT, C30 scores were equal to or higher than the baseline scores. In this prospective study, it has been shown that after IMRT, it is possible for patients to return to their baseline QoL levels at one-year post-IMRT, while the complaints of xerostomia and sticky saliva persist for more extended periods (Tribus et al., 2015).

Voice and speech quality is another function that is affected after radiotherapy of non-laryngeal head and neck cancers. In a study including 73 patients with unknown primary or oropharyngeal tumours who underwent IMRT, voice changes were assessed using the patient-reported Functional

Assessment of Cancer Therapy-Head and Neck Scale (FACT-HN) questionnaire; it was determined that the voice changes were frequent but mild. Keeping the mean dose of the uninvolved larynx below 50Gy has been recommended to minimise the voice changes (Sanguineti et al., 2014). Similarly, in another study in which 91 patients were followed for 24 months, glottic larynx dose was an independent predictive factor affecting voice quality. In the study, before and during the follow-up, the Communication Domain of the Head and Neck Quality of Life (HNQOL-C) instrument and the Speech question of the University of Washington Quality of Life (UWQOL-S) instrument were applied to oropharyngeal cancer patients who underwent definitive chemoradiotherapy. In univariate analyses, neck dissection, time since chemoradiotherapy, oral cavity dose, and N stage were also factors affecting voice quality. The authors recommended that the mean glottic larynx dose should be limited to as low as possible in the treatment of non-laryngeal cancers and should be below 20Gy if possible (Vainshtein et al., 2014). It is emphasised that in patients with nasopharyngeal cancer, careful delineation of the target volumes in the most optimised way will be effective in preserving swallowing functions (Pi et al., 2018).

5. QoL after Breast Cancer IMRT

In treating breast cancer, adjuvant radiotherapy and breast-conserving surgery can have the same results as mastectomy (Fisher et al., 2002). Breast-conserving has many psychosocial positive effects on women, such as body image, sexual functions, and ease of dressing (Rowland et al., 2000). The better the cosmetic result after surgery and radiotherapy, the better the breast protection approach will achieve its goal. Acute and late side effects of whole breast radiotherapy are induration, desquamation, telangiectasia, fibrosis and hyperpigmentation (Kelemen et al., 2012). Due to dose inhomogeneity and the inability to avoid hot spots in 2D radiotherapy techniques, these side effects were common. In a study in which patients treated by 2D radiotherapy or IMRT were followed photographically for five years, the risk of changes in breast appearance with 2D radiotherapy was 1.7 times higher. In the same study, no difference was found between the two groups regarding patient-reported breast discomfort or QoL (Donovan et al., 2007). Although IMRT provides homogeneous dose distribution, especially in large breasts, its long-term benefits have not been demonstrated clearly. A Canadian study published after an extended follow-up of 10 years comparing 241 patients treated with

IMRT or 2D radiotherapy found no difference in chronic breast pain, cosmesis, or QoL. Young age and pain during radiotherapy were associated with chronic breast pain (Pignol et al., 2016).

Another advantage of IMRT in whole breast radiotherapy is that tumour bed boost can be applied with the simultaneous integrated boost (SIB) technique, thus shortening the total treatment time. In a randomised phase III study comparing IMRT-SIB with 3D conformal radiotherapy + sequential boost techniques, IMRT-SIB was found to be non-inferior in terms of local control and cosmesis. Considering QLQ-C30 and QLQ-BR23 scores in the second year, it was shown that the QoL of IMRT-SIB patients was better than the other arm. Post-RT 6 weeks, pain and arm symptoms were also less common in the IMRT-SIB arm (Forster et al., 2021).

Tomotherapy provides a homogeneous dose distribution in target volumes and extensive protection in normal tissues. It facilitates radiotherapy, especially in the treatment of breast cancers where normal tissue constraints cannot be achieved due to anatomical disadvantages. In a study reporting the results of 288 patients treated with tomotherapy after breast-conserving surgery or mastectomy, grade 2 acute radiodermatitis was reported in 35.4% of patients, grade 2 acute esophagitis in 6.3%, and grade 2 breast fibrosis in 5.4%. 84.6% of the patients commented as "good" or "excellent" cosmetically at the end of the 1-year follow-up (Bataille et al., 2020).

Accelerated partial breast (APB) RT is an effective and shorter treatment option of 5 fractions in selected early-stage cases instead of conventional fractionated whole breast radiotherapy lasting 30 fractions. The QoL results of the APBI-IMRT-Florence phase 3 randomised trial, in which patients treated by IMRT to tumour bed were compared with those treated by conventional whole breast radiotherapy, were published at the end of the 2-year follow-up period. EORTC QLQ-C30 and BR23 questionnaires were applied to the patients before and in the first and second years after radiotherapy. While there was no difference in QoL between the two arms before treatment, the APBRT arm was significantly superior in overall health, functional and symptomatic scales at the end of the first year. The same results continued in the second year, and body image and future perspective were better in the accelerated partial breast group (Meattini et al., 2017).

6. QoL after Rectum Cancer IMRT

Rectal cancer surgery was a treatment that had high morbidity, and patients had to continue their lives with probable urinary and sexual dysfunctions caused by pelvic nerve damage, ileostomy, or bowel dysfunctions, even if a cure was possible (Engel et al., 2003; Juul et al., 2014). Preoperative approaches aimed to preserve the anal sphincter and the health-related QoL. Preoperative chemoradiotherapy has become the standard approach in locally advanced rectal cancer, as randomised trials have also indicated the advantages in local control and survival (Giunta et al., 2021). Rectal cancer is treated with a multimodal approach, including surgery, chemotherapy, and radiotherapy. Apart from local excision, it is inevitable that the patients' bowel, urinary and sexual functions will be affected by combined treatments (Jones et al., 2020). Therefore, the evolution of the radiotherapy technique from the conventional box technique to IMRT is not likely to improve the QoL of the patients, so this issue has not been a subject of much research. The QoL results of 106 patients, 70 of whom were treated with IMRT and 36 with conformal radiotherapy, 86 with neoadjuvant, and 20 with adjuvant approaches, performed in a centre in Turkey, were published in 2022. EORTC QLQ-C30 and CR29 questionnaires were used in the evaluation. It has been indicated that at the end of radiotherapy, both functional and symptomatic scores of the patients worsened compared to baseline but returned to pre-treatment levels in the third-month controls (Benli et al., 2022).

The neoadjuvant radiotherapy dose prescription can be as 5x5Gy (short-course) or 25x2Gy (long-course). The Stockholm III study compared the survival outcomes of immediate surgery after short RT, surgery at 4-8 weeks after short RT, and surgery at 4-8 weeks after long RT. This study's 5-year adverse effects and QoL results were reported in 2021. There was no statistically significant difference in survival, local control, functional or symptomatic QoL between the three arms. In this study, as in similar studies, no evaluation was made in terms of radiotherapy technique (conformal or IMRT) (Erlandsson et al., 2021).

7. QoL after Gynaecological Cancers IMRT

The disease-free survival favour of adjuvant pelvic radiotherapy in operated cervical and endometrial cancers with risk factors such as deep invasion, large tumour size, and lymphovascular invasion is well known (Nout et al., 2010; Peters et al., 2000). However, radiotherapy over pelvic surgery increases late effects by up to 25%, predominantly on the gastrointestinal system (Creutzberg et al., 2001). In post-hysterectomy pelvic irradiation, several studies have been published indicating that IMRT decreases the small bowel and bladder doses and reduces acute and late toxicities (Mundt et al., 2002; Mundtet al., 2003; Taylor and Powell, 2008). It has been reported that pelvic irradiation with IMRT has fewer grade 2 gastrointestinal side effects, and antidiarrheal drugs are used rarer during radiotherapy (Taylor and Powell 2008). In another study involving patients with gynaecological cancer who received postoperative radiotherapy, 45% of the conformal radiotherapy arm and 16% of the IMRT arm were reported to have late toxicity in the third follow-up year ($p = 0.004$) (Chen et al., 2015). A randomised controlled trial, including 300 cervical cancer patients undergoing postoperative radiotherapy, was published in 2021. Patients were randomised to 3D conformal radiotherapy (3DCRT) and image-guided IMRT (IG-IMRT) arms. The 3-year cumulative gastrointestinal grade 2 and higher late toxicity was 42.4% in the 3DCRT arm and 21.1% in the IG-IMRT arm ($p < 0.001$). Cumulative overall grade 2 and higher late toxicity were also less in the IG-IMRT arm. Patients in the IG-IMRT arm reported significantly less diarrhoea, loss of appetite, and bowel complaints (Chopra et al., 2021). In the publication in which the side effects and patient-reported symptoms were compared according to the radiotherapy technique of the patients in the PORTEC-3 study, it was reported that grade 2 and higher diarrhoea and haematological side effects were significantly lower in the patients who underwent IMRT. The patient-reported abdominal pain, bowel urgency, and diarrhoea were also less common in the IMRT arm than in the conformal radiotherapy arm throughout treatment (Wortman et al., 2022).

Considering all this literature, it can be concluded that preferring IMRT in pelvic irradiation of gynaecological cancers is necessary for less acute and late toxicity.

Conclusion

In addition to its dosimetric advantages in radiotherapy, there is strong evidence that IMRT, which has been corroborated to have similar survival outcomes to conventional methods, contributes to health-related QoL. The lower incidence of late effects in patients treated with IMRT has been demonstrated by evidence-based medicine, especially in head and neck cancers, prostate cancer, and gynaecological cancers. The symptomatic and functional evaluation of acute and late toxicities of radiotherapy should not be only physician-reported but should be patient-reported through cancer-site-specific QoL questionnaires. In addition, the progress of QoL can be revealed by comparing baseline status before treatment with that at follow-up. Thus, a more objective clinical examination is provided. It is among the responsibilities of radiation oncology practitioners to follow any clinical and technological developments that may improve the long-term QoL of cancer survivors.

References

Aaronson, N. K., Ahmedzai, S., Bergman, B., Bullinger, M., Cull, A., Duez, N. J., ... & Takeda, F. (1993). The European Organization for Research and Treatment of Cancer QLQ-C30: a quality-of-life instrument for use in international clinical trials in oncology. *JNCI: Journal of the National Cancer Institute*, *85*(5), 365-376.

Alemozaffar, M., Regan, M. M., Cooperberg, M. R., Wei, J. T., Michalski, J. M., Sandler, H. M., ... & Sanda, M. G. (2011). Prediction of erectile function following treatment for prostate cancer. *Jama*, *306*(11), 1205-1214.

Alterio, D., Gugliandolo, S. G., Augugliaro, M., Marvaso, G., Gandini, S., Bellerba, F., ... & Jereczek-Fossa, B. A. (2021). IMRT versus 2D/3D conformal RT in oropharyngeal cancer: A review of the literature and meta-analysis. *Oral Diseases*, *27*(7), 1644-1653.

Alterio, D., Marvaso, G., Ferrari, A., Volpe, S., Orecchia, R., & Jereczek-Fossa, B. A. (2019, June). Modern radiotherapy for head and neck cancer. In *Seminars in oncology* (Vol. 46, No. 3, pp. 233-245). WB Saunders.

Bataille, B., Raoudha, B., Le Tinier, F., Basson, L., Escande, A., Langin, H., ... & Pasquier, D. (2020). Prospective Study of Intensity-Modulated Radiation Therapy for Locally Advanced Breast Cancer. *Cancers*, *12*(12), 3852.

Bauman, G., Rumble, R. B., Chen, J., Loblaw, A., Warde, P., & IMRT Indications Expert Panel. (2012). Intensity-modulated radiotherapy in the treatment of prostate cancer. *Clinical Oncology*, *24*(7), 461-473.

Benedict, C., Traeger, L., Dahn, J. R., Antoni, M., Zhou, E. S., Bustillo, N., & Penedo, F. J. (2014). Sexual bother in men with advanced prostate cancer undergoing androgen deprivation therapy. *The journal of sexual medicine*, *11*(10), 2571-2580.

Benli Yavuz, B., Aktan, M., Kanyilmaz, G., & Demir, L. S. (2022). Assessment of Quality of Life Following Radiotherapy in Patients with Rectum Cancer. *Journal of Gastrointestinal Cancer*, 1-9.

Bian, X., Song, T., & Wu, S. (2015). Outcomes of xerostomia-related quality of life for nasopharyngeal carcinoma treated by IMRT: based on the EORTC QLQ-C30 and H&N35 questionnaires. *Expert Review of Anticancer Therapy*, *15*(1), 109-119.

Bittner, M. I., Grosu, A. L., & Brunner, T. B. (2015). Comparison of toxicity after IMRT and 3D-conformal radiotherapy for patients with pancreatic cancer–a systematic review. *Radiotherapy and Oncology*, *114*(1), 117-121.

Bruner, D. W., Hunt, D., Michalski, J. M., Bosch, W. R., Galvin, J. M., Amin, M., ... & Sandler, H. M. (2015). Preliminary patient-reported outcomes analysis of 3-dimensional radiation therapy versus intensity-modulated radiation therapy on the high-dose arm of the Radiation Therapy Oncology Group (RTOG) 0126 prostate cancer trial. *Cancer*, *121*(14), 2422-2430.

Cella, D. F., Tulsky, D. S., Gray, G., Sarafian, B., Linn, E., Bonomi, A., ... & Bonomi, P. (1993). The Functional Assessment of Cancer Therapy scale: development and validation of the general measure. *J Clin Oncol*, *11*(3), 570-579.

Chen, A. Y., Frankowski, R., Bishop-Leone, J., Hebert, T., Leyk, S., Lewin, J., & Goepfert, H. (2001). The development and validation of a dysphagia-specific quality-of-life questionnaire for patients with head and neck cancer: the MD Anderson dysphagia inventory. *Archives of Otolaryngology–Head & Neck Surgery*, *127*(7), 870-876.

Chen, L. A., Kim, J., Boucher, K., Terakedis, B., Williams, B., Nickman, N. A., & Gaffney, D. K. (2015). Toxicity and cost-effectiveness analysis of intensity modulated radiation therapy versus 3-dimensional conformal radiation therapy for postoperative treatment of gynecologic cancers. *Gynecologic Oncology*, *136*(3), 521-528.

Chopra, S., Gupta, S., Kannan, S., Dora, T., Engineer, R., Mangaj, A., ... & Shrivastava, S. K. (2021). Late toxicity after adjuvant conventional radiation versus image-guided intensity-modulated radiotherapy for cervical cancer (PARCER): a randomized controlled trial. *Journal of Clinical Oncology*, *39*(33), 3682-3692.

Creutzberg, C. L., van Putten, W. L., Koper, P. C., Lybeert, M. L., Jobsen, J. J., Wárlám-Rodenhuis, C. C., ... & PORTEC Study Group. (2001). The morbidity of treatment for patients with Stage I endometrial cancer: results from a randomized trial. *International Journal of Radiation Oncology* Biology* Physics*, *51*(5), 1246-1255.

Daly, P. E., Dunne, M. T., O'Shea, C. M., Finn, M. A., & Armstrong, J. G. (2012). The effect of short term neo-adjuvant androgen deprivation on erectile function in patients treated with external beam radiotherapy for localised prostate cancer: an analysis of the 4-versus 8-month randomised trial (Irish Clinical Oncology Research Group 97-01). *Radiotherapy and Oncology*, *104*(1), 96-102.

Davy, C., & Heathcote, S. (2021). A systematic review of interventions to mitigate radiotherapy-induced oral mucositis in head and neck cancer patients. *Supportive Care in Cancer*, *29*(4), 2187-2202.

Delouya, G., & Taussky, D. (2018). Pelvic radiotherapy in prostate cancer: An unresolved question. *The Lancet. Oncology*, *19*(11), 1428-1429.

Dirix, P., Haustermans, K., Junius, S., Withers, R., Oyen, R., & Van Poppel, H. (2006). The role of whole pelvic radiotherapy in locally advanced prostate cancer. *Radiotherapy and oncology*, *79*(1), 1-14.

Donovan, E., Bleakley, N., Denholm, E., Evans, P., Gothard, L., Hanson, J., ... & Yarnold, J. (2007). Breast Technology Group. Randomised trial of standard 2D radiotherapy (RT) versus intensity modulated radiotherapy (IMRT) in patients prescribed breast radiotherapy. *Radiother Oncol*, *82*(3), 254-264.

Donovan, J. L., Hamdy, F. C., Lane, J., Mason, M., Metcalfe, C., Walsh, E., ... & Neal, D. E. (2016). Patient-reported outcomes after monitoring, surgery, or radiotherapy for prostate cancer. *N Engl J Med*, *375*, 1425-1437.

Ebert, M. A., Foo, K., Haworth, A., Gulliford, S. L., Kennedy, A., Joseph, D. J., & Denham, J. W. (2015). Gastrointestinal Dose-Histogram Effects in the Context of Dose-Volume–Constrained Prostate Radiation Therapy: Analysis of Data From the RADAR Prostate Radiation Therapy Trial. *International Journal of Radiation Oncology* Biology* Physics*, *91*(3), 595-603.

Engel, J., Kerr, J., Schlesinger-Raab, A., Eckel, R., Sauer, H., & Hölzel, D. (2003). Quality of life in rectal cancer patients: a four-year prospective study. *Annals of surgery*, *238*(2), 203.

Erlandsson, J., Fuentes, S., Radu, C., Frödin, J. E., Johansson, H., Brandberg, Y., ... & Martling, A. (2021). Radiotherapy regimens for rectal cancer: long-term outcomes and health-related quality of life in the Stockholm III trial. *BJS open*, *5*(6), zrab137.

Ferreira, M. R., Thomas, K., Truelove, L., Khan, A., Parker, C., Dearnaley, D. P., & Gulliford, S. (2019). Dosimetry and gastrointestinal toxicity relationships in a phase II trial of pelvic lymph node radiotherapy in advanced localised prostate cancer. *Clinical Oncology*, *31*(6), 374-384.

Firkins, J., Hansen, L., Driessnack, M., & Dieckmann, N. (2020). Quality of life in "chronic" cancer survivors: a meta-analysis. *Journal of Cancer Survivorship*, *14*(4), 504-517.

Fisher, B., Anderson, S., Bryant, J., Margolese, R. G., Deutsch, M., Fisher, E. R., ... & Wolmark, N. (2002). Twenty-year follow-up of a randomized trial comparing total mastectomy, lumpectomy, and lumpectomy plus irradiation for the treatment of invasive breast cancer. *New England Journal of Medicine*, *347*(16), 1233-1241.

Fonteyne, V., Sadeghi, S., Ost, P., Vanpachtenbeke, F., Vuye, P., Lumen, N., & De Meerleer, G. (2015). Impact of changing rectal dose volume parameters over time on late rectal and urinary toxicity after high-dose intensity-modulated radiotherapy for prostate cancer: A 10-years single centre experience. *Acta Oncologica*, *54*(6), 854-861.

Forster, T., Hommertgen, A., Häfner, M. F., Arians, N., König, L., Harrabi, S. B., ... & Hörner-Rieber, J. (2021). Quality of life after simultaneously integrated boost with intensity-modulated versus conventional radiotherapy with sequential boost for adjuvant treatment of breast cancer: 2-year results of the multicenter randomized IMRT-MC2 trial. *Radiotherapy and Oncology*, *163*, 165-176.

Ge, X., Liao, Z., Yuan, J., Mao, D., Li, Y., Yu, E., ... & Ding, Z. (2020). Radiotherapy-related quality of life in patients with head and neck cancers: a meta-analysis. *Supportive Care in Cancer*, *28*(6), 2701-2712.

Giunta, E. F., Bregni, G., Pretta, A., Deleporte, A., Liberale, G., Bali, A. M., ... & Sclafani, F. (2021). Total neoadjuvant therapy for rectal cancer: Making sense of the results from the RAPIDO and PRODIGE 23 trials. *Cancer treatment reviews*, *96*, 102177.

Hamstra, D. A., Mariados, N., Sylvester, J., Shah, D., Gross, E., Hudes, R., ... & Michalski, J. (2018). Sexual quality of life following prostate intensity modulated radiation therapy (IMRT) with a rectal/prostate spacer: Secondary analysis of a phase 3 trial. *Practical radiation oncology*, *8*(1), e7-e15.

Hamstra, D. A., Mariados, N., Sylvester, J., Shah, D., Karsh, L., Hudes, R., ... & Michalski, J. (2017). Continued benefit to rectal separation for prostate radiation therapy: final results of a phase III trial. *International Journal of Radiation Oncology* Biology* Physics*, *97*(5), 976-985.

Jensen, S. B., Vissink, A., Limesand, K. H., & Reyland, M. E. (2019). Salivary gland hypofunction and xerostomia in head and neck radiation patients. *JNCI Monographs*, *2019*(53), lgz016.

Jones, H. J., Al-Najami, I., & Cunningham, C. (2020). Quality of life after rectal-preserving treatment of rectal cancer. *European Journal of Surgical Oncology*, *46*(11), 2050-2056.

Juul, T., Ahlberg, M., Biondo, S., Espin, E., Jimenez, L. M., Matzel, K. E., ... & Christensen, P. (2014). Low anterior resection syndrome and quality of life: an international multicenter study. *Diseases of the Colon & Rectum*, *57*(5), 585-591.

Kaidar-Person, O., Roach III, M., & Créhange, G. (2013). Whole-pelvic nodal radiation therapy in the context of hypofractionation for high-risk prostate cancer patients: a step forward. *International Journal of Radiation Oncology* Biology* Physics*, *86*(4), 600-605.

Kelemen, G., Varga, Z., Lázár, G., Thurzó, L., & Kahán, Z. (2012). Cosmetic outcome 1–5 years after breast conservative surgery, irradiation and systemic therapy. *Pathology & Oncology Research*, *18*(2), 421-427.

Klopp, A. H., Yeung, A. R., Deshmukh, S., Gil, K. M., Wenzel, L., Westin, S. N., ... & Bruner, D. W. (2018). Patient-reported toxicity during pelvic intensity-modulated radiation therapy: NRG Oncology–RTOG 1203. *Journal of clinical oncology*, *36*(24), 2538.

Lardas, M., Liew, M., van den Bergh, R. C., De Santis, M., Bellmunt, J., Van den Broeck, T., ... & Bourke, L. (2017). Quality of life outcomes after primary treatment for clinically localised prostate cancer: a systematic review. *European urology*, *72*(6), 869-885.

Lee, N., Puri, D. R., Blanco, A. I., & Chao, K. C. (2007). Intensity-modulated radiation therapy in head and neck cancers: an update. *Head & Neck: Journal for the Sciences and Specialties of the Head and Neck*, *29*(4), 387-400.

Marta, G. N., & Silva, V. (2014). de andrade Carvalho, h., de arruda. *FF, hanna, Sa, Gadia, r., Silva, JL F., Correa, SFM, abreu, CECV and riera, r*, 9-15.

Meattini, I., Saieva, C., Miccinesi, G., Desideri, I., Francolini, G., Scotti, V., ... & Livi, L. (2017). Accelerated partial breast irradiation using intensity modulated radiotherapy versus whole breast irradiation: Health-related quality of life final analysis from the Florence phase 3 trial. *European Journal of Cancer*, *76*, 17-26.

Michalski, J. M., Gay, H., Jackson, A., Tucker, S. L., & Deasy, J. O. (2010). Radiation dose–volume effects in radiation-induced rectal injury. *International Journal of Radiation Oncology* Biology* Physics*, *76*(3), S123-S129.

Mundt, A. J., Mell, L. K., & Roeske, J. C. (2003). Preliminary analysis of chronic gastrointestinal toxicity in gynecology patients treated with intensity-modulated whole pelvic radiation therapy. *International Journal of Radiation Oncology* Biology* Physics*, *56*(5), 1354-1360.

Mundt, A. J., Lujan, A. E., Rotmensch, J., Waggoner, S. E., Yamada, S. D., Fleming, G., & Roeske, J. C. (2002). Intensity-modulated whole pelvic radiotherapy in women with gynecologic malignancies. *International Journal of Radiation Oncology* Biology* Physics*, *52*(5), 1330-1337.

Murthy, V., Maitre, P., Bhatia, J., Kannan, S., Krishnatry, R., Prakash, G., ... & Mahantshetty, U. (2020). Late toxicity and quality of life with prostate only or whole pelvic radiation therapy in high risk prostate cancer (POP-RT): A randomised trial. *Radiotherapy and Oncology*, *145*, 71-80.

Nakai, Y., Tanaka, N., Anai, S., Miyake, M., Asakawa, I., Morizawa, Y., ... & Fujimoto, K. (2018). Quality of life worsened the most severely in patients immediately after intensity-modulated radiotherapy for prostate cancer. *Research and Reports in Urology*, *10*, 169.

Nguyen, N. T. A., & Ringash, J. (2018). Head and neck cancer survivorship care: a review of the current guidelines and remaining unmet needs. *Current treatment options in oncology*, *19*(8), 1-20.

Noone, A. M., Howlader, N., Krapcho, M. A., Miller, D., Brest, A., Yu, M., ... & Cronin, K. A. (2018). SEER cancer statistics review, 1975–2015. *Bethesda, MD: National Cancer Institute*, *4*.

Nout, R. A., Smit, V. T. H. B. M., Putter, H., Juergenliemk-Schulz, I. M., Jobsen, J. J., Lutgens, L. C. H. W., ... & PORTEC Study Group. (2010). Vaginal brachytherapy versus pelvic external beam radiotherapy for patients with endometrial cancer of high-intermediate risk (PORTEC-2): an open-label, non-inferiority, randomised trial. *The Lancet*, *375*(9717), 816-823.

Peters III, W. A., Liu, P. Y., Barrett, R. J., Stock, R. J., Monk, B. J., Berek, J. S., ... & Alberts, D. S. (2000). Concurrent chemotherapy and pelvic radiation therapy compared with pelvic radiation therapy alone as adjuvant therapy after radical surgery in high-risk early-stage cancer of the cervix. *Obstetrical & Gynecological Survey*, *55*(8), 491-492.

Petersen, S. E., Thorsen, L. B., Hansen, S., Petersen, P. M., Lindberg, H., Moe, M., ... & Bentzen, L. (2022). A phase I/II study of acute and late physician assessed and patient-reported morbidity following whole pelvic radiation in high-risk prostate cancer patients. *Acta Oncologica*, *61*(2), 179-184.

Pi, G. L., Bi, J. P., He, H. P., Li, Y., Cheng, T. C., & Li, Y. P. (2018). The protective effect of optimized target delineation in intensity modulated radiation therapy on swallowing function in patients with different TNM staging of nasopharyngeal carcinoma. *Lin Chuang er bi yan hou tou Jing wai ke za zhi= Journal of Clinical Otorhinolaryngology, Head, and Neck Surgery*, *32*(8), 617-620.

Pignol, J. P., Truong, P., Rakovitch, E., Sattler, M. G., Whelan, T. J., & Olivotto, I. A. (2016). Ten years results of the Canadian breast intensity modulated radiation therapy (IMRT) randomized controlled trial. *Radiotherapy and oncology*, *121*(3), 414-419.

Pignon, J. P., Le Maitre, A., Maillard, E., Bourhis, J., & Mach-Nc Collaborative Group. (2009). Meta-analysis of chemotherapy in head and neck cancer (MACH-NC): an update on 93 randomised trials and 17,346 patients. Radiotherapy and oncology, 92(1), 4-14.

Pisansky, T. M., Pugh, S. L., Greenberg, R. E., Pervez, N., Reed, D. R., Rosenthal, S. A., ... & Bruner, D. W. (2014). Tadalafil for prevention of erectile dysfunction after radiotherapy for prostate cancer: the Radiation Therapy Oncology Group [0831] randomized clinical trial. *Jama*, *311*(13), 1300-1307.

Roach III, M., Nam, J., Gagliardi, G., El Naqa, I., Deasy, J. O., & Marks, L. B. (2010). Radiation dose–volume effects and the penile bulb. *International Journal of Radiation Oncology* Biology* Physics*, *76*(3), S130-S134.

Rosenthal, D. I., Lewin, J. S., & Eisbruch, A. (2006). Prevention and treatment of dysphagia and aspiration after chemoradiation for head and neck cancer. *Journal of clinical oncology*, *24*(17), 2636-2643.

Rowland, J. H., Desmond, K. A., Meyerowitz, B. E., Belin, T. R., Wyatt, G. E., & Ganz, P. A. (2000). Role of breast reconstructive surgery in physical and emotional outcomes among breast cancer survivors. *Journal of the National Cancer Institute*, *92*(17), 1422-1429.

Sanguineti, G., Ricchetti, F., McNutt, T., Wu, B., & Fiorino, C. (2014). Dosimetric predictors of dysphonia after intensity-modulated radiotherapy for oropharyngeal carcinoma. *Clinical oncology*, *26*(1), 32-38.

Scherr, D., Swindle, P. W., & Scardino, P. T. (2003). National Comprehensive Cancer Network guidelines for the management of prostate cancer. *Urology*, *61*(2), 14-24.

Schmidt, S., Garin, O., Pardo, Y., Valderas, J. M., Alonso, J., Rebollo, P., ... & Ferrer, M. (2014). Assessing quality of life in patients with prostate cancer: a systematic and standardized comparison of available instruments. *Quality of Life Research*, *23*(8), 2169-2181.

Siglin, J., Kubicek, G. J., Leiby, B., & Valicenti, R. K. (2010). Time of decline in sexual function after external beam radiotherapy for prostate cancer. *International Journal of Radiation Oncology* Biology* Physics*, *76*(1), 31-35.

Schover, L. R., van der Kaaij, M., van Dorst, E., Creutzberg, C., Huyghe, E., & Kiserud, C. E. (2014). Sexual dysfunction and infertility as late effects of cancer treatment. *European journal of cancer supplements*, *12*(1), 41-53.

Speyer, R. (2013). Oropharyngeal dysphagia: screening and assessment. *Otolaryngologic Clinics of North America*, *46*(6), 989-1008.

Taylor, A., & Powell, M. E. B. (2008). Conformal and intensity-modulated radiotherapy for cervical cancer. *Clinical oncology*, *20*(6), 417-425.

Thong, M. S., Koch-Gallenkamp, L., Jansen, L., Bertram, H., Eberle, A., Holleczek, B., ... & Arndt, V. (2019). Age-specific health-related quality of life in long-term and very long-term colorectal cancer survivors versus population controls–a population-based study. *Acta oncologica*, *58*(5), 801-810.

Tribius, S., Raguse, M., Voigt, C., Münscher, A., Gröbe, A., Petersen, C., ... & Singer, S. (2015). Residual deficits in quality of life one year after intensity-modulated radiotherapy for patients with locally advanced head and neck cancer. *Strahlentherapie Und Onkologie*, *191*(6), 501-510.

Ursino, S., D'angelo, E., Mazzola, R., Merlotti, A., Morganti, R., Cristaudo, A., ... & Lohr, F. (2017). A comparison of swallowing dysfunction after three-dimensional conformal and intensity-modulated radiotherapy. *Strahlentherapie und Onkologie*, *193*(11), 877-889.

Ware Jr, J. E., & Sherbourne, C. D. (1992). The MOS 36-item short-form health survey (SF-36): I. Conceptual framework and item selection. *Medical care*, 473-483.

Ward, M. C., Adelstein, D. J., Bhateja, P., Nwizu, T. I., Scharpf, J., Houston, N., ... & Koyfman, S. A. (2016). Severe late dysphagia and cause of death after concurrent chemoradiation for larynx cancer in patients eligible for RTOG 91-11. *Oral oncology*, *57*, 21-26.

Weber, D. C., Bieri, S., Kurtz, J. M., & Miralbell, R. (1999). Prospective pilot study of sildenafil for treatment of postradiotherapy erectile dysfunction in patients with prostate cancer. *Journal of clinical oncology*, *17*(11), 3444-3449.

Wijers, O. B., Levendag, P. C., Braaksma, M. M., Boonzaaijer, M., Visch, L. L., & Schmitz, P. I. (2002). Patients with head and neck cancer cured by radiation therapy: A survey of the dry mouth syndrome in long-term survivors. *Head & neck*, *24*(8), 737-747.

Wortman, B. G., Post, C. C., Powell, M. E., Khaw, P., Fyles, A., D'Amico, R., ... & de Boer, S. M. (2022). Radiation Therapy Techniques and Treatment-Related Toxicity in the PORTEC-3 Trial: Comparison of 3-Dimensional Conformal Radiation Therapy Versus Intensity-Modulated Radiation Therapy. *International Journal of Radiation Oncology* Biology* Physics*, *112*(2), 390-399.

Xu, D., Li, G., Li, H., & Jia, F. (2017). Comparison of IMRT versus 3D-CRT in the treatment of esophagus cancer: a systematic review and meta-analysis. *Medicine*, *96*(31).

Vainshtein, J. M., Griffith, K. A., Feng, F. Y., Vineberg, K. A., Chepeha, D. B., & Eisbruch, A. (2014). Patient-reported voice and speech outcomes after whole-neck intensity modulated radiation therapy and chemotherapy for oropharyngeal cancer: prospective longitudinal study. *International Journal of Radiation Oncology* Biology* Physics*, *89*(5), 973-980.

Zelefsky, M. J., Shasha, D., Branco, R. D., Kollmeier, M., Baser, R. E., Pei, X., ... & Mulhall, J. P. (2014). Prophylactic sildenafil citrate improves select aspects of sexual function in men treated with radiotherapy for prostate cancer. *The Journal of urology*, *192*(3), 868-874.

About the Editor

Sibel Karaca
Department of Radiation Oncology, Akdeniz University Faculty of Medicine, Antalya, Turkey

Sibel Karaca received her doctorate degree in 2016 from Atatürk University. She worked as a Medical Physicist in the Radiotherapy Department for about 15 years. She is currently working as an assistant professor at Medical Faculty, Department of Radiation Oncology, Akdeniz University, Antalya, Turkey. She has dosimetric and clinical studies especially in the field of radiotherapy physics. Her other work is focused on radiation awareness. She published papers in well-known medical physics and radiation oncology journals, of which she is the first author and co-author.

E- mail: sibeltuzlaci@gmail.com; sibelkaraca@akdeniz.edu.tr

List of Contributors

Sibel Karaca
Kadriye Aysenur Karacam
Ercan Balci
Meltem Kirli Bolukbas
Taylan Tuğrul
Esma Didem Nasuhbeyoglu
Mehmet Ertugrul Erturk
Cemile Ceylan
Nural Ozturk
Aydin Cakir
Murat Okutan
Murat Koylu
Ayse Gulbin Kavak
Serap Çatlı Dinç
Menekşe Turna
Emel Haciislamoglu
Hamit Basaran
Hakan Eren
Zumrut Arda Kaymak

List of Abbreviations

2D two-dimensional
3D CRT three-dimensional conformal radiation therapy
3D three-dimensional
4D four-dimensional
6D six-dimensional
AAPM American association of physicists in medicine
ABC active-breathing control
ACMP American college of medical physicians
ALARA as low as reasonably achievable
APB accelerated partial breast
API application programming interfaces
ART adaptive radiation therapy
ASTRO American society for radiation oncology
BM brain metastasis
CBCT cone-beam computed tomography
CCD charge-coupled device
CI conformity index
Cm centimeter
CNS central nervous system
CRT chemoradiotherapy
CT computer tomography
CTCAE common terminology criteria for adverse events
CT-Sim CT-Simulator
CTV clinical target volume
DAO direct aperture-based optimisation
DC direct current
DD dose difference
DIBH deep inspiration breath-hold
DICOM digital imaging and communications in medicine
DIR deformable image registration

Dmean mean dose
DMLC dynamic MLC
DNA deoxyribonucleic acid
DRR digitally reconstructed radiograph
DTA distance to agreement
EAR excess actual risk
EBRT external beam radiotherapy
ECOG Eastern cooperative oncology group
EDR exposure data recogniser
EORTC European organisation for research and treatment of cancer
EPIC expanded prostate cancer index composite
EPID electronic portal imaging device
ERR excess relative risk
ESTRO European society for radiotherapy and oncology
EU European union
EUD equivalent uniform dose
FACT functional assessment of cancer therapy
FDG fluorideoxyglucose
FFF flattening filter-free
FMO flexible mask optimisation
gEUD generalized equivalent uniform dose
GPA graded prognostic assessment
GTV gross tumour volume
Gy Gray
HDR high dose rate
HDR-BRT high-dose rate brachytherapy
HI homogeneity index
HNC head and neck
HU Hounsfield Unit
ICRP international commission on radiation protection
ICRU international commission on radiation units and measurements
IDR instantaneous dose rate
IAEA international atomic energy agency
IGRT image guided radiotherapy
IMAT intensity-modulated arc therapy
IMPT Intensity-modulated proton therapy
IMRT intensity modulated radiation therapy
IP inverse planning
IR infared

IRLEDs infrared light-emitting diodes
ITV Internal target volume
JROSG Japanese working group on radiation oncology
KPS Karnofsky performance status
kV kilovoltage
LAR lifetime attributable risk
LDR low dose rate
LINAC linear accelerator
LNT linear-no-threshold
LQ linear quadratic
MAR metal artifact reduction
MC Monte Carlo
MCO multi-criteria optimisation
MeV mega electron volt
MF modulation factor
MHz megahertz
MIMiC multi-leaf intensity-modulating collimator
MIP maximum intensity projection
ml millilitre
MLC multileaf collimator
Mm millimetre
mpMRI multiparametric magnetic resonance imaging
MRgRT magnetic resonance-guided radiotherapy
MRI magnetic resonance imaging
mSv millisievert
MU monitor unit
MV megavoltage
MVCT megavoltage computed tomography
MW megawatt
NCRP National Council on Radiation Protection
NSCLC non-small cell lung cancer
NTCP normal tissue complication probability
OAR organs at risk
OED organ equivalent dose
OS overall survival
OTT overall treatment time
PBRT proton beam radiotherapy
PDD percentage depth dose
PDR pulsed dose-rate

PET positron emission tomography
PF pitch factor
PFS progression-free survival
PRISMA preferred reporting items for systematic reviews and meta-analyses
PRV planning organ-at-risk volume
PTV planning target volume
QA quality assurance
QMS quality management system
QoL quality of life
RCT respiratory-controlled therapy
RF radiofrequency
RIR rigit image registration
RPA recursive partitioning analysis
RPM real-time position management
RT radiotherapy
RTOG radiation therapy oncology group
RVR remaining volume at risk
SAD source-axis distance
SBRT stereotactic body radiation therapy
SD standard deviation
SEER surveillance, epidemiology, and end results
SIB simultaneous integrated boost
SM set-up margin
SMLC static MLC
SPECT single photon emission computed tomography
SRS stereotactic radiosurgery
SS step-and-shoot
SSD source skin distance
SW sliding window
TAR tissue air ratio
TCP tumour control probability
TG task group
TMR tissue maximum ration
TPR tissue phantom ratio
TPS treatment planning system
TROG radiation therapy oncology group
TV treated volume
UTCP uncomplicated tumour control probability
VMAT volumetric modulated arc therapy

WBRT whole brain radiotherapy
WHO world health organisation
XQ xerostomia questionnaire

Index

I

L

M

N

O

P

Q